Strength and Conditioning for Team Sports

Strength and Conditioning for Team Sports is designed to help devise more effective high-performance training programmes for team sports. This textbook remains the only evidence-based study of sport-specific practice to focus on team sports and features all-new chapters, including one on neuromuscular training, and dedicated chapters exploring injury prevention and the specific injury risks for different team sports. Fully revised and updated throughout, the new edition also includes the addition of over 200 new references to the research literature in the field.

This book addresses the core science underpinning different facets of physical preparation, covering all aspects of training prescription and the key components of any degree course related to strength and conditioning, including:

- physiological and performance testing;
- strength training;
- metabolic conditioning;
- power training;
- agility and speed development;
- training for core stability;
- training periodisation;
- training for injury prevention.

Bridging the traditional gap between sports science research and practice in the field, each chapter features guidelines for evidence-based best practice, as well as recommendations for approaches to physical preparation to meet the specific needs of team sports players. This new edition also includes an appendix that provides detailed examples of training programmes for a range of team sports. Fully illustrated throughout, it is essential reading for all serious students of strength and conditioning, and for any practitioner seeking to extend their professional practice.

Paul Gamble has worked in high-performance sport for over a decade, during which time he has coached elite athletes in an array of sports and at all ages and stages of development. Paul began his career working in professional rugby with English Premiership side London Irish, and has since worked in a range of sports, most recently serving as National Strength and Conditioning Lead for Scottish Squash. He has published a number of articles in peer-reviewed journals, chapters in edited textbooks and has previously written two textbooks as sole author.

STRENGTH AND CONDITIONING FOR TEAM SPORTS

Sport-specific physical preparation for high performance, second edition

Paul Gamble

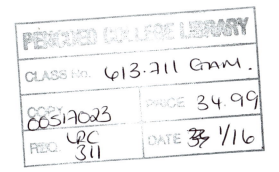
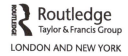
Routledge
Taylor & Francis Group

LONDON AND NEW YORK

First published 2009 by Routledge
This edition published 2013
2 Park Square, Milton Park, Abingdon, Oxon OX14 4RN

Simultaneously published in the USA and Canada
by Routledge
711 Third Avenue, New York, NY 10017

Routledge is an imprint of the Taylor & Francis Group, an informa business

British Library Cataloguing in Publication Data
A catalogue record for this book is available from the British Library

Library of Congress Cataloging in Publication Data
Gamble, Paul.
Strength and conditioning for team sports : sport-specific physical preparation for
high performance / by Paul Gamble. -- 2nd ed.
   p. cm.
   1. Sports--Physiological aspects. 2. Sports teams--Physiological aspects.
   3. Physical education and training. 4. Athletes--Training of. I. Title.
   GV711.5.G345 2012   613.7'11--dc23
   2012016560

ISBN: 978-0-415-63792-3 (hbk)
ISBN: 978-0-415-63793-0 (pbk)
ISBN: 978-0-203-08425-0 (ebk)

Typeset in Bembo and ITC Stone Sans
by Bookcraft Ltd, Stroud, Gloucestershire

CONTENTS

TABLES

FIGURES

ACKNOWLEDGEMENTS

I am keenly aware what a privileged position it is to be able to work in performance sport, and I must thank all those coaches and athletes I have been fortunate enough to work with and learn from. Equally, I strongly believe the responsibility of training athletes is a right that must be earned and I hope the information presented in this book assists aspiring strength and conditioning specialists in that quest.

Once more this book is for Sian.

1

PRINCIPLES OF SPECIFICITY AND TRANSFER OF TRAINING EFFECTS

Introduction

Specificity of training is increasingly acknowledged as fundamental in shaping training responses (Kraemer *et al.* 2002). Training specificity encapsulates two key concepts. The first is that the nature of acute training responses will be dependent upon – hence *specific to* – the nature of the particular training stimulus. The second, a corollary of the first, is that the degree to which training resembles – is *specific to* – conditions faced during competition influences the degree to which training effects will transfer to performance in the short term. These two concepts therefore relate to all aspects of physical preparation.

The essence of training specificity is that training responses elicited by a given exercise mode are directly related to the physiological elements involved in coping with the specific exercise stress (Kraemer *et al.* 2002). Accordingly, the strength and conditioning specialist can expect very little impact upon muscles and metabolic pathways that are not directly engaged during the particular exercise (Millet *et al.* 2002b).

The degree of carry-over from training to competition is described in terms of transfer of training effect (Stone *et al.* 2000). In the short term, this is heavily influenced by the level of mechanical and bioenergetic (energy systems) specificity of training in relation to competition. The probability that a training intervention will be reflected in performance changes therefore depends upon the degree to which training replicates the constraints of that aspect of athletic performance (Gamble 2006).

The impact that training specificity has on training outcomes also grows with exposure to training (Young 2006). With advances in training experience, training specificity influences the athlete's training responses to an increasing degree. Hence, factors relating to specificity assume increased relevance and importance at later stages of development. Training specificity therefore becomes a critical consideration as athletes approach elite levels of performance.

Presented is an outline of general principles of specificity, and a discussion of how they relate to training. Brief examples of the ways in which specificity is manifested are also given. Finally, the implications of this information for coaches and athletes and how this should be implemented when designing training plans will be discussed.

Principle of individuality

Inherited traits will influence athletes' performance capacities and trainability for a particular physiological property (Beunen and Thomis 2006). The 'internal training load' exerted upon the athlete and the timeframe and magnitude of training responses are therefore to some extent specific to the individual.

Genotype influences the individual athlete's responsiveness to a particular form of training, and also effectively sets the ceiling for any training effect (Smith 2003). These factors will impact upon both the rate of development and also the upper ceiling for training adaptation for each individual. The athlete's genotype exerts considerable influence upon athletic capabilities such as speed, power, strength and cardiorespiratory endurance, and their propensity for developing these qualities (Beunen and Thomis 2006). For example, hereditary factors are reported to account for 47 per cent of the variability in an individual's trainability with respect to the relative VO_2max response to training (Bouchard 2011).

Although genetic potential may be beyond the control of the coach and athlete, the training performed and the environment the athlete is exposed to will influence the degree to which inherited traits are expressed (Beunen and Thomis 2006). This is the *phenotype* of the athlete, which will be specific to the history of the individual and other environmental factors (Smith 2003). Phenotypic expression of physical qualities is thus determined by the interaction of genetics, the athlete's training and other environmental factors (Beunen and Thomis 2006). In a squad setting, even with a fixed external training load, such factors will determine the specific 'internal load' placed upon each athlete, which in turn will define their individual training response to the training prescribed (Impellizzeri *et al.* 2005).

The degree to which athletes' inherited traits translate into performance abilities in the competition arena will depend not only upon the quality of the training prescribed, but also athletes' motivation and dedication when undertaking training. Likewise, the key technical and tactics elements that determine success in skill sports are teachable (Smith 2003). The quality of coaching and the coach–athlete interaction are thus important factors. The athlete's personality traits will further determine the effectiveness of physical preparation as well as both athletic and sports skill acquisition. Self-discipline, appetite for work and willingness to learn are all important in determining whether the athlete fulfils the many hours of quality training and practice required for elite-level performance (Smith 2003).

Process of training adaptation

Broadly, the process of training adaptation is that exposure to an effective training stimulus prompts the physiological and/or neuromuscular systems affected to respond by increasing their capacities in order to be better able to cope if faced with a similar challenge in the future. The original theoretical basis of training adaptation is the general adaptation syndrome (GAS) proposed by Hans Seyle (Seyle 1956), which describes a generic response of an organism to a stressor (Wathen *et al.* 2000). According to this model, the first phase of response to any stressor is characterised as *shock* or *alarm* (Brown and Greenwood 2005). Following this is a *supercompensation* phase, whereby the body adapts to increase the specific capabilities affected by the particular stressor. Over time if the stressor continues the organism may enter a terminal phase, termed *maladaptation* (Brown and Greenwood 2005).

However, each individual physical capacity has its own individual window of adaptation:

•   the rate of adaptation varies according to the individual athlete (genetic factors) and also depends upon their training history – that is, how much adaptation has already taken place;

- the total degree of adaptation that is possible is dependent on genetic aspects, which effectively set the ceiling for adaptation of a particular physical capacity for each athlete.

Accordingly, this GAS paradigm has since been refined by the fitness–fatigue model (Chiu and Barnes 2003; Plisk and Stone 2003). A key distinction is that the fitness–fatigue model differentiates between the actions of a given stressor on individual neuromuscular and metabolic systems (Chiu and Barnes 2003). A corollary of this is that there are effectively individual windows for adaptation for each physical capacity. Particular acute adaptive responses are described as being restricted and specific to the systems employed in the training stimulus. The fitness–fatigue model also stipulates that the extent and length of any short-term effects following training are specific to the training stimulus – rather than a generic response (Chiu and Barnes 2003).

The other major advancement of the fitness–fatigue model is that it describes a dual adaptive response – resulting in both fitness and fatigue after-effects, as opposed to the single common response described by GAS. These fitness and fatigue responses exert opposing effects on performance and are described as having defined characteristics: there are distinct differences in both magnitude and duration of fitness versus fatigue responses (Chiu and Barnes 2003). The athlete's physiological status is effectively determined by the net effect of these two opposing factors at that given time (Chiu and Barnes 2003).

Specificity in relation to training experience and athletic status

The extent to which specificity principles apply appears to vary according to initial training status and degree of training experience (Young 2006). In untrained individuals, training specificity does not exert the same level of influence as that observed with trained individuals. This is illustrated by the responses of untrained subjects to endurance training. Following training, untrained and recreationally trained individuals often demonstrate improved endurance scores on other exercise modes (Millet *et al.* 2002). This is not the case with elite athletes; what limited cross training effects have been observed in trained athletes fall far short of performance improvements elicited by mode-specific training (Millet *et al.* 2002).

The limiting factor in terms of oxygen transport also appears to vary between untrained individuals and athletes (Hoff 2005). The muscles of untrained subjects are not fully able to utilise available oxygen delivered via the blood. Conversely, the locomotor muscles of trained individuals have the capacity to handle significantly more oxygenated blood than the heart is able to pump. Hence, for athletes during dynamic activity utilising large muscles – as occurs in team sports – the limiting factor is their cardiac output (Hoff 2005).

There is also evidence that the relationship between stroke volumes and VO_2 is also different for well-trained versus moderately and untrained individuals (Hoff 2005). What occurs in the untrained and moderately trained is the classical textbook pattern of a levelling off in stroke volume as workloads increase beyond around 60 per cent VO_2max (Hoff 2005). However, it is apparent that well-trained athletes continue to increase stroke volume with increasing workloads up to VO_2max (Hoff 2005).

A similar scenario is evident with strength training. Almost any training represents a novel stimulus to the untrained neuromuscular system. As a result, untrained individuals demonstrate an array of training effects, regardless of the nature of the training (Newton and Kraemer 1994). Consequently, a wide variety of training interventions will produce favourable adaptations in a given aspect of neuromuscular performance with untrained individuals (Kraemer *et al.* 2002). Again, this is not the case in advanced lifters and elite strength-trained athletes.

There is increasing evidence that the dose – response relationships pertaining to volume, frequency and intensity of strength training are specific to the level of training experience and athletic status of the individual (Peterson *et al.* 2004; Rhea *et al.* 2003). The optimal strength training prescriptions differ for untrained individuals and those with strength training experience. Examination of training studies reveals that subject groups comprising strength-trained athletes differ markedly on all three of these training variables in comparison to both untrained and trained non-athletes (Peterson *et al.* 2004; Rhea *et al.* 2003). The trends in each training parameter between groups appear to form a continuum of optimal levels of volume, frequency and intensity with progression in training experience and athletic status.

Specificity of training

A foundation of training is described by the acronym SAID: *specific adaptation to imposed demands* (Baechle *et al.* 2000). Simply, any physiological adaptation produced is dependent on the specific form of overload provided by the training stimulus (Stone *et al.* 2000).

Metabolic specificity

Metabolic specificity of training adaptations applies to the energy systems mobilised during exercise. The amount of muscle mass involved and overall exercise intensity dictate the scope of central and peripheral training effects. For example, these factors will determine whether training responses are limited to adaptations at muscle level, or if central cardiovascular changes are elicited (Millet *et al.* 2002).

Training mode specificity can also be observed with metabolic conditioning. The running and cycling training completed by elite triathletes are shown to be unrelated to their swim performance (Millet *et al.* 2002). Accordingly, improved performance measured via a swimming test mode following swim training is not reflected in treadmill test scores. In trained non-athletes, cross training (swimming) is likewise shown to be inferior to running training in improving running performance parameters (Foster *et al.* 1997).

Adaptations following purely anaerobic training are mainly restricted to increased activity of enzymes involved in anaerobic metabolism (Wilmore and Costill 1999). Conversely, continuous submaximal aerobic training is reflected in improved oxidative enzymes, whilst the anaerobic enzyme profile remains largely unchanged (Wilmore and Costill 1999). Eliciting anaerobic adaptations requires anaerobic training, whereas improvements in oxidative capacity can only be derived using conditioning activities that stress the aerobic system.

It has been suggested that high-intensity sprint interval training methods defy the principles of specificity on the basis that this approach is observed to produce gains in oxidative capacity despite the fact that this form of training consists of maximal 30-second sprints, with extensive rest between, and greatly reduced overall training volume (Burgomaster *et al.* 2008). However, this form of training does in fact engage and stress oxidative metabolic systems, and the contribution from aerobic metabolism increases markedly during succes-sive work bouts (Bogdanis *et al.* 1996a; Ross and Leveritt 2001). Equally, the training adaptations remain specific to the form of training. The nature of the training response differs between high-intensity interval training, which elicits predominantly peripheral adaptations, and conventional endurance training, which is associated with both central and peripheral adaptations (Bishop *et al.* 2004).

Depending on the format, interval training with shorter (that is, incomplete) rest inter-vals may maximally stress both aerobic and anaerobic systems (Tabata *et al.* 1996, 1997). This training format can thus exhibit a combined training response. The specific training adaptation elicited, however, remains dependent upon the format of interval training, and factors such as the intensity of work intervals and the particular work:rest ratios employed (Spencer *et al.* 2005).

Biomechanical specificity

Biomechanical specificity concerns parameters of training that include range of motion and joint angles (Stone *et al.* 2000a). This is applicable both to dynamic and isometric training, with superior strength gains observed within the range of motion and at the joint angles featured in training (Morrissey *et al.* 1995). Based upon these observations, it follows that exercise selection should reflect the full range of motion and joint angles featured in the sport or athletic activity. This is particularly important for certain muscle groups such as the hip extensors, especially the hamstrings. For these muscles the profile of peak torque versus joint angle is identified as being critical for healthy function and protecting against injury (Heiderscheidt *et al.* 2010). Accordingly it is very important that the training for these muscles replicates the joint ranges of motion required during athletic activities, for example running and sprinting.

Biomechanical specificity also extends to aspects such as posture and limb position. Consequently, greatest strength responses are manifested during closed kinetic chain movements following closed kinetic chain training, whereas the opposite applies to open kinetic chain exercises (Stone *et al.* 2000). Similarly, a lift performed in a standing position (for example, barbell squat) has greater carry-over to most types of athletic performance than a similar movement performed in a seated or supine position (for example, leg press).

Biomechanical specificity is also evident in the relationship between unilateral (single-limb) and bilateral (both limbs working simultaneously) strength measures (Enoka 1997; Newton and Kraemer 1994). Cyclists are shown to exhibit greater overall strength when single-leg press scores are summed in comparison to their bilateral leg press score – an effect known as 'bilateral deficit' (Enoka 1997). This reflects the fact that cyclists work unilaterally – alternately exerting force with each leg – during training and competition. Conversely, athletes for whom training is bilateral can exhibit bilateral facilitation (Enoka 1997). For example, it is reported that rowers' bilateral leg press scores are greater than the sum of their single-leg press scores (Enoka 1997; Newton and Kraemer 1994). It follows that exercise selection should emphasise either bilateral or unilateral movements, corre-sponding to what occurs during competition in the sport or athletic event.

Finally, training effects are specific to the muscle contraction type employed in the training exercise (that is, concentric, eccentric or isometric) (Morrissey *et al.* 1995). Consequently, superior strength scores post-training are observed in measures that feature the same mode of contraction as that employed in training (Morrissey *et al.* 1995). For example, isometric training elicits greater isometric strength improvement (registered under static conditions) than dynamic strength training (Morrissey *et al.* 1995). Contraction-type specificity is also observed in the finding that eccentric training interventions are associated with training responses, such as changes in torque – joint angle relationships (Brockett *et al.* 2001), which are not seen with concentric training modes (Rees *et al.* 2009).

Kinetic and kinematic specificity

In addition to biomechanical factors, other aspects of movement including relative force, velocity and timing characteristics are also important. Such considerations include magnitude and duration of loading, acceleration/deceleration profile of the movement, and movement velocity.

The duration and rate of force generation for a particular athletic task have a major bearing on the degree of statistical relationship observed with other measures, despite similarities in biomechanics between tasks (Cronin and Sleivert 2005). For example, jump squat training was reported to produce gains in jump height that were not seen in the subject group trained with traditional barbell squat and leg press, despite the two training modes having very similar biomechanical characteristics (Newton *et al.* 1999). Differences in acceleration and rate of force development between the two training modes were suggested to account for the difference in training effects observed.

Contraction-type specificity is also observed and this serves to determine the nature of training responses elicited by particular strength and speed-strength training modes. For example, changes in the eccentric phase of activities such as jumping that are preceded with a countermovement and improvements in coupling of eccentric–concentric components are only observed with training modes that feature these elements (Cormie *et al.* 2010a).

Velocity specificity is evident in that strength gains will tend to be restricted to the velocities at which the muscles are trained (Morrissey *et al.* 1995). It appears that there is a greater degree of velocity specificity in training responses at the higher end of the training velocity spectrum (Morrissey *et al.* 1995). At slower contraction speeds there may be some carry-over to velocities at and below the training velocity. In contrast, within the upper region of the force–velocity curve, strength improvements are typically only registered within the narrow range of velocities used in training (Morrissey *et al.* 1995).

Psychological specificity

Physiological capabilities are manifested in a sports setting as part of co-ordinated and skilled movements. A corollary of this is that strength and conditioning specialists should consider the context in which physiological training is performed (Siff 2002). Specificity considerations therefore also include psychological aspects of performance conditions. Cognitive and perceptual elements of performance conditions should likewise be accounted for in training design (Ives and Shelley 2003).

The principles of specificity thus also apply to psychological aspects. For athletes in team sports in particular, physical and mental capabilities are irrevocably linked. Three crucial interrelated components that are identified as influencing training responses are attention, mental effort and intention (Ives and Shelley 2003):

Attention is a key factor in perception–action coupling and the superior decision-making of elite performers. Elite athletes attend to relevant cues from the competition environment and process them better as the basis for their movement responses (Ives and Shelley 2003). During competition and practices, attention is also crucial to anticipatory responses and associated postural and motor control. The athlete's locus of attention, in terms of whether it is externally or internally focused, is shown to impact upon motor learning and performance (Ives and Shelley 2003).

It is recognised that directed mental effort has the potential to directly affect the magnitude of training responses (Ives and Shelley 2003). Conscious effort to exert maximal force has been found to significantly influence gains in strength and power (Jones *et al.* 1999). It has been reported that greater gains in strength are manifested when subjects were specifically instructed to focus on maximally accelerating the barbell for every repetition, as opposed to lifting without specific focus or instruction (Jones *et al.* 1999).

Intent is integral to neural factors associated with adaptations in high-velocity strength and rate of force development (Behm and Sale 1993; Ives and Shelley 2003). Recruitment and firing of muscles during training are in part dictated by what is anticipated prior to the movement (Behm and Sale 1993; Behm 1995). An illustration of this is that training effects associated with ballistic training can be derived with isometric training under certain conditions. If the lifter trains with the conscious intention of moving the static resistance explosively, significant improvements in rate of force development can take place – despite the fact that no movement actually takes place (Behm and Sale 1993). Physiological adaptations are thus specific to and partially determined by the intention and corresponding neuromuscular patterns during training (Ives and Shelley 2003).

It is important therefore to consider not only mechanical and metabolic specificity, but also to address other aspects of the training environment. Imposing sport-specific constraints may help appropriately shape training movement responses. It is suggested this approach may encourage more adaptive learning and likewise develop decision-making (Ives and Shelley 2003).

Conversely, excessively restricting training either by mechanically fixing the planes and range of movement or through overtly prescriptive coaching intervention will tend to discourage development of directed mental effort, task-specific attention, and sport-specific intent (Handford *et al.* 1997). Conducting physiological training in isolation from the athletic performance the athlete is training for is likely to hinder transfer of training effects (Ives and Shelley 2003).

The paradox of specificity and transfer of training effects

Theoretically, the most 'sport-specific' or 'functional' form of training is to perform the actual movement(s) of the sport (Siff 2002), although this assertion does neglect the element of overload required to elicit a training response. That said, the major implication of training specificity is that training modes which correspond most closely to the target activity can be expected to result in the greatest direct transfer of training effects in the short term. However, the paradox of training design is that over the long term the most task-specific training employed in isolation is unlikely to provide the development of the foundation qualities required to ultimately achieve optimal performance (Bondarchuk 2007).

An example from strength training is that 'non-specific' heavy resistance training modes are required initially in order to best develop underlying contractile properties and morphological aspects for high-intensity performance (such as sprinting). This is also the case for metabolic conditioning: whilst performing repetitions over 200m with complete rest between might seem the most 'specific' approach for a 200m runner, during the earlier stages of the training year these athletes will in fact benefit more from performing a range of sessions over various distances, with varying (incomplete) rest intervals. Although these sessions appear on the surface to be less specific to the constraints of a performing a 200m race in competition, this approach will over time provide the foundation development of oxidative capacities and anaerobic capacity that will allow the athlete to train and compete at high intensity later in the competition season.

It is therefore critical that the strength and conditioning specialist is mindful of both short-term and long-term training adaptation and the underlying processes involved (Bondarchuk 2007). As has been described in the previous sections, specificity is a key factor that governs training responses in the short term; however, a longer-term perspective is also required in order to best organise training to ultimately take full advantage of transfer of training at the critical periods of the competition phase in the calendar.

As will be discussed in a later chapter, is equally important that there is variation in exercise selection throughout the training year in order to avoid plateaus in training adaption. It would appear, therefore, that what will be required is a coherent progression during the course of the training macrocycle through a range of exercises that span the specificity spectrum (Gamble 2011d).

Accounting for specificity in training programme design

The first step in deriving the benefits of training specificity is a thorough needs analysis. One aspect of this is identifying the biomechanics and bioenergetics associated with the particular sport or playing position. By defining the specific demands of competition it will be possible to account for the relevant parameters in the design of players' training. Another aspect of the needs analysis process involves identifying the individual profile of each athlete in terms of different aspects of physical preparedness.

Considerations for biomechanical specificity include direction and range of movement, type of muscle contraction, movement velocity and the rate and duration of force development (Stone *et al.* 2000). Exercise selection should cater for the full range of motion identified from competition, as well as the conditions under which movements are initiated (Sheppard 2003). The degree of loading that is appropriate will vary according to the movement. In the case of fine motor skills, excessive loading may interfere with the proper execution of the movement (van den Tillar 2004).

Applying metabolic specificity basically requires that the format of conditioning reflects the parameters of competition. One approach used in other sports and athletic events involves setting target training paces, based upon actual or desired competition performance (Plisk and Gambetta 1997). Identifying such parameters (work rates, movement patterns, work:rest ratios) in order to design sport-specific conditioning programmes for team sports poses a greater challenge. This will be explored further in a later chapter.

Performance benefits may be derived by accounting for psychological aspects in the training environment. There are early indications that incorporating practice-related cognitive strategies during training leads to greater carry-over of training effects to sports performance (Ives and Shelley 2003). For example, visual and verbal cueing has been suggested to enhance the effectiveness of plyometric jump training for volleyball players (Ives and Shelley 2003). In the case of strength training, psychological interventions may take the form of mental imagery or specific cueing to lift explosively from the strength coach whilst lifting (Jones *et al.* 1999).

Coaches must also recognise that skill level and training experience influence the training parameters that will be effective in developing athletic performance (Cronin *et al.* 2001b; Peterson *et al.* 2004; Rhea *et al.* 2003). With progression in training status, training specificity assumes further importance. It would appear to follow that programme design must ultimately become increasingly specific to elicit the desired response when addressing a particular aspect of performance (Newton and Kraemer 1994).

Finally, training should be tailored to the specific needs and constraints of the individual. The delivery of training should be responsive to the relative stresses placed upon each individual, and coaches should recognise that the time course and magnitude of gains will also vary between athletes. Each athlete will also have different relative strengths and weaknesses, both of which should be accounted for in their individual training programme. Players will also vary in terms of their tolerance and responsiveness to different forms of training.

2

ASSESSING PHYSIOLOGICAL AND PERFORMANCE PARAMETERS

Introduction

The principles of training specificity have implications when assessing athletic performance (Abernethy *et al.* 1995). Fundamentally, in order to be relevant, any physiological tests selected must match the specific capabilities identified as contributing to performance in the sport (Bosquet *et al.* 2002). For team sports this requires consideration of not only the sport but also the playing position.

It follows that physiological tests selected should therefore be specific to the sport the player is training for (Murphy and Wilson 1997). Tests that are most game-specific tend to be given greatest credence by those involved in the sport. In basketball, the vertical jump test is shown to be the best predictor of playing time given to players of any athletic performance test (Hoffman *et al.* 1996). This is a reflection of the specificity – and hence relevance to performance – of vertical jump testing for basketball players.

Test specificity is again manifested in the observation that the greatest degree of improvement in muscle function following training is registered with the test modality that most closely matches the training movement (Morrissey *et al.* 1995). It follows that testing should be specific to the movement patterns and velocity used in training in order to be sensitive to training-induced changes in muscle function (Abernethy *et al.* 1995).

Fundamentally, training is aimed at improving the player's performance. From this point of view, physiological tests should ultimately be judged upon the extent that they reflect changes in sports performance (Murphy and Wilson 1997). In order to be relevant, tests must not only be sensitive to adaptations elicited by the training intervention but also capable of registering any resulting improvements in performance (Murphy and Wilson 1997).

One consideration with test specificity is taking account of the conditions under which tests of muscle function are measured. For example, neuromuscular properties such as rate of force development (RFD) and high-velocity strength are relevant to dynamic performance (Newton and Kraemer 1994). However, the corresponding test measures for these capabilities are only related to athletic performance if they are measured under appropriate conditions (Wilson *et al.* 1995).

Rationale for testing team sports players

Testing in sport is typically undertaken with one of three broad aims in mind:

1   The first of these is to evaluate the abilities or current state of preparedness of the player in the context of the demands of their sport (Impellizzeri *et al.* 2005); this may be:

- from a talent identification viewpoint (Abernethy *et al.* 1995), or
- in order to identify specific strengths and weaknesses of the players assessed in order to prioritise different training goals for the individual (Lemmink *et al.* 2004).

2   The second application of testing is to monitor progression and evaluate the effectiveness of training prescribed (Abernethy *et al.* 1995, Impellizzeri *et al.* 2005).

3   Finally, testing can be undertaken for training prescription purposes – for example, setting individualised training intensity parameters based on the evaluated capacities of each player (Buchheit 2008).

Application of testing in team sports

There are notable cases in sport where players' scores on a particular battery of performance tests are given a great deal of credence by those involved in the sport. Possibly the best example of this is the National Football League Combine – the standard battery of tests that is employed for selection in professional American football. Performance on these tests has been identified as a significant factor that distinguishes players successful in being drafted onto NFL teams from those who were unsuccessful (Sierer *et al.* 2008). In recognition of this, some authors have advocated targeted training to improve a player's performance specifically for particular tests that hold a lot of weight in the sport, with the aim of improving their prospects of selection – and the prospective financial rewards of signing professional contracts (McGee and Burkett 2003). Indeed, the degree to which players' performance on these tests apparently influences players' chances of selection has led entrepreneurial strength coaches to adopt the approach of training players specifically for the NFL Combine assessments, as opposed to preparing them to compete in the sport. Increasingly this is becoming standard practice in the strength and conditioning 'industry'.

The application of testing to guide training goals in the context of strength and power training has been described as 'strength diagnosis' (Wilson and Murphy 1996). In this way a player's relative scores on different measures of muscular performance, in relation to the demands associated with the sport, provide a means to identify deficits in particular areas. Addressing the areas of relative weakness identified then becomes the priority in the player's subsequent training block.

As mentioned in the previous section, testing is also employed directly to prescribe training intensity. Examples include strength training where intensity for a given exercise may be prescribed as percentages of a player's one-repetition maximum for that lift. Similarly, intensity for endurance training can be prescribed as percentage of the player's recorded maximum oxygen uptake (VO_2max), heart rate maximum (HRmax), or more commonly, their maximum aerobic speed derived from testing (Buchheit 2008).

Testing is also widely used to track improvements in players' fitness and performance, and as a means to assess the effectiveness of training prescribed (Impellizzeri *et al.* 2005). One consideration with team sports is that the individual stimulus provided by training prescribed to a group of players will vary for each player. Even if the external load in terms of intensity and volume prescribed is constant, genetic endowment and training background will both influence the magnitude of the 'internal load' imposed upon each player, which will in turn affect their individual training response (Impellizzeri *et al.* 2005). In view of this, testing will only provide a partial reflection of the effectiveness of the training prescribed, unless accompanied by ongoing monitoring and manipulation of players' individual daily training load. By extension, it follows that evaluating the day-to-day training process is as important as periodic assessment of the training outcome in order to determine the effectiveness of the training programme (Impellizzeri *et al.* 2005).

Utility and practical relevance of physiological and performance tests

Whether testing is carried out in the laboratory or in the field, both reliability and validity are key issues (Reilly *et al.* 2009). Reliability pertains to how consistent the scores of the given test are – hence how repeatable the test is. Validity concerns the extent to which the test actually measures the physical capability it is intended to assess. Both criteria must be met for any given test to be of any value as a means for assessing players' performance. It is possible to have a reliable test – one that gives highly consistent scores – that may not necessarily be a valid test, in terms of its ability to measure the particular aspect of motor performance the coach wishes to assess. Conversely, a highly valid test from the point of view of closely reflecting the movement or aspect of performance the test is designed to measure is of little value if it is not reliable in terms of producing consistent scores. In the latter case, the tester cannot be confident that any measured change over time is due to actual change in performance rather than just the error inherent in the test measure.

A good illustration of this comes from basketball, where a sport-specific test battery was designed to measure performance capabilities, which the authors named the Performance Index Evaluation (PIE) (Barfield *et al.* 2007). The tests chosen appeared highly specific to the sport of basketball; however, further investigation of the validity and reliability of the PIE with male and female collegiate players revealed it to have unacceptable test–retest reliability. Furthermore, the PIE showed scores that also appeared to lack criterion-related validity on the basis that they failed to correlate to playing time allocated to these collegiate players (Barfield *et al.* 2007).

In order to provide a framework within which players can then be evaluated, it is important to identify the specific parameters that influence performance for the particular sport (Muller *et al.* 2000). Once identified, tests that are sensitive enough to discern changes in the particular parameter should be sought. Specificity considerations have a major bearing on both these aspects. In order to be relevant, the parameter must be specific to performance of the sport in question, and correspondingly the test measure must be specific and therefore sensitive to the parameter the coach wishes to test.

One approach is to identify potentially important aspects of motor performance based upon qualitative assessment of the sport and then identify tests that are designed to measure each of these areas (Muller *et al.* 2000). The next step is for players competing at different levels to undergo the battery of motor performance tests derived. The degree to which each test correlates to players' level of performance can be taken as an indication of the importance of the corresponding parameter to success in the sport (Muller *et al.* 2000). In this way the tests that appear most strongly associated with success in the sport can be identified. However, one major caveat to this approach is that it is not safe to assume a causal relationship based solely on an apparent statistical relationship from a single set of measurements. Whilst two measures may show an apparent correlation from a one-off measurement, it has been demonstrated that with repeated measurement the relationship between performance measures may diverge over time (Nimphius *et al.* 2010). A better, albeit more time-consuming, approach may therefore be to assess the relationship between measures over time, via periodic repeated assessment.

Biomechanical specificity is a key factor with respect to test specificity, but it is only part of the equation. Other elements such as acceleration–deceleration profiles may be equally important. An illustration of this is the difference between barbell squat repetition maximum and barbell jump squat assessments, and their relationship with dynamic measures of performance such as sprint times with team sports players. In the case of the barbell squat 3-repetition maximum (3-RM) test, no relation to sprint performance was found over any distance, whereas barbell jump squat test scores were observed to be significantly correlated to 5m, 10m, and 30m speed of professional and semi-professional rugby league players (Cronin and Hansen 2005). Players' 3-RM squat and jump squat scores were also not related to each other in this study, despite the fact that the two movements are biomechanically very similar.

If the objective of testing is to evaluate the effectiveness of players' training, then specificity with regard to the training used must be considered. Greatest effects are observed during testing at velocities in the range featured in training (Morrissey *et al.* 1995). It follows that testing should be specific to the movement patterns and velocity used in training in order to be sensitive to training-induced changes in muscle function (Abernethy *et al.* 1995). However, it is not sufficient for test measures to be specific only to the type of training employed. Testing to monitor training effects must also bear relation to the sport in order to be sensitive to sports performance. When these conditions are not met, improvements in neuromuscular and athletic performance (maximum strength and sprint scores) can be observed following training despite the chosen test measures registering no change (Murphy and Wilson 1997). The particular test mode and outcome measures chosen must therefore be selected carefully in order to meet the objective of monitoring the effectiveness of players' physical preparation (Cronin and Hansen 2005).

Practicality of test modes for athletic assessment

Two major issues concerning modes for physiological and performance assessment are cost (expense of test apparatus and skilled personnel to operate it) and time demand. Considering both these factors – aside from concerns regarding specificity and relevance – individual laboratory assessment for large squads of players is not likely to be affordable or practical. Field-based tests are generally more conducive to team sports testing as these can be conducted in the field (avoiding the related travel and cost implications of using a laboratory) and also enable larger numbers to be tested in a relatively shorter time than tends to be possible with laboratory-based testing.

Whatever the mode of assessment, subject motivation is a crucial factor. Field tests have more obvious relevance from the players' viewpoint, and also benefit from context specificity: field tests are conducted in a setting where the players habitually train and perform as opposed to the more alien environment of a laboratory. In addition, field tests can be carried out with larger numbers of players, which allows those conducting the test to incorporate a competitive element. Because of these factors, field-based tests are therefore likely to engender greater compliance and motivation among team sports players, which improve the chance of consistent and maximal effort when testing is repeated over a period.

Design of field-test protocols are often modified in an attempt to make them more specific to the sport. Many sport-specific field tests are described in the literature (Barfield *et al.* 2007; Graham *et al.* 2003; Mirkov *et al.* 2008). With any 'sport-specific' field test there is inevitably a trade-off between replicating game conditions and standardising test conditions to obtain a reliable measure. Likewise, with any novel test protocol there is a need for sufficient normative data for the sporting population in question to provide a reference for comparison.

Scheduling of testing

Testing is only useful to the extent that it is repeated at regular intervals. Only in this way can progress be monitored or issues affecting performance be identified (for example, errors in training design, competition and other stressors). From this viewpoint it is very important that the test battery is carefully selected in order to be time-efficient, and can therefore be undertaken on a regular basis without excessive disruption to the training schedule. That said, the full battery of tests need not be undertaken at every test session: an abridged version of the test battery can be used during most regular test sessions and the full array of tests reserved for key points in the training year.

Strength assessment

Maximum strength

Strength is generally defined as maximal force or torque generated during a maximal voluntary contraction under a given set of conditions. Key parameters include posture, nature of the movement employed (single-joint versus complex multi-joint movements), contraction type and movement velocity (Abernethy *et al.* 1995). Broadly, strength qualities can be categorised in terms of static, concentric and eccentric modes of contraction. In recognition of the force–velocity curve, authors similarly make a distinction between low-velocity maximum strength and strength expressed at high movement velocities.

Modes of strength assessment can be categorised as 'isometric', 'isokinetic' or 'isoinertial'.

Isometric strength assessment

Isometric assessment typically uses a force transducer integrated into fixed apparatus against which the player (statically) applies force. This can also be undertaken using a force platform in a squat rack or other rigid structure for static actions performed standing: measuring the force applied to the ground through the feet (Wilson and Murphy 1996). In either case the defining aspect of isometric assessment is that force is applied against immovable apparatus and that there is no change in joint angle (Abernethy *et al.* 1995). By definition, isometric assessment measures strength qualities under static conditions, hence it provides little information regarding concentric or eccentric strength capabilities. Measurements with this form of assessment also vary considerably with changes in joint angle.

Isokinetic strength

Isokinetic assessment uses a dynamometer to control the velocity of movement while the subject exerts maximal force against the moving lever arm. These assessments therefore typically involve *open kinetic chain* movement – that is, the limb(s) applying force is moving. A common example of isokinetic strength assessment involves knee extension and/or flexion, performed seated with the subject's torso and other limbs secured in place. This mode of testing assesses the players' ability to generate torque through a fixed range of motion for a restricted single-joint movement at a constant angular velocity (Abernethy *et al.* 1995). The controlled conditions under which isokinetic strength measures are recorded assist in producing reliable (that is, repeatable) measurements. Conversely, the controlled and restricted nature of isokinetic dynamometry renders this mode of strength assessment less applicable to athletic movements. In most sports, strength is expressed during movements that are commonly performed in a weight-bearing posture (not performed seated) and involve complex rather than single-joint actions. In accordance with this, isokinetic strength measures are typically not reported to be sensitive to changes in measures of athletic performance (Murphy and Wilson 1997).

Isoinertial strength

Isoinertial strength assessment employs free weights or fixed resistance machines to quantify the greatest resistance the player can lift for a specified range of motion. Common machine-based assessments include leg press, chest press or shoulder press fixed resistance machines. Strength assessment involving fixed resistance machines share similar issues of biomechanical specificity to those described for isokinetic testing. Isoinertial strength assessment that employs free weight resistance is therefore the preferred method of assessment for athletic populations. This form of testing typically involves maximal efforts with one of the powerlifting competition lifts: barbell squat, deadlift and bench press. Isoinertial testing with free weights allows strength to be assessed for weight-bearing tasks, including closed kinetic chain movements, and also features the coupling of eccentric and concentric actions. Furthermore, these tests require the player to balance both themselves and the resistance whilst generating force, as opposed to having the plane of movement fixed and the body supported in a sitting or lying position, as occurs during fixed resistance machine assessments.

As such, isoinertial assessment with free weights is considered the testing mode that bears closest resemblance to what occurs during athletic movements (Newton and Dugan 2002). By definition, players' isoinertial test scores will to some extent be limited by their level of skill in performing the given strength exercise movement (Abernethy *et al.* 1995). However, such issues will likewise influence a player's ability to express their strength capabilities during sports skill and athletic movements.

Repetition maximum (RM) testing is widely used in physical assessment in sports: a player's one-repetition maximum (1-RM) for a particular lift is defined as the highest weight they are able to lift for one repetition through the full range of motion of that lift (Morales and Sobonya 1996; Harman and Pandorf 2000). In terms of practicality, 1-RM testing can be carried out in the weights room as it does not require specialised equipment and so can be undertaken at the team's training facility. Free weights 1-RM testing does demand a level of technical competence. From a safety viewpoint it is important that lifting form and posture does not break down under the maximal loads used, particularly in the case of barbell squat and deadlift.

An alternative to one-repetition maximum (1-RM) testing that attempts to avoid such issues involves the use of submaximal strength testing at lower repetition maximum loads, from which 1-RM values can be predicted (Morales and Sobonya 1996). One such approach is to assess the maximum load the player can lift for a specified number of repetitions, for example 3-RM or 5-RM testing. The number of repetitions chosen for submaximal RM testing influences the accuracy of the 1-RM prediction. The submaximal repetition test that most closely predicts 1-RM load reportedly also appears to vary according to the lift. A study of collegiate power athletes (football players and athletics field event throwing athletes) identified that 95 per cent 1-RM loads best predicted 1-RM values for bench press, which equates to a 2-RM test (Morales and Sobonya 1996). In contrast, the best prediction for power clean lifts were made at 90 per cent 1-RM (equating to a 4-RM test), whereas for barbell back squat the best prediction was made using 80 per cent 1-RM (8-RM test) in these athletes.

Assessing eccentric strength

Assessment of eccentric strength has traditionally been undertaken using isokinetic devices; that is, the player resists with maximal force the movement of the lever arm of the dynamometer as it moves in the opposite direction at a set angular velocity. This mode of eccentric strength testing carries the same biomechanical and postural specificity issues as described for concentric isokinetic strength assessment. Isoinertial assessments of eccentric strength do also exist, although they are not currently widely used (Meylan et al. 2008). Assessments of this type include protocols employing variations of standard strength exercises that impose a 3-second eccentric phase; that is, evaluating the maximum weight the subject is capable of lowering for a duration of three seconds through the full eccentric range of motion for the particular lift. Other forms of isoinertial eccentric-strength assessment employ a force platform and measure ground reaction forces during high-load or high-velocity eccentric movements. The use of these latter protocols will be restricted by access to the force platform equipment required and availability of trained staff to operate the apparatus.

Maximum force developed under eccentric (lengthening) conditions will always exceed maximum voluntary force developed during concentric or isometric contractions. As such the loads involved during eccentric strength testing exceed those used during isometric or concentric strength testing (Meylan et al. 2008). The higher level of loading imposed raises concerns over the safety of this form of assessment for some players. This is particularly the case with young players who are still maturing physically, and conversely older players who also may not tolerate the physical stresses involved.

Strength-endurance

Strength-endurance is identified as an independent aspect of neuromuscular performance, as opposed to just a derivative of other strength properties (Yessis 1994). This capability is commonly assessed by evaluating the number of repetitions the player is capable of completing at a given submaximal load. The load used is usually set as a percentage of their 1-RM for the particular strength exercise or body weight (for example, maximum chin up test). The number of repetitions through the full range of motion the player is able to complete with the predetermined load is then used as the outcome measure.

One notable example of a commonly administered strength-endurance test is the 225lb bench press repetition test that is performed as part of the NFL Combine. This is categorised as a test of strength-endurance for these American football players on the basis that the average number of repetitions completed by eligible players tested in the NFL Combine is reported to be 10 repetitions or above (Sierer *et al.* 2008). This may not be the case for other players in other sports, however.

Assessing 'speed-strength' or explosive power

Testimony to the high perceived importance of 'explosive' power or speed-strength with respect to sports performance (Abernethy *et al.* 1995), numerous different testing modalities exist to assess this particular quality.

Isokinetic dynamometry

Isokinetic testing using higher angular velocities on the dynamometer have been used as a measure of both high-velocity strength and speed-strength. In the same way as discussed for strength assessment, the validity of this form of testing for evaluating speed-strength performance is questionable. Isokinetic measures of speed-strength, in the form of hamstring and quadriceps torques, show no relation to sprint times over any distance (5m, 10m, or 30m) in team sports players (professional and semi-professional rugby league players) (Cronin and Hansen 2005). This finding is in keeping with the lack of biomechanical specificity with respect to the co-ordinated multi-joint movements that feature in athletic performance of the single-joint open kinetic chain movements involved in this form of assessment.

Tests of rate of force development

Rate of force development (RFD) is identified as a key component of speed-strength performance (Newton and Kraemer 1994). However, in accordance with test specificity, the conditions under which this aspect of neuromuscular function is measured have a major bearing on its validity. When measured under isometric (static) conditions, RFD scores showed no change in response to either ballistic, plyometric or strength-oriented lower-body training, even though improvements were demonstrated in measures of dynamic athletic performance (Wilson *et al.* 1993). A concentric measure of RFD was, however, shown to be capable of discriminating between good and poor performers on a sprint test, where the isometric RFD test failed to do so (Wilson *et al.* 1995).

The measure of RFD selected is shown to be important in terms of reliability. Specifically, peak RFD values are subject to a high degree of random error as it represents a single point on the force–time curve, whereas mean RFD is a far more reliable and robust measure as it is derived via integration of the whole of the force–time curve. Measurement of RFD does also require expensive and not easily portable equipment: typically a force plate. For these reasons, assessments of this type tend to share the same issues of cost and practicality as other forms of laboratory-based testing.

Isoinertial assessment of power output

Isoinertial assessments of power output against resistance loads have typically employed apparatus such as a Smith machine that consists of a barbell mounted on vertical runners. In this way, isoinertial resisted movements can be performed, albeit in a single vertical plane, and position transducers built into the device can be used to quantify barbell velocity and acceleration; hence mechanical power output can be derived via the following formula:

$$P = \text{force (barbell mass} \times \text{acceleration)} \times \text{velocity}$$

The barbell jump squat is most commonly employed for isoinertial assessment; however,the barbell bench throw has also been used to evaluate upper-body power expression. The barbell bench throw does, however, require either specialised apparatus or spotters to assist with catching the bar after it has been projected to avoid endangering the athlete.

Assessment of maximal power P_{max} load

Much attention has been given to the load at which peak power output is achieved, termed P_{max} from both a training and testing viewpoint. Athletes' power outputs across a spectrum of loads for a ballistic speed-strength exercise (typically barbell jump squat or bench throw) have been used to identify both this P_{max} value and athletes' power output curves (plotted against load) (Harris et al. 2007). Similarly, an increasingly common practice when testing an athlete's speed-strength capabilities is to plot their individual load versus power output curve for the jump squat. One proposed application of this method is to serve as a diagnostic tool to guide athletes' training prescription in order to shift their load/power curve in a certain direction.

However, it has been highlighted that the apparatus (Cormie et al. 2007a) and method of calculation (Cormie et al. 2007b) commonly employed in fact produce grossly inaccurate power output values. This results in a warped load versus power output plot, which is not reflective of the true relationship (Cormie et al. 2007b). When the correct apparatus is employed and power output values are calculated correctly it has been shown that the load which maximises power output for the barbell jump squat in fact equates to zero per cent 1-RM: that is, the player's own body mass without any external load. This result has been reported for both adolescent (Dayne et al. 2011) and college-aged male athlete subjects (Cormie et al. 2007b).

Furthermore, a number of authors increasingly question the practical importance of this P_{max} value, and such application of the load/power output curve is also debated. A study of senior elite rugby union players reported that the difference in power outputs either side of the calculated P_{max} value were minimal: loads 10 per cent and 20 per cent above or below the player's identified P_{max} load on average affected power outputs by only 1.4 per cent and 5.4 per cent respectively (Harris *et al.* 2007). In terms of practical application, P_{max} values also appear to relate only to the training movement tested and thus cannot be generalised to other training exercises.

Jump squat testing

As discussed above, jump squat assessments of speed-strength performance are often conducted over a range of loads. From a methodological point of view, it appears that the use of apparatus such as a Smith machine may impact upon the relationship between jump squat power output and measures of athletic performance (Cronin and Hansen 2005). Scores on an unrestricted squat jump using a free weight Olympic barbell were found to correlate with sprint performance in rugby league football players (Cronin and Hansen 2005), whereas absolute squat jump scores measured in restricted apparatus reportedly did not (Baker and Nance 1999a). By restricting the plane of motion of the bar it may be that this apparatus affects the functionality of the test by reducing the degree of specificity to sports movements, such as balance and co-ordination aspects (Cronin and Hansen 2005).

Devices are now commercially available that allow free weight barbell jump squats to be used for the same form of assessment to evaluate power output. However, preliminary data indicate that these accelerometer apparatuses may not provide accurate values for peak velocity or power when performing unrestricted jumping movements (McMaster *et al.* 2011). These findings are in support of a previous study which reported systematic bias and large random error in measurement of peak power and peak force with commercially available accelerometer and linear position transducer devices (Crewther *et al.* 2011). It also appears that measurements are affected by where the accelerometer device is mounted: that is, whether it is affixed to the athlete or on the barbell. The greatest accuracy of measurement seems to be associated with peak force values derived when the device is mounted directly on the hip of the athlete (McMaster *et al.* 2011).

Olympic weightlifting repetition-maximum testing

Another common measure of speed-strength capabilities against greater resistance involves repetition-maximum (RM) testing using Olympic weightlifting movements. The power clean is generally chosen due to the familiarity of this lift for most players and the fact that it has a distinct end point – essentially the player either fails or succeeds to catch the bar at the top of the lift. In much the same way as for free weight isoinertial strength tests, players' scores will tend to be limited by their technical proficiency with the lift. To avoid such limiting factors, some practitioners employ the pulling derivatives of the Olympic lifts for RM assessments: that is, without the catch portion of the movement at the top of the lift. This may help to offset issues relating to lifting skill associated with the 'catch'. However, there may be other issues using the Olympic pulling derivatives for RM testing. In the absence of the catch as a distinct end point, there are challenges standardising how high the barbell must be raised in order to deem that the player has successfully completed the pulling lift with a given weight.

Repetition-maximum testing using the hang power clean (that is, a power clean initiated with the bar at the 'hang' position at mid-thigh) is also often used to assess maximum speed-strength capabilities. Australian rules football players' scores on the 1-RM hang power clean were found to be related to their vertical jump, maximum strength (squat 1-RM) and sprint performance (Hori et al. 2008). Similarly, the power clean 1-RM scores of college American football players, expressed relative to body mass, were reported to show a significant statistical relationship with measures of acceleration and straight-line sprint performance (Brechue et al. 2010).

Vertical jump assessment

Variations of the vertical jump are the most commonly employed measure of lower-body 'explosive power' or speed-strength performance for both athletic and non-athletic populations (Klavora 2000). Some have questioned the validity of using vertical jump as a specific measure of lower-body power given that multiple segments, including both lower and upper limbs, contribute to the movement and that motor skill and co-ordination aspects also influence vertical-jump performance (Young et al. 2001b). Regardless of these debates, from the point of view of assessing athletic performance the vertical jump is a common action in most sports and is biomechanically similar to various acceleration and game-related dynamic movements. It would therefore appear valid to include some form of vertical-jump assessment in a battery of tests to assess speed-strength expression and athletic performance of team sports players.

The standard test for concentric power production is the squat jump, executed from a set squat depth, and initiated without any countermovement. The countermovement jump, with eccentric and concentric movements performed rapidly and without a pause, is the standard test of combined concentric and 'slow' stretch-shortening cycle performance. The difference between (concentric-only) squat jump and countermovement jump height has been used to evaluate the contribution of the eccentric phase or 'slow' stretch-shortening cycle to the player's performance. Drop vertical jumps may also be used in a similar way to evaluate the 'fast' stretch-shortening cycle component (Ford et al. 2005); this form of assessment does, however, also comprise reactive strength qualities (discussed in the following section).

One study reported that of a range of field-based vertical jump tests the squat (concentric-only) and countermovement jump tests executed with hands on hips had the greatest reliability with recreationally active subjects (physical education students), in terms of producing consistent scores across trials (Markovic et al. 2004). However, restricting the use of arm swing would appear to compromise the biomechanical specificity of the jump movement – very few jumping movements in sport are executed without using the arms. Removing arm swing also has the effect of reducing jump height (in comparison to the corresponding test performed with arm swing) (Feltner et al. 1999; Markovic et al. 2004). Arm swing is shown to augment torque generation at hip and knee joints during the propulsive phase of the vertical jump (Feltner et al. 1999). Another related methodological consideration is that jumping (with arm swing) to reach a target overhead has been shown to influence both movement mechanics and jump height (Ford et al. 2005). It follows that an overhead goal should be a feature of the field test apparatus used to measure jump height where possible – and that arm swing (and reach) should be permitted during the test movement.

In accordance with the methodological and specificity considerations discussed, a field testing device using a jump and reach protocol (with arm swing and reaching up to touch measurement vanes positioned overhead) was reported to have the highest correlation with selection in a sample of elite ice hockey players (Burr et al. 2007). This study examined both squat (concentric-only) and countermovement jumps and compared correlations with the respective tests performed using a contact mat system and performed without arm swing. Jump and reach scores using the overhead measuring vane apparatus correlated more closely with the order of players' eventual order of selection in the National Hockey League draft than the corresponding squat and countermovement jump (no arm swing) scores on the contact mat system (Burr et al. 2007). The authors of this study concluded that the overhead measurement vane apparatus using a jump and reach protocol – in particular the concentric-only squat jump and reach – was the most appropriate for off-ice testing for elite ice hockey players.

It has been shown that a one-step initiation movement before executing a (bilateral) countermovement jump increases jump height (Lawson et al. 2006). The one-step lead in technique also alters the biomechanics and kinematics of the movement (joint angles and ground reaction forces) despite the fact that the jump is still executed from two legs (bilateral stance). A study of male and female volleyball players found that players preloaded their lead leg during the step close version of the test, resulting in greater hip, knee and ankle torques and ground reaction forces measured in lead leg versus trail leg (Lawson et al. 2006). Assessing both dominant and non-dominant leg as the lead leg during step close jumps can also indicate bilateral differences in performance between lower limbs. Single-leg variations of the standard vertical jump tests can be used in the same way (Newton et al. 2006). Likewise, vertical jumps with run-up of various distances (1-step, 3-step, 5-step) have also been used to assess power and athletic performance (Young et al. 2001b).

Horizontal jump tests

Standing long jump and standing triple jump are also used to measure lower-body power in a horizontal movement, in contrast to most forms of assessment which evaluate only movement in a vertical direction. The fact that horizontal jump tests require generation of horizontal and vertical ground reaction forces is identified as beneficial in terms of replicating running and locomotion activities that feature in sport (Holm et al. 2008). The greater specificity of this mode of assessment is reflected in positive statistical relationships reported with measures of acceleration, speed and change of direction (Brughelli et al. 2008; Peterson et al. 2006). The single-leg countermovement horizontal jump in particular is identified as a good predictor of speed and change of direction performance (Meylan et al. 2009).

In addition to strength and power qualities of the locomotor muscles, this form of assessment also demands co-ordination and balance, particularly when the test involves multiple jumps, hops or bounds (Hamilton et al. 2008). Consequently, one methodological consideration with these horizontal jump tests is that subjects' familiarity with the movement will tend to influence the reliability of scores between trials (Markovic et al. 2004). Specifically, a motor learning effect has been observed with physical education students during a single test session – so that performance tended to improve with consecutive trials (Markovic et al. 2004). For this reason practice trials are recommended prior to assessing performance, particularly during the initial stages when these tests are first introduced.

Assessing reactive (speed-)strength and stretch-shortening cycle performance

Reactive strength concerns the coupling of eccentric and concentric muscle actions; this form of assessment typically requires the athlete to decelerate their own momentum in a negative direction, before reversing the movement to initiate a concentric propulsion action in a positive direction (Newton and Dugan 2002). As such, these measures comprise both eccentric and concentric speed-strength qualities, in addition to stretch-shortening cycle (SSC) components. Assessment of reactive strength for 'slow' SSC movements that feature longer ground contact are derived from the difference between concentric-only jumping measures (for example, squat jump) and countermovement jump height. Lower limb reactive strength and fast SSC performance are typically assessed via drop jump testing. Drop jump height is also often expressed with respect to the player's corresponding countermovement jump height score. When conducting drop jump tests to measure reactive strength, participants are instructed to maximise jump height whilst minimising the time in contact with the ground – so that the participant aims to initiate the jump as soon as they touch down after dropping down from the box.

If drop tests are carried out using a force platform or contact mat, a 'reactive strength index' can also be derived from the ratio between contact time and flight time (elapsed time between take-off and landing) (Newton and Dugan 2002). The validity of the drop jump height measure is supported by the observation that drop jump height index scores correlated with sprint performance in female high school sprinters (Hennessy and Kilty 2001). This form of assessment often involves multiple drop jumps executed from various box heights: drop height can then be plotted against heights jumped to provide a profile of the player's drop jump and fast SSC reactive strength capabilities. Players with a plyometric training background will tend to jump higher from a drop jump – so that the box height used in training can be increased until they reach a drop jump height that exceeds their fast SSC reactive strength capabilities. A study assessing athletes from different sports using a drop jump test from a relatively large height (60cm) showed that team sports (soccer, volleyball, handball and basketball) players employed different motor strategies to track and field athletes and rowers when performing the drop jump test (Kollias *et al.* 2004). Like other types of jump, the presence of a vertical goal during vertical drop jump testing appears to influence movement mechanics, lower limb biomechanics, contact time and even jump height (Ford *et al.* 2005).

Single-leg variations of the vertical jump test also exist which allow the reactive speed-strength and SSC performance of dominant and non-dominant limbs to be assessed independently. Likewise, horizontal drop jump tests have also been investigated (Holm *et al.* 2008). These tests involve dropping (vertically) from a box of specified height and immediately jumping for distance in a horizontal direction upon touchdown. Horizontal drop jump testing also includes both bilateral and unilateral variations. The single-leg horizontal drop jump test has reported positive statistical relationships with measures of acceleration and speed performance with team sports players (Holm *et al.* 2008).

Triple-hop testing offers another means to assess reactive speed-strength performance in a horizontal direction (Hamilton *et al.* 2008). In addition to reactive speed-strength and stretch-shortening cycle qualities, executing repeated hops requires considerable athleticism, balance and postural stability. Triple jump or hop performance is therefore likely to demonstrate a marked familiarisation effect (Markovic *et al.* 2004). Performance on the triple hop test was shown to be related to vertical jump performance in male and female collegiate soccer players, which led the authors of this study to conclude that the triple hop test was a valid measure of power performance in these players (Hamilton *et al.* 2008). The unilateral nature of repeated hop tests allows comparison of performance between limbs. A five-hop variation of this test was shown to identify differences in performance between dominant and non-dominant limbs among collegiate female softball players (Newton *et al.* 2006). Accordingly, single-leg repeated hop tests of this type have seen application in a rehabilitation setting to evaluate functional performance of injured versus uninjured legs (Hamilton *et al.* 2008).

Evaluating endurance performance

One approach when assessing endurance capabilities of athletes is to test the individual physiological parameters that underpin endurance performance (Jones and Carter 2000). Traditionally, the standard measure of endurance capacity has been the measured maximal oxygen uptake or VO_2max, which is typically evaluated in the laboratory using a variety of incremental test protocols performed to failure. The running velocity or work intensity at which VO_2max is attained (also known as 'vVO_2max') can also be used as an index of aerobic endurance capacity. This parameter has traditionally been assessed using laboratory protocols with direct measurement of expired air. Other approaches to assessing vVO_2max or maximal aerobic speed (MAS) evaluate this parameter using a maximal incremental test performed to volitional failure; these protocols may or may not record oxygen uptake or heart rate given that vVO_2max or MAS is the criterion measure. These protocols were originally devised to be performed on a running track (Leger and Boucher 1980); however, shuttle-running based field test protocols that allow an analogue measure of MAS to be derived have also since been developed for application with team sports players.

In addition to maximal oxygen uptake, a player's aerobic endurance is also determined by their capacity to sustain a high percentage of their maximum aerobic output without lactate accumulation. This parameter is termed the lactate threshold (LT) or maximum lactate steady state (MLSS), and is in turn linked to the athlete's muscle buffering capacity as well as their propensity to metabolise and clear lactate. Similarly, given the intermittent nature of activity team sports, anaerobic capacity and repeated sprint ability are also critical factors that determine sport-specific endurance capacities. The final factors that contribute to endurance performance are running economy or work efficiency. This can be viewed as the neuromuscular component of endurance. In the context of team sports, it follows that any test should aim to replicate the types of locomotion that features during a game in order to fully address this movement economy factor when assessing aerobic endurance (Aziz *et al.* 2005).

Laboratory assessments

Laboratory testing requires specialised equipment that is expensive and requires trained personnel to operate it. Given these cost issues, as well as the time demands of testing each player individually, laboratory testing is not generally amenable to application with squads of players (Impellizzeri *et al.* 2005). In the case of intermittent sports, and particularly team sports, the use of laboratory-based assessment is therefore typically restricted to a research setting. In addition to these issues of practicality, the validity of laboratory-based measures that are typically derived from continuous protocols performed on a treadmill has also been questioned for team sports players (Carey *et al.* 2007).

Field tests have therefore been developed that offer a more practical and potentially more valid alternative for use with players who compete in intermittent sports. As the field-test protocols are often closer to what occurs in intermittent sports, these tests are often considered more relevant to players and coaches in these sports than laboratory tests (Bosquet *et al.* 2002). Scores with these field tests generally report high correlations with laboratory test measurements (Bosquet *et al.* 2002). Regression equations do also exist that can be used to derive estimated scores for standard 'laboratory' measures, such as VO_2max (Impellizzeri *et al.* 2005).

Field-based maximal tests of cardiorespiratory fitness

Incremental protocols for over-ground running

Protocols such as the Université de Montréal track test were originally devised for over-ground running on a running track in order to assess athletes' vVO_2max, and thereby provide an indirect estimate of maximal aerobic capacity without direct measurement of expired air (Leger and Boucher 1980). However, a strong relationship has emerged between vVO_2max and endurance performance in competition, so that vVO_2max has to some extent replaced VO_2max as the criterion measure. In recent years a modified version of the original Université de Montréal track test has been developed, named the Vam-eval protocol. This test is performed on a running track and the pace is controlled using audio signals: the starting velocity is $8ms^{-1}$ and running speed is increased by $0.5ms^{-1}$ each minute (Chtara *et al.* 2005).

Measures of vVO_2max and MAS have been identified as key parameters of endurance for team sports players. Despite this, vVO_2 scores derived from the Vam-eval incremental track test protocol were not reported to correlate well with running performance recorded during a match for the majority of playing positions in youth soccer (Buchheit *et al.* 2010c). This lack of relationship may be a consequence of the lack of specificity of this mode of assessment; continuous running around a track is not reflective of the intermittent nature of exertion or the frequent changes in direction that occur during a match.

Twenty-metre multistage shuttle test

In order to improve the specificity of assessment modes, various shuttle run protocols have been developed for use with team sports players (Castagna *et al.* 2006). The 20m multi-stage fitness test has become a standard field test for aerobic endurance (Flouris *et al.* 2005; Wilkinson *et al.* 1999). Measured VO_2max during the 20m multistage shuttle test (MST) has shown to correspond well with laboratory measured VO_2max during a maximal tread-mill test for team sports players (rugby players and field hockey players) (Aziz *et al.* 2005). The fact that endurance athletes (triathletes and runners) showed different VO_2max scores between the field and treadmill tests points to the greater familiarity and specificity of the shuttle run test mode for team sports players as opposed to endurance athletes.

The 20m MST has been adapted for other sports: an on-ice version of the test was devised and validated for ice hockey players (Leger *et al.* 1979). Variations of the original 20m MST have also been proposed. These include a modified incremental 20m shuttle test that increases running speed after each shuttle (Wilkinson *et al.* 1999), as opposed to increasing velocity at 1-minute intervals as occurs with the original version of the test. The authors of this study argue that such an approach avoids the tendency for players to drop out at the start of a given level, as can happen with the original test protocol (Wilkinson *et al.* 1999). Such a scenario may make the original 20m MST less sensitive to changes in training status, as players may voluntarily drop out once they have achieved their target level rather than continuing to volitional fatigue.

Yo-Yo intermittent test

Other field tests of aerobic endurance that are widely used in team sports include the Yo-Yo intermittent fitness test, which has become particularly popular in soccer (Metaxas *et al.* 2005). The most striking feature of the Yo-Yo intermittent test protocol is that players do not run continuously. The test requires subjects to perform repeated bouts of running (two sets of 20m shuttle runs) at increasing intensity; these work intervals are interspersed with 10-second rest periods (Bangsbo *et al.* 2008). A correlation study concluded that, although the two measures were correlated, this intermittent test protocol assessed physiological qualities additional to the continuous 20m shuttle test (Castagna *et al.* 2006). The Yo-Yo intermittent test protocol would appear to more closely resemble the intermittent nature of exertion that players engage in during competition. Two versions of the Yo-Yo intermittent test protocol exist: Yo-Yo intermittent recovery level 1 (IR1) begins at a slower running velocity and so features more progressive increases in running speed; level 2 (IR2) starts at a faster velocity so that subjects engage in high-intensity exertion much sooner (Bangsbo *et al.* 2008). Both versions of the test have been found to have acceptably high levels of test–retest reliability with various groups of subjects.

Regression equations also exist to predict VO_2max from both IR1 and IR2 Yo-Yo test performance. However, some studies have found that the Yo-Yo intermittent field test offers a less accurate measure of VO_2max than laboratory-based treadmill tests that directly measure oxygen consumption (Metaxas *et al.* 2005). From a practical viewpoint it should be borne in mind that obtaining a measure of VO_2max is of less relative importance than providing an assessment of the endurance capacity of players competing in intermittent sports, which will inevitably feature an anaerobic component.

In support of this, a study of Australian rules football reported that players' VO_2max scores showed no difference between starting players and substitutes, whereas Yo-Yo IR2 test scores were able to differentiate between starting and non-starting players (Young *et al.* 2005). Another study, this time in soccer, found that Yo-Yo IR1 test scores recorded by soccer players were shown to correlate to their on-field performance (quantity of high-intensity running total undertaken during games), whereas their treadmill VO_2max scores did not (Krustrup *et al.* 2003). These studies indicate that it is beneficial for field tests of endurance to feature an anaerobic component in order to be reflective of the specific endurance capabilities required by intermittent sports. Accordingly, scores on the Yo-Yo IR1 test reported positive statistical relationships with a variety of physical performance measures recorded by elite youth soccer players during a match (Castagna *et al.* 2010).

The Yo-Yo intermittent recovery level 2 (IR2) protocol is intended for use specifically by trained athletes: it is run at faster cadence – hence test duration is shorter – and is demonstrated to have a large anaerobic component based upon lactate profiles and muscle biopsy samples (Bangsbo *et al.* 2008). For this reason it has been suggested that the IR2 protocol has greater scope for discriminating between elite players and those competing at lower levels, given the greater demand for high-intensity exertion during matches at elite level. Crucially, both IR1 and IR2 tests also appear sensitive to changes in fitness elicited by training and associated improvements in on-field performance (time spent engaged in high-intensity running and maximum distance covered in five-minute interval during a match) (Bangsbo *et al.* 2008).

30–15 intermittent fitness test

The 20m multistage shuttle run test and Yo-Yo test described previously can be used to provide an indirect measure of the (shuttle) running speed associated with VO_2max or maximum aerobic speed (MAS). It has, however, been identified that the values provided by the Yo-Yo test particularly do not correlate well with direct measures of MAS or vVO_2max and therefore it has been argued that the Yo-Yo test scores should not be used for prescribing training intensity. An alternative protocol, the 30–15 intermittent fitness test ($30–15_{IFT}$), has been developed specifically for the purpose of evaluating an analogue measure of MAS in the field.

The measure derived from the final running speed achieved in this protocol, termed V_{IFT}, in fact equates to an intensity above vVO_2max. Typically, V_{IFT} scores are ≈20 per cent higher than MAS scores from a continuous over-ground running test, such as the Vam-eval, and ≈35 per cent higher than the final shuttle running speed recorded on the 20m MST (Buchheit 2008). Players' V_{IFT} scores do, however, correlate well with both these measures. Furthermore, due to the reliability and accuracy of the V_{IFT} measure for individualising players' training intensity, the $30–15_{IFT}$ protocol is becoming widely used when undertaking interval running conditioning in team sports (Buchheit 2008).

The $30–15_{IFT}$ protocol is intermittent in nature, in a similar way to the Yo-Yo test. Subjects run shuttles for 30 seconds at a given velocity interspersed with 15 seconds active recovery bouts; running velocity for the work bouts is progressively increased with each run. However, the course consists of two cones spaced 40 metres apart: subjects perform an initial 40m run, followed by a 180-degree turn and a run of a specified distance in the opposite direction. The calculated distances for each run are corrected for the time required to complete the necessary 180-degree turns (Buchheit 2008). During the later levels when the pace increases and the distance for the return shuttle exceeds 40m, the player makes a final 180-degree turn and runs a specified distance in the original direction. The $30–15_{IFT}$ has been validated against vVO_2max directly measured in the laboratory and MAS measures derived from standard field tests involving continuous over-ground running. Scores on the $30–15_{IFT}$ also correlated well with other tests of speed (10m sprint) and power (vertical) in young team sports players (Buchheit 2008). An on-ice version of the $30–15_{IFT}$ has also recently been developed and validated for ice hockey players (Buchheit *et al.* 2011b).

Sport-specific test protocols

An alternative approach to assessing endurance performance for sports is to test players' scores on specific tests designed to replicate the endurance demands of the sport (Hoff 2005; Impellizzeri *et al.* 2005). Both treadmill (laboratory-based) (Sirotic and Coutts 2007) and field-based (Hoff 2005) sport-specific endurance tests of this type have been developed. Such tests aim to simulate movement patterns and even incorporate technical skills that feature in the sport in order to increase the level of specificity of the test measure (Impellizzeri *et al.* 2005). The integrated approach used by such sport-specific protocols thus attempts to assess endurance performance in a way that reproduces the bioenergetics of the sport. As such, these tests do not offer insight into individual physiological components; rather energy systems and performance abilities are assessed in combination (Impellizzeri *et al.* 2005). However, serious limitations to this approach exist. One major issue is the difficulty in standardising conditions in order to obtain a reliable and repeatable test measure. Similarly, the challenge with these sport-specific test protocols is accumulating sufficient normative data to provide reference values against which to evaluate players' scores. In the case of treadmill 'sport-specific' simulations, the usual practical issues with regard to laboratory-based testing for large numbers of players also arise.

Submaximal tests of endurance fitness

When performing serial measurements with players, repeated use of maximal tests may engender motivation and compliance issues. Progressive tests to exhaustion are dependent upon the motivation of players to perform maximally (Lemmink *et al.* 2004). In view of this, attention has been given to submaximal tests for endurance performance. Submaximal tests would seem to be more conducive to repeated testing at regular intervals given that they avoid such complications with respect to motivation and compliance (Impellizzeri *et al.* 2005; Krustrup *et al.* 2003; Lemmink *et al.* 2004).

Such submaximal tests are often modified versions of existing progressive maximal test protocols; essentially the test is terminated at a predetermined submaximal workload. The test scores recorded are generally based upon measurement of physiological responses (for example, heart rate) during and/or following the standardised final (submaximal) workload (Lemmink *et al.* 2004). In the laboratory ventilatory and heart rate responses can be recorded to provide a measure of how taxing the submaximal workload was for the player on a given test occasion. A notable example of an equivalent field-based test is the submaximal 'non-exhaustive' version of the Yo-Yo test of aerobic fitness (Bangsbo *et al.* 2008). The protocol used is identical to the maximal version of the test – up until the point when it is terminated 'early' at a submaximal workload. One practical issue with field-based submaximal tests is that these tests do still require that physiological responses (typically heart rate) are monitored – consequently all participating players must have access to relevant equipment, such as heart rate monitors (Krustrup *et al.* 2003).

It appears that submaximal test protocols must exceed a minimum threshold duration in order to ensure that the outcome measure does show the desired relationship with maximal performance. A 3-minute submaximal version of the Yo-Yo test was reported to be insufficient, whereas a 6-minute protocol did show correlation to maximal Yo-Yo test scores (Bangsbo *et al.* 2008). Similarly, the data suggest that the higher the final workload (running speed) chosen for the final stage of the submaximal test the greater the reliability of the physiological measure, particularly in the case of heart rate (Lemmink *et al.* 2004). It has been identified that the final workload should aim to elicit exercise intensities in the range 86–93 per cent of players' HR_{max} in order to reduce measurement error and improve sensitivity in detecting meaningful changes (Lamberts *et al.* 2011). This final test workload might be determined via baseline testing for the squad of players; however, for consistency the protocol would thereafter need to remain the same for the duration of a season of testing. As these tests involve serial measurements, each player essentially acts as his/her own reference against which scores are evaluated.

Assessment of running economy or work efficiency

Exercise economy is typically assessed as the oxygen uptake (VO_2) at a given work intensity (Jones and Carter 2000). Running economy is therefore commonly assessed in the laboratory by measuring the athlete's oxygen uptake at a reference running velocity on the treadmill. Similarly, gas analysis can be used in the same way with cycle or rowing ergometer at a reference work intensity to evaluate the same parameter for cycling or rowing performance. Portable gas analysis equipment does exist that can allow similar assessments to be made in the field, implementing appropriate pacing on the track to standardise velocity; however, this tends to be less widely used. Running economy and work efficiency measures will be highly specific to both the mode (Millet *et al.* 2002a) and velocity of locomotion (Jones and Carter 2000) used in testing. Measuring work economy for team sports players would therefore require that both the different modes and velocities of locomotion that feature in a game are accounted for. To date no such protocol exists for team sports players.

Assessments of lactate-handling capacity

Although lactate-handling capacity may be relevant to endurance performance with team sports players, the measure used to assess this parameter has a major bearing in terms of comparing players' scores. Classically, the criterion for 'onset of blood lactate' (OBLA) or lactate threshold (LT) has been a fixed concentration of blood lactate, typically 4mmol/l (Bosquet *et al.* 2002). Deflection point(s) in the curve between running velocity and measured blood lactate are also used as a measure of lactate threshold. Such tests are typically carried out in the laboratory to allow running velocity to be standardised and facilitate blood lactate sampling.

Methods for indirect evaluation (without taking blood lactate samples) of LT or the equivalent 'anaerobic threshold' (AT) also exist, which are based upon changes detected in ventilatory or heart rate responses (Bosquet *et al.* 2002). The validity of the 'ventilatory threshold' (VT) model has been questioned on the basis that its determination is highly subjective and also highly variable, as well as being dependent on the criteria chosen. It has also been demonstrated that the LT and VT can be manipulated independently under different conditions (Bosquet *et al.* 2002). Similarly, heart rate-based procedures are undermined by serious doubts about whether such a physiological deflection point in heart rate responses actually exists, and if it does whether it bears any relation to LT (Bosquet *et al.* 2002).

Lactate threshold

Classically, this lactate threshold has been taken to correspond to a concentration of blood lactate (BLa) of $4mmol.l^{-1}$ – this has been widely used to denote the 'onset of blood lactate' (OBLA). However, over recent years it has been documented that the actual concentration of BLa that corresponds to the maximum steady-state workload varies widely between individuals, falling between a broad range of values from $2mmol.l^{-1}$ to $8mmol.l^{-1}$ (Billat et al. 2003). This $4mmol.l^{-1}$ OBLA value thus appears to be an arbitrary figure, which bears little resemblance to the actual BLa concentration at steady state for many individuals. For the same reasons, comparing absolute values of BLa concentration sampled within and between studies would also appear spurious without the appropriate reference MLSS BLa concentration values for each subject.

Serial measurement of LT has been used to track fitness among junior professional soccer players via repeated measurements at pre-season and periodically during the subsequent playing season (McMillan et al. 2005b). The only significant change in these measures was observed between baseline pre-season scores and the in-season test scores – there were no changes subsequent to the start of the playing season. These serial LT measures were therefore only sensitive to the gross changes in fitness between pre-season (which players entered in a relatively detrained state following a five-week off-season period without structured training) and the start of the playing season (McMillan et al. 2005b). This apparent lack of sensitivity combined with the lack of specificity and aforementioned practical issues of laboratory testing a squad of players, in addition to the methodological concerns regarding lactate threshold measurement, would seem to call into question the validity of this form of testing for team sports players.

Maximum lactate steady state assessment

Maximum lactate steady state (MLSS) has been proposed as an alternative form of assessment of lactate handling for athletes. MLSS is defined as the maximum intensity at which lactate clearance matches lactate production – that is, the highest workload that can be sustained without accumulation of BLa (Billat et al. 2003). From this point of view, MLSS is equivalent to the theoretical upper lactate threshold at the deflection point in the curve of lactate concentration plotted against exercise intensity.

Given these methodological and theoretical concerns regarding traditional lactate threshold measures, the MLSS measure would appear to be a more robust and valid marker for use as a parameter of endurance performance. However, determination of MLSS involves a time-consuming protocol typically involving repeated visits to a laboratory. Direct measurement of MLSS is also invasive in the sense that it relies upon repeated blood lactate sampling. Such considerations raise questions about the practicality of including assessment of MLSS in a standard battery of performance tests for a squad of players.

Field tests of 'anaerobic capacity'

The standard measure of anaerobic capacity in the laboratory evaluates maximally accumulated oxygen deficit (MAOD), which represents the difference between estimated oxygen demand and measured oxygen uptake during a maximal exercise test (Moore and Murphy

2003). As discussed previously, such laboratory-based physiological testing is generally impractical for routine assessment of team sports players.

Field tests have been developed to assess anaerobic capacity for single maximal efforts performed at supramaximal intensity. For example, the Wingate test performed on a cycle ergometer has often been used to assess anaerobic capacity, based on average power output maintained during the 30-second all-out effort (Popadic Gacesa et al. 2009). Fatigue effects observed and associated decrements in work output are shown to differ between test modes, and are typically more pronounced for repeated cycling exercise versus running protocols (Girard et al. 2011a). There is also some question whether this form of assessment is relevant or valid for running-based sports, particularly at elite level (Legaz-Arrese et al. 2011).

A running-based protocol that has been reported to correlate well with MAOD measured in the laboratory involves a maximal 20m shuttle running test over a total distance of 300 metres (Moore and Murphy 2003). The time taken to cover this distance is the outcome measure, and typical values reported are in the range of 62–70 seconds.

Tests of repeated sprint ability

Repeated sprint ability (RSA) is widely recognised as a critical parameter of endurance for team sports players (Impellizzeri et al. 2008). While measures of RSA demonstrate moderate statistical relationships with both speed and MST endurance measures, this capacity is found to be a discrete quality and should therefore be assessed independently (Pyne et al. 2008). Players' scores on an RSA test have reported positive statistical relationships with measures of high-intensity running and sprinting distance recorded during matches in soccer (Rampinini et al. 2007a).

Field-based RSA tests commonly evaluate performance on a series of maximal efforts. Protocols can be divided into two categories: those which feature all-out efforts involving relatively longer distance or duration; and protocols that involve sprint efforts of shorter duration (≤10 seconds) or distance (generally 40m or less). The majority of test protocols fall into the former category, with most tests employing sprint bouts of 5–6 seconds duration or 30–40m in the case of over-ground running protocols. A range of selected assessments of RSA is presented in Table 2.1.

The rest intervals employed between sprint bouts vary with different assessments of RSA. This is a factor which strongly influences metabolic and physiological responses and associated effects on sprint performance in successive work bouts (Oliver et al. 2009; Spencer et al. 2005). Manifestation of fatigue effects and any corresponding deterioration in sprint performance observed also appears to depend to a large degree on the sprint distance or duration assessed. An investigation by Balsom and colleagues (1992) employed 15 sets of 40m sprints with different recovery intervals (30-secs, 1-min or 2-min). The common finding whatever the recovery duration employed was that 30–40m split times were most consistently affected in the latter sprints (Balsom et al. 1992). In contrast, the fatigue effects on sprint performances over shorter distances were less apparent. Indeed, changes in 0–15m split times were only seen with the shortest 30-second rest interval protocol, and the decrements in performance were only minor (Balsom et al. 1992).

In order to provide a specific measure of RSA for the sport there is an argument that sprint distances and rest intervals selected should reflect what occurs during a match (Bishop et al. 2001). Sprint distances and durations most commonly observed during

Table 2.1 Selected repeated sprint ability test protocols

Test mode	Distance/ duration	Protocol	Outcome measure	Reference
Cycle ergometer	6-second bouts	Repeated every 30 seconds (i.e. 6 seconds work, 24 seconds rest)	Work output scores	Bishop *et al.* 2001
			Power output values expressed relative to body mass	Bishop *et al.* 2004
Non-motorised treadmill	5-second sprints	7 × 5-second sprints with 20 seconds recovery between	Maximum speed recorded in 1-second interval each sprint Combined mean speed (all sprints) Total work (all sprints) Mean work each sprint trial	Oliver *et al.* 2009
Over-ground straight-line running	30-metre sprints	6 × 30-metre sprints departing every 20 seconds	Sum of sprint times Percentage change in times from first to last sprint	Pyne *et al.* 2008
Over-ground straight-line running	30-metre sprints	6 × 30-metre sprints departing every 25 seconds	Sum of sprint times	Spencer *et al.* 2006
Over-ground shuttle running	40-metre shuttle sprints – 2 × 20m	6 × 40m shuttle sprints with 20-seconds recovery between	Mean sprint time Best sprint time % decrement score (mean sprint time divided by best sprint time)	Impellizzeri *et al.* 2007
Over-ground shuttle running	30-second duration shuttle sprints	Shuttle sprints over 5 metres and 10 metres, alternately, for 30s 6 sets performed in total, with 35 seconds rest between each set	Sum of distances covered during each 30-second bout	Boddington *et al.* 2001

matches in field-based team sports equate to 10–20 metres or 2–3 seconds, which contrasts with most RSA assessment protocols (Spencer *et al.* 2005). Equally, it could be argued that the distance or duration of sprint bouts and the duration of rest intervals employed should represent the extremes of what the player might face during competition, in order both to provide a sufficiently challenging assessment, and also to ensure that fatigue effects will be elicited during successive sprints.

Assessments of RSA generally provide two different indices of performance: the sum of all sprint efforts (combined distance covered or sprint times recorded); and a measure of the relative decrement in performance across repeated sprint bouts. The way that the latter measure is calculated appears to be a critical factor (Spencer *et al.* 2005; Girard *et al.* 2011a).

For example, some protocols employ a simple *fatigue index* measure: that is, a percentage score derived from the calculation:

(best sprint trial score − worst sprint trial score) / best sprint trial score

It is argued that this fatigue index measure generally does not provide a good measure of repeated sprint ability (Oliver 2009; Pyne *et al.* 2008; Spencer *et al.* 2006). Therefore an alternative measure, termed the percentage decrement score or S_{dec}, has been recommended as a more valid and reliable measure of fatigue for repeated sprint ability tests (Glaister *et al.* 2008). The calculation of S_{dec} takes into account performance for all sprint trials in the repeated sprint test:

$$S_{dec} (\%) = \left\{ \frac{(S_1 + S_2 + S_3 \ldots + S_{Final})}{S_{Best} \times \text{number of sprints}} - 1 \right\} \times 100$$

Assessing speed components

In the context of team sports, speed comprises the ability to move at high velocity in a variety of directions, and often not in a straight line; equally critical is the player's ability to change direction at pace. Players' scores on straight-line sprinting and tests of change of direction performance typically show only limited statistical relationship. A study of professional soccer revealed that players' acceleration, maximum speed and change of direction test scores shared low statistical relationships (Little and Williams 2005). The authors concluded that these are distinct and separate abilities: accounting for the fact that the corresponding scores were relatively unrelated in these players (Little and Williams 2005). Furthermore, correlations between measures of these abilities reportedly decrease markedly when any sport skill component is incorporated in the agility test (Young *et al.* 2001b). This appears to reflect the dissimilarity of movement mechanics between straight-line running and the locomotion employed during change of direction tasks (Sheppard and Young 2006, Young *et al.* 2001a).

A number of electronic timing gates systems are commercially available that offer high degrees of accuracy (to nearest hundredths or thousandths of a second) and reliability. Such timing gates are amenable to both straight-line sprinting tests and change of direction tests, and this equipment is also portable so is suitable for field testing. Access to timing gate devices is almost a prerequisite if the strength and conditioning specialist aims to conduct speed or change of direction testing with any confidence, in terms of accuracy and reliability (Brown *et al.* 2004). The inaccuracy of results reported when timing using handheld stopwatches is compounded by the finding that, while handheld stopwatch-recorded times are generally faster than those recorded using electronic timing, this is not a consistent outcome (Hetzler *et al.* 2008). As a result, it is not possible to apply a correction factor in order to convert stopwatch-recorded times. Based on these findings, it seems that when testing is conducted with a handheld stopwatch, the times recorded should be used only as a guide and the coaches should be made aware of the random measurement error with this method.

From a context specificity viewpoint, it would appear advantageous that testing should take place on a similar surface and setting to that upon which players train and perform (Handford *et al*. 1997). One caveat for sports that are played outdoors on a grass surface is that weather and pitch conditions may vary, which can influence serial measurements over time. From the point of view of standardisation it may therefore be preferable to use an all-weather artificial surface or indoor artificial turf facility for field-based running speed assessments in these outdoor field sports.

Measures of straight-line acceleration abilities

Speed scores over 5m have been employed as a measure of 'first-step quickness' (Cronin and Hansen 2005). Players' split times over 10m or 15m are likewise often used to evaluate acceleration ability. Whereas the 'first-step quickness' time over 5m and 'acceleration' 10m time correlated closely in semi-professional and professional rugby league players, their 5m times were much less closely related to their maximal speed scores over 30m (Cronin and Hansen 2005). These findings indicate that acceleration and maximal speed are quite distinct abilities in team sports players, and should therefore be evaluated as such.

Assessment of straight-line running speed

Assessments of running speed commonly used in team sports typically employ total distances of 30 or 40 metres, depending largely on the convention for the sport (Gamble 2011b). In North America it is customary to assess speed over a distance of 40 yards; for example, the NFL Combine features the 40-yard dash (Sierer *et al*. 2008). In addition, these tests often include split times over specified distances in order to evaluate players' sprint performance for different phases within the speed test (Brown *et al*. 2004). This will also allow the tester to concurrently assess measures of acceleration, as described above. Another method of evaluating maximal speed capabilities that is employed by some in the field is to derive the maximum speed measure from the fastest split time within the overall sprint. Commercially available electronic timing gate systems are required, particularly if attempting to evaluate split times.

Testing agility performance

Commonly employed 'agility tests' in fact assess only change of direction performance: 'agility' is defined in terms of change of direction or velocity in response to a stimulus (Sheppard and Young 2006). This stipulates that there must be some element of reaction and/or decision-making in any true assessment of agility. Some change of direction tests do incorporate simple reaction cues, such as responses to lights or similar. However, this does not represent a valid measure of the game-related information-processing and decision-making factors that contribute to team sports agility performance (Sheppard and Young 2006).

Regardless of these issues, change of direction tests are of relevance: change of direction abilities are a foundation of agility performance. As such, tests of change of direction performance do provide important information, which justifies their inclusion in any battery of tests for team sports players.

Tests of change of direction performance

A wide variety of tests that measure change of direction ability are employed in different sports (Brughelli et al. 2008; Little and Williams 2005; Sheppard and Young 2006; Young et al. 2001a). Protocols differ in terms of both complexity and duration, and the statistical relationship between scores on different change of direction measures varies accordingly (Sporis et al. 2010). Two major considerations when selecting a test protocol are the extent to which the protocol resembles the movement demands required in competition, and also how much normative data exist for the test to provide a reference against which to evaluate players' scores. Factors such as whether the protocol requires change of direction movements to be executed with the dominant or non-dominant leg are also found to influence results (Meylan et al. 2009). As with speed tests, these assessments are most reliable when conducted with electronic timing gates.

The most basic change of direction tests comprise simple 180-degree turns. For example, in the 5–0–5 test the player turns once to sprint 5m back to the start line (Sheppard and Young 2006). The pro agility shuttle is a test that features in the NFL Combine and is essentially an extended version of the 5–0–5 test protocol (Sierer et al. 2008). The player sprints 5 yards, pivots 180-degrees to sprint 10 yards in the opposite direction before executing a final 180-turn to sprint 5 yards back to the start line. The 9–6–3–6–9 test described by Sporis et al. (2010) is run on a straight-line course that extends over a total distance of 18m and comprises a total of five sprints of varying distances and four 180-degree turns. The protocol consists of an initial sprint of 9m before executing a 180-degree turn to sprint 3m in the opposite direction followed by another 180-degree turn and sprint 6m in the original direction, then another 180-degree turn and 3m sprint before a final 180-degree turn and 9m sprint to the finish line.

The '9–6–3–6–9 test with backwards and forwards running' is a modification to the above test which covers the same course, and involves changing direction at the same points; however, the adaptation to the protocol is that the test features only forwards and backwards running – so that the athlete faces in the same direction (towards the finish line) throughout the test. This version of the test was found to differentiate the particular change of direction abilities of defenders and midfield players versus attackers in soccer (Sporis et al. 2010). A number of shuttle change of direction tests also exist in the literature that involve running a prescribed number of shuttle sprints over varying distances. Examples include the 10 yard (9m) shuttle, 6 × 5m shuttle and 4 × 5.8m shuttle tests (Brughelli et al. 2008).

Other change of direction assessments feature a combination of 90-degree and 180-degree turns – one such example is the L-run test or the 3-cone drill featured in the NFL Combine (Sierer et al. 2008) The course players run features a cone placed 5 yards in front of the start/finish cone, with a third cone placed 5 yards to the right of the second cone. The course thus features a 90-degree cut to the right, a 180-degree pivot and turn, and a 90-degree cut to the left before the player returns to the start/finish cone. Of all the change of direction tests employed in the NFL Combine, performance on the L-run test was found to have the greatest correlation to draft pick ranking of American football players selected for professional teams (Sierer et al. 2008).

The 4 × 5m sprint test described by Sporis and colleagues (2010) features a set-up similar to the L-run test course, with the addition of another cone. The protocol is identical to the one described above with an additional 90-degree turn before a final 180-degree turn and 5m sprint to the finish line. The T-test is a widely employed test of change of direction performance, which consists of a 10m sprint forwards to a cone placed at the centre of the 'T', followed by 90-degree lateral cuts to reach cones placed 5m away to the left and right of the centre cone before sprinting 10m back from the centre cone to the start/finish cone. Different versions of this test also exist with modifications to the distances between cones and the movement constraints imposed during the test.

More complex and arguably more relevant change of direction protocols consist of multiple cuts of varying degrees. For example, there are a variety of zigzag run protocols, usually involving cutting change of direction movements around three cones placed between the start and finish cones. The usual cutting angle between successive cones is 100 degrees, and cones are typically placed 5m apart (Mirkov *et al.* 2008). The Slalom test described by Sporis *et al.* (2010) consists of a slalom course through six cones placed on a straight line at 2m intervals – the distance between the start line and the final cone is 11m so the athlete covers a total distance of 22m. The athlete begins on the start line with the first cone of the six-cone slalom course one metre away; the athlete completes a slalom course through each cone in a forwards direction, then performs a 180-degree turn after the final cone to complete the slalom course in the opposite direction to finish back at the start line. The Illinois agility test (Sheppard and Young 2006) is a well-established protocol that features multiple slalom cuts through cones and 180-degree turns. Of all of the standard change of direction tests the Illinois has possibly the greatest complexity of movement, and the time required to complete the test is also among the longest.

Change of direction tests that incorporate a sports skill component have also been studied. For example, the reliability of a range of field-based tests of change of direction, sprinting ability, and power for soccer players have been investigated. Comparison of performance (that is, run time) on a change of direction course when performed without a ball and whilst dribbling a ball have also been used in order to provide a 'skill index' measure (Mirkov *et al.* 2008). While such tests may be useful for comparing scores of players within a squad, a lack of adequate normative data for different populations makes further interpretation difficult.

Assessments of 'reactive agility'

Change of direction tests have been modified to incorporate a simple reaction component to the movement task, so that the movement is executed in response to an external cue. The time recorded by the athlete on tests of this type therefore represents a combination of both reaction time and the time taken to subsequently complete the movement task. Some commercially available timing gate devices provide the facility for reactive tests, so that when the athlete breaks a designated gate one of a selection of 'finish' gates illuminates to indicate which direction the athlete must run to. Alternatively, more simple field-based protocols involve the tester initiating the movement response by performing a sidestep motion in the direction that the athlete is required to move (Sheppard *et al.* 2006). More technologically advanced protocols that have been employed in a research setting use a video display so that the athlete is required to initiate the movement in response to movement of players on the screen (Farrow *et al.* 2005).

Different reactive agility protocols have been investigated with various groups of field team sports athletes. One study compared the same test protocol, performed under both pre-planned conditions (the athlete was told which gate to sprint to before the trial) and reactive conditions cued by a video projection of a player passing the ball in the direction of the gate the athlete was to sprint to (Farrow *et al.* 2005). Movement times are on average slower in the reactive condition due to the perceptual component. However, the difference between split times for pre-planned versus reactive conditions were less for both highly skilled (national institute) and moderately skilled (state-level) netball players, resulting in faster reactive agility times compared to lesser skilled players (B-grade club players) (Farrow *et al.* 2005). As a result, test measures recorded under reactive conditions also appear to be superior in differentiating elite competitors from sub-elite players in these sports.

An investigation of the reactive agility test (RAT) protocol originally described by Sheppard *et al.* (2006), which involves the athlete starting from a stationary position and the movement response being triggered by movement of the tester, reported similar results in Australian rules football players. Players' scores on the RAT protocol differentiated between players of different playing standard, whereas a similar change of direction test under pre-planned conditions was unable to do so. Very similar findings with respect to superior reactive agility times as well as movement response accuracy have also been reported for elite versus sub-elite rugby league players using the same RAT protocol (Gabbett and Benton 2009).

Balance and stability testing

Single-leg balance and stabilisation

Static postural balance

Postural balance is defined as the ability of an individual to maintain their centre of mass within their base of support (Hrysomallis 2007). Practically, balance ability involves input from visual, vestibular, and somatosensory systems (Hamilton *et al.* 2008). When assessing balance it is important therefore to account for each of these subsystems that contribute to balance ability. For example, an eyes-closed variation of a test removes visual system input. Similarly, balance tests involving turning, or raising or lowering the head, attempt to isolate vestibular system input.

Standard tests of balance ability commonly measure time that the player is able to maintain equilibrium under a given set of conditions (for example, stable/labile surface, eyes closed/open). Alternatively, the number of attempts taken to balance under a given set of conditions for a specified time period is recorded (Hrysomallis 2007). A field test of single-leg balance performed standing with eyes closed for ten seconds was employed with collegiate players competing in (men's) American football, men's and women's soccer and women's volleyball (Trojian and McKeag 2006). Players' scores on this test were reportedly predictive of subsequent ankle injury incidence during the playing season. Equipment such as ankle discs, foam mats and wobble boards are also widely used for balance testing. Some balance board apparatuses are built with contact sensors incorporated into the device in order to detect loss of equilibrium, thereby providing a quantitative measure when scoring the test (Hrysomallis 2007).

Force platforms (both laboratory-based and portable systems for field testing) are commercially available that allow postural sway to be measured by recording movement of the subject's centre of pressure. Such equipment can similarly be used to assess (static) postural control under given conditions (bilateral/unilateral stance, eyes open/closed, etc.). Instrumented testing of this type appears to be more sensitive in detecting deficits in postural control that are predictive of injury risk (McKeon and Hertel 2008). In a research setting, force plate centre of pressure and ground reaction force measurement has been used in combination with tibial motor nerve stimulation, in order to create 'external' disruption of balance and derive a 'time to stabilisation' measure (Brown and Mynark 2007). However, such testing involving costly equipment and specialist staff to interpret the data is unlikely to be feasible for routine testing of healthy players.

Dynamic postural balance

A popular field-based assessment of 'dynamic' postural balance is termed the star excursion balance test (SEBT) (Bressel *et al.* 2007). This protocol requires the athlete to balance on one leg while reaching out in various directions for maximal distance with the opposite leg. The athlete is only permitted to touch down lightly when marking their maximal reach distance in each direction – the trial is discarded and repeated if they shift their weight onto the reaching leg. The athlete is scored for distance reached in each direction and these scores are corrected for limb length, in order to allow comparisons between athletes (McKeon *et al.* 2008). Athletes' scores on the SEBT were reported to differ from their corresponding scores on a standard static balance test, which led the authors of this study to conclude that this test assesses different balance abilities (Bressel *et al.* 2007). This test also reports high sensitivity in detecting deficits in sensorimotor function of the previously injured lower limb in those who suffer from recurrent ankle injury (McKeon *et al.* 2008). Preliminary data indicate that team sports players appear to exhibit superior SEBT performance, based on comparisons between scores recorded by female collegiate soccer players and healthy non-athlete female subjects (Thorpe and Ebersole 2008). This would appear to support the contention that this test evaluates relevant capacities for team sports players.

Tests of postural balance ability described above are commonly used as part of screening prior to beginning a programme of physical preparation – see section below. Scores on postural balance are frequently used to identify players with chronic ankle instability (Brown and Mynark 2007). The other common application is during rehabilitation – particularly following knee or ankle injury – providing a tool to guide progression and to serve as a basis to make judgements regarding readiness to return to full training or competitive play (Wikstrom *et al.* 2006).

Dynamic stabilisation

Dynamic stabilisation can be defined as the athlete's ability to maintain equilibrium during movement (Brown and Mynark 2007). This capacity comprises multiple aspects, including neuromuscular control and the integrated function of various systems that provide dynamic stability to the lower limb joints (Wikstrom *et al.* 2006). It has been identified that dynamic stabilisation and static postural balance are discrete abilities, on the basis that measures of the two abilities are not strongly related to each other (Brown and Mynark 2007). Tests of dynamic stabilisation typically assess the player's ability to make the transition from movement to a stationary posture, for example jumping or hopping onto either a stable or labile surface and holding the landing.

Assessments of dynamic stabilisation in a laboratory or clinical setting commonly involve hopping or landing from a box onto a force plate. Measures recorded include postural sway, ground reaction force and time to stabilisation (Wikstrom et al. 2006). Another assessment that has been used in clinical and research settings uses electromyography (EMG). Surface EMG electrodes are used to detect muscle recruitment and activity during preparatory and reactive phases when subjects perform movement tasks or respond to challenges in balance (Wikstrom et al. 2006). Such laboratory and clinical assessments do, however, require specialised equipment and appropriately trained personnel to interpret the test data. Given the cost, time and access to specialised staff and equipment involved, these tests are therefore likely to be impractical for routine testing for a squad of players.

Lumbopelvic 'core' stability

The particular combination of muscles that contribute to providing lumbar spine stabilisation varies depending on posture and nature of the activity (Juker et al. 1998). Furthermore, in a weight-bearing posture, the position in which lumbopelvic stability is most commonly exhibited during sports performance, the hip musculature that helps stabilise the pelvis and supporting lower limb(s) also play a critical role. As such, during weight-bearing, lumbopelvic stability has elements in common with postural balance and dynamic stabilisation. There is therefore inevitably some cross-over into postural balance and dynamic stabilisation when attempting to assess lumbopelvic stability during upright stance or weight-bearing movements.

Given the complex and multidimensional nature of lumbopelvic stability described, no standard test for core stability currently exists. Standard endurance tests for the trunk muscles measure the time an athlete is able to maintain a given position or posture (McGill 2007d). Examples of such tests include the side bridge, flexor endurance test and static back extension 'Biering-Sorensen' endurance test (Carter et al. 2006). Normative data have been published for these tests with healthy subjects as a reference for comparison from the perspective of identifying low back injury risk (McGill 2007d). Ratios of flexor versus extensor scores and comparisons between sides (in the case of side bridge) are suggested to be most useful in identifying low back pain and injury risk. Data for these tests for athlete subjects have also recently been published (Evans et al. 2007). In contrast to the data for non-athletes, the female and male athletes studied had comparable flexor and extensor endurance times. However, side bridge endurance times were significantly lower among the female athletes compared to male athletes (Evans et al. 2007).

Another test more typically performed in a laboratory or clinic assesses the player's ability to maintain trunk muscle activation during challenged breathing. The laboratory version of the test involves the player maintaining a quarter squat position with weights held in the hands while breathing a lowered oxygen and raised CO_2 mixture – activity of core muscles is assessed via EMG recordings (McGill 2007d). In a field-based clinical version of the test, the player first performs a prior bout of exercise to raise their respiration rate and the clinician then assesses their ability to maintain muscle activation by palpating the player's oblique abdominal muscles. The laboratory test carries the usual issues of time, cost, equipment and need for specialist staff common to all laboratory-based assessments – for this reason it is unlikely to be included in a standard battery of tests for a large squad of players. The field-based version of the test, while more practical and less costly, is subjective and relies upon the judgement of a suitably trained clinician (physiotherapist or athletic trainer).

Field-based clinical tests of torsional stability are becoming routinely employed in functional screening protocols (see next section). Two examples are the 'push up test' (of which there are two variations) and the 'back bridge test' (McGill 2007d). The push up test is performed in an extended plank (push up) position with the player alternately lifting off each supporting arm while attempting to maintain a static posture (McGill 2006b). A variation of this test involves alternately raising the supporting foot from the same extended plank position. The back bridge is performed from a full bridge position (player is supine supported on their heels and shoulders, knees flexed, hips raised off the ground); while maintaining a stable position the player attempts to raise each foot off the ground alternately (McGill 2007b). These tests are qualitative: they are subjectively scored by the assessor upon set criteria (Cook 2003a).

Similarly, tests of torque generation involving projecting a medicine ball from a seated posture have been used as a measure of the concentric 'power' of the core stabiliser muscles (Cowley and Swensen 2008). Variations of the seated medicine ball throw in a sideways and backwards direction have also been proposed (Shinkle et al. 2012). While preliminary data suggest that scores on these tests may satisfy reliability criteria, the relationship with athletic performance and/or injury risk remains to be established.

In much the same way as for postural balance, devices have also been converted in order to measure ability to maintain equilibrium while holding a core stability exercise posture. One study examined subjects' core stability by evaluating their attempts to maintain core stability postures on a stability platform device commonly used to assess postural balance in standing (Liemohn et al. 2005). There did appear to be a considerable learning effect associated with this form of testing. Subjects were studied on four consecutive days with the device: the data recorded on day three were found to be the most reliable (Liemohn et al. 2005). Whilst this appears a promising area of study, there is currently a paucity of published data with such testing apparatus.

Musculoskeletal profiling and movement screening

Traditional musculoskeletal assessment protocols comprise static measurements and clinical examinations of joint integrity and range of motion, which mainly comprise passive assessment (Ford et al. 2003). There are limitations to assessing neuromuscular and musculoskeletal factors in this way: joints and muscles respond during passive tests in such a way that limited information is provided on how the body behaves under dynamic conditions. Another issue is that there is commonly inadequate follow-up to screening: it has been reported that although musculoskeletal problems are identified via such tests in 10 per cent of athletes, appropriate intervention is typically undertaken in only 1–3 per cent (Ford et al. 2003).

That said, some clinical tests of musculoskeletal function have been shown to be predictive of intrinsic (athlete-related) injury risk. Tests of joint range of motion and muscle flexibility are recommended as a means to identify players at risk of muscle strain injury. Pre-season baseline scores on quadriceps and particularly hamstring flexibility were shown to be predictive of subsequent muscle strains in Belgian professional soccer players during the following playing season (Witvrouw et al. 2003). The authors concluded that scores below 90 degrees on a passive test of hamstring muscle flexibility assessed in a supine position identified players at risk of hamstring injury. A similar relationship was reported with reduced ROM scores and adductor muscle strains in a study of soccer players in Iceland (Arnason et al. 2004). Clinical tests of joint integrity also typically identify joint laxity in the majority of players who have suffered previous joint strains (Arnason et al. 2004). Previous injury is often identified as a significant risk factor, so injury history and such clinical tests of joint laxity are important to identify players at risk.

Although the application of isokinetic testing and training has been questioned from a performance viewpoint, it does have applications for injury prevention and monitoring rehabilitation. Isokinetic assessment of strength ratios can help identify muscle strength imbalances that can predispose players to injury; for example, comparisons of isokinetic internal and external rotation strength measures for the shoulder have been used this way. Comparison of isokinetic measures between previously injured and healthy contralateral limbs appears to identify players at risk of recurrent hamstring injury. These isokinetic scores and ratios (particularly eccentric and mixed eccentric:concentric ratio measures) show potential for use as a test for readiness to return to competition following a programme of rehabilitation (Croisier et al. 2002). Similarly, isokinetic testing profiles assessing the optimal angle (knee angle at the highest recorded concentric knee flexor torque) are also shown to differentiate between injured limb and uninjured contralateral limb in players with a history of recurrent hamstring injury (Brockett et al. 2004).

There are a number of dynamic tests of neuromuscular function and control that are used in clinical settings for the purposes of screening for injury risk. These are described in detail in Chapter 3. In addition, movement-based screening protocols are seeing increasing use in the field, alongside or even in place of standard clinical musculoskeletal assessments. These commonly comprise active tests of mobility and stability, alongside qualitative assessment of fundamental movement skill tasks – such as variations of squat and lunge movements. The most commercially successful of these is the Functional Movement Screen (FMS) devised by Gray Cook (Cook 2003a). The use of these methods has become widespread in recent years, particularly in the field of strength and conditioning.

Evaluating motor patterns and fundamental movement abilities is an area of athletic assessment that is identified as having implications both for performance and injury prevention (Cook 2003a). The rationale for this approach is that players will tend to compensate for imbalances or areas of poor mobility and reduced stability by adopting altered movement mechanics. By their nature, these compensatory movement patterns are less efficient, and are likely to inhibit performance and predispose the player to injury (Cook 2003a).

The rationale presented by Gray Cook for the FMS protocol and 'functional' assessment methods in general appears sound in theory, and anecdotally many practitioners have used this form of assessment with some success. Nevertheless, where possible each of the movement-based 'screens' selected in a battery of assessments should have been validated in the literature. Currently, there remains a lack of published data validating the FMS assessment. One of the few investigations to date reported that individuals' scores on the FMS showed only weak statistical relationships with selected measures of athletic performance

(Okada *et al.* 2011). Another study investigated the relationship between FMS measures and a variety of standard assessments of athletic performance (vertical jump, 20m sprint times and T-test performance) and a sports skill task in collegiate athletes (golfers) (Parchmen and McBride 2011). This study failed to find any significant statistical relationships with any of the performance measures examined for either the subjects' combined FMS scores or their scores on the individual FMS assessments. To conclude, there is currently insufficient evidence to support the hypothesised relationship between FMS and athletic performance. There also remains a need for studies to provide evidence in support of the postulated link between the FMS assessment and incidence of injury.

There are examples in the literature of clinical tests designed to assess functional performance that were not subsequently found to be predictive of injury risk. Performance on a balance board test was found to have no relation to ankle sprain injury incidence among high school athletes (McHugh *et al.* 2006). The rationale for assessing proprioception and postural stability in this way would appear to be sound in theory from the point of view of injury prevention, given that these are risk factors for ankle injury. However, the lack of correlation found reinforces the fact that a causal relationship cannot just be assumed and that tests must be validated to provide confidence in their relevance. Given this, the inclusion of such tests in players' musculoskeletal screening and movement profiling would have to be considered until their efficacy has been demonstrated.

3

NEUROMUSCULAR TRAINING

Introduction

Conceptually, neuromuscular training can be considered to comprise any exercise mode that challenges a particular aspect of neuromuscular control and co-ordination. As such, this type of training can take a variety of forms. For example, neuromuscular training modes include strength training exercises that impose various postural control and intermuscular co-ordination demands. Conversely, exercises that require balance and stabilisation requiring postural and lower and/or upper limb control performed without any external resistance – that is, body weight exercises – comprise another form of neuromuscular training. In the latter case, exercises of this type might also be performed on a stable surface, or alternatively may incorporate a labile supporting surface or equipment such as stability balls or other balance devices.

It is therefore evident that there are a large number and wide variety of exercise modes that may be employed for neuromuscular training. Whatever form it takes, the emphasis of neuromuscular training is on qualitative aspects – such as the quality of movement. Accordingly, this type of training necessitates a quite different approach to other forms of training. Specifically, training parameters such as intensity, volume and frequency will be quite different. With respect to intensity, rather than focusing on performing a given movement against the highest resistance possible, progression of training is achieved by manipulating the stability and mobility challenge posed by the exercise. Similarly, volume for each session in terms of repetitions and sets will be quite modest, as opposed to aiming to train to fatigue. Conversely, the frequency of training is quite high, in order to reinforce motor patterns and facilitate motor learning.

The necessity for neuromuscular training for athlete populations

The fundamental movement capabilities of the athlete will help to determine their proficiency in performing the specific movement skills required by the sport (Gamble 2011c). The fundamental movements identified as being common to most sports include variations of squatting and/or lifting movements, pushing and/or pulling, lunging, gait (for example, running), twisting movements and balance activities (McGill 2006c). In order to execute these fundamental movements efficiently, the athlete must demonstrate the requisite neuromuscular capabilities which underpin these movements. In this way, different aspects of neuromuscular control and co-ordination ultimately represent a limiting factor in the athlete's abilities to execute the movements of their sport effectively and efficiently. This relationship is depicted in Figure 3.1.

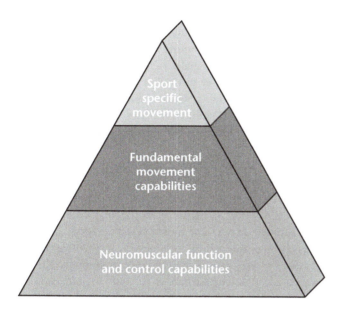

Figure 3.1 The role of neuromuscular function schematic

In addition to the general benefits of appropriate neuromuscular training described with respect to enhancing the performance capabilities of the athlete, certain populations have been identified as having a particular need for corrective neuromuscular training. Specifically, young athletes (of both sexes) and female athletes warrant particular attention and for both these groups neuromuscular training should be considered a priority.

There is a strong interaction between motor skill development and the processes of growth and maturation throughout the developmental years until late adolescence–early adulthood (Naughton *et al.* 2000). The importance of specific neuromuscular and movement skill training has therefore been emphasised during critical phases before, during and after puberty (Barber-Westin *et al.* 2005; Philippaerts *et al.* 2006). This is underlined by the reported effectiveness of corrective neuromuscular training interventions with these young athletes in reducing injuries sustained during youth sports (Emery and Meeuwisse 2010).

Studies report improvements in strength scores and measures of lower limb alignment in young males during the period spanning puberty and adolescence (Schmitz *et al.* 2009) and this is reflected in an improved ability to dissipate landing forces (Quatman *et al.* 2006). These naturally occurring changes observed with young males during maturation are attributed to a phenomenon known as the 'neuromuscular spurt', and are associated with concomitant hormonal changes (Quatman *et al.* 2006). The continuing need for neuromuscular training for young males should not be ignored, however, as there are data to indicate that despite the neuromuscular spurt phenomenon, some young males will still exhibit deficits in neuromuscular control following puberty (Barber-Westin *et al.* 2006).

Female athletes do not benefit from the 'neuromuscular spurt' phenomenon: the same growth and maturation-related improvements in strength and motor performance reported for males are not observed with young female athletes. Studies report that deficits in measures of lower limb control shown by female athletes are not corrected during growth and maturation, and even appear to become more pronounced as these athletes reach adolescence (Schmitz *et al.* 2009). As a result, significant differences in neuromuscular performance are evident between males and females following puberty that are not present among prepubescent boys and girls (Ford *et al.* 2010). For example, when compared to males, adolescent and adult female athletes are shown to demonstrate different lower limb kinematics and kinetics during drop-jump (Quatman *et al.* 2006) and stop-jump tasks (Chappell *et al.* 2002), and sidestep cutting movements under both planned (Hanson *et al.* 2008) and unanticipated conditions (Landry *et al.* 2007).

These gender differences in various indices of proximal control of the lower limbs are identified as contributing to the increased incidence of lower limb injury observed with female athletes (Mendiguchia *et al.* 2011). For example, the injury surveillance data indicate that knee injuries are in the range of 2–10 times more prevalent in females (depending on the sport) compared to males who compete in the same sport (Agel *et al.* 2005). This trend is apparent from adolescence and continues into adulthood (Hewett *et al.* 2006b; Murphy *et al.* 2003). Again, the effectiveness of corrective neuromuscular training interventions in reducing injury incidence among female athletes (Gilchrist *et al.* 2008; Mandelbaum *et al.* 2005), and normalising reported rates of injury towards the same range as those reported for male athletes (Hewett *et al.* 1999), points to the necessity of implementing preventative neuromuscular training for all female athletes.

Dose–response relationship and retention of neuromuscular training effects

Preliminary data indicate that neuromuscular training interventions show a dose–response relationship. In particular, the *frequency* of training appears to be a critical factor with respect to producing greater adaptations in neuromuscular co-ordination (Carroll *et al.* 2001). For example, a study that employed neuromuscular training intervention for injury prevention identified a positive trend between the number of training sessions performed and the degree of the protective effect observed in terms of reductions in (non-contact) injury incidence (Kraemer and Knobloch 2009).

Similarly, the relative duration of a neuromuscular training intervention appears to strongly influence the retention of neuromuscular training effects. A recent study by Padua and colleagues (2012) assessed the retention of positive changes to lower-limb control and mechanics resulting from a neuromuscular training intervention with young team sports athletes (soccer players). When assessed three months post-training, the group that had performed the training for a nine-month period demonstrated better retention of improved lower-limb mechanics and control compared to a group that had performed the same training intervention for three months (Padua *et al.* 2012).

It is also apparent that compliance is critical in order to take advantage of the beneficial effects of neuromuscular training (Soligard *et al.* 2010). While this has been a major issue for some earlier studies, more recent studies that have reported positive results often achieve good compliance by integrating the neuromuscular training intervention into the players' normal training, such as during the warm-up (Kraemer and Knobloch 2009; Gilchrist *et al.* 2008). Education of coaches and players with regard to the necessity and benefits of neuromuscular training interventions is also identified as a key factor for achieving compliance (Soligard *et al.* 2010).

Identifying deficits in neuromuscular control

In much the same way as for other forms of training, testing serves an important function when undertaking neuromuscular training interventions. Appropriate assessment provides a means to initially evaluate the athlete, and subsequently can serve as a tool to monitor the athlete and thereby guide training progression. A variety of assessments exist in the literature that are designed to assess a particular aspect of neuromuscular control and dynamic function. These assessment modes essentially fall into two categories:

* Assessments of balance or ability to maintain equilibrium under a given set of conditions;
* Tests that qualitatively evaluate lower limb alignment and mechanics during movement-based tasks.

Assessing balance abilities

Balance involves a host of sensorimotor capacities, comprising input from visual, vestibular and somatosensory systems (Bressel *et al.* 2007). Definitions are important for clarity: discrete types of balance ability have been identified and these are relatively independent of each other. Definitions of balance are typically described with respect to a base of support, for example the 'ability to maintain centre of mass within base of support'. However, balanced movement often comprises instances where the athlete is airborne. Examples include the flight phase when running, which can comprise close to 75 per cent of the gait cycle at maximal speeds (Yu *et al.* 2008), and also the flight phase prior to landing movements. It would therefore appear necessary to refine the global term 'balance', by describing this ability in terms of maintaining equilibrium without specific reference to the base of support (if any) involved.

Discrete abilities within the global term 'balance' have been identified in the literature: *static postural balance*, *dynamic postural balance*, and *dynamic stabilisation*; the distinctions between these abilities are detailed below.

Static balance	Ability to maintain centre of mass over a static base of support and stationary supporting surface (Bressel *et al.* 2007)
Dynamic balance	Capacity to maintain centre of mass over a fixed base of support under a movement challenge; specifically, motion of other limbs and body segments, or unanticipated disturbance to the supporting surface (DiStefano *et al.* 2009)
Dynamic stabilisation	Ability to maintain equilibrium during the transition from motion to a stationary position, such as a landing movement (Myer *et al.* 2006a)

Various forms of neuromuscular assessment also exist to evaluate each of these different balance abilities. Essentially these balance testing modes assess the athlete's ability to retain their equilibrium under a given set of conditions. This can be evaluated in a variety of ways, depending on the type of balance ability assessed and the equipment employed during testing.

In an applied or clinical setting, *static balance* is typically assessed as the number of attempts required to balance for a predetermined time duration under a given set of conditions (eyes open/closed, head movements in various directions), possibly alongside some subjective assessment, such as the degree of effort and amount of corrective action the athlete displayed during the assessment. Assessments of *dynamic balance* typically challenge the athlete to reach the other limb(s) as far away from their base of support as possible while retaining their balance – the most commonly used test is the star excursion balance test (Bressel *et al.* 2007). Tests of *dynamic stabilisation* typically involve jumping or hopping onto either a stable or labile surface; upon landing the athlete attempts to maintain their equilibrium – that is, 'stick' the landing without taking a step or losing balance. To date, the use of these tests has been largely restricted to a research setting, employing specialised apparatus to quantify measures such as postural sway. In a field or clinical setting more subjective assessment criteria will be need to be implemented.

Movement-based assessments of neuromuscular function and control

A number of assessment modes are employed to evaluate neuromuscular function and dynamic control during closed kinetic chain movements from a fixed base of support, as well as landing, pivoting and cutting movements. These 'neuromuscular assessment' modes vary in terms of the level of sophistication of the measurement and equipment employed, reflecting their application in research versus applied settings. A number of simplified versions of these assessment modes have been developed for use as a screening and monitoring tool that can be conducted by those staff who work closely with the athlete.

One such example is the single-leg squat, which is widely used in a clinical setting to evaluate neuromuscular control and function of muscles of the hip complex (Crossley *et al.* 2011). In particular, this test is designed to assess proximal control of lower limb alignment – that is, positioning and movement of pelvis, hip and knee in relation to the athlete's supporting foot and torso. The single-leg squat exercise is typically performed with body weight resistance only; however, versions of this assessment mode performed with external resistance also appear in the literature (Shields *et al.* 2005). Preliminary data indicate that clinicians' ratings of performance on this test based upon specified criteria are indicative of measured differences in hip muscle activation as well as differences in selected measures of hip and trunk muscle function between subjects (Crossley *et al.* 2011).

Drop jump screening is another assessment method that has become a well-established tool in a clinical setting to evaluate neuromuscular function and control under more dynamic conditions. In much the same way as the single-leg squat, this test is employed to assess proximal lower limb control during a relatively basic movement-based task. In particular, this mode of testing examines the athlete's ability to maintain lower limb alignment during both landing and take-off, and additionally the ability to resist knee abduction moments of force during these movements. The drop jump test in its original format as employed in a research setting has likewise recently been adapted for use in a clinical and applied setting (Myer *et al.* 2010). This version of the test requires only a digital camera and a standard laptop or desktop personal computer. Furthermore, capturing the relevant images at landing and take-off from the video recording and the subsequent analysis can be conducted using software that is available free of charge via the internet.

Importantly, this clinical or field version of the drop jump test has reported close agreement with laboratory-based measurements, which indicates that it is a similarly valid tool for evaluating frontal plane lower limb alignment in order to detect neuromuscular control deficits (Myer *et al.* 2010). Likewise, assessments of this type do appear to be sufficiently sensitive to register improvements in neuromuscular control elicited by neuromuscular training interventions (Noyes *et al.* 2005). A limitation of this field or clinical version of the drop-jump test is that as it only provides a picture of lower limb alignment in a single plane of motion (frontal plane). One caveat therefore is that it does not provide a true representation of neuromuscular control during more complex multi-planar movements (Noyes *et al.* 2011).

There are various examples in the sports medicine literature of assessments which evaluate neuromuscular function during more complex athletic movements, such as pivoting and cutting change of direction movements. At this stage the application of these assessments has been limited to a research setting, and these laboratory-based protocols require specialised apparatus and trained technicians to operate the equipment and analyse the data. However, there is the potential for field-based versions of these tests to be developed and validated to provide a clinical tool that is readily accessible to those who work with the athlete. One such example is the bound and cut test that featured in a recent study by Imwalle and colleagues (2009).

Neuromuscular training for postural control and balance

Static balance training

In the case that the athlete's screening has identified a deficiency in their static balance abilities there is a clear need for dedicated training to improve this capacity. In general it would also appear prudent to incorporate some form of static balance activities in the day-to-day training of all athletes. Static balance training is also likely to be beneficial for young athletes, particularly at critical stages in their growth and development. Similarly, static balance training is highly relevant to female athletes of all ages, given the prevalence of lower limb injury and associated neuromuscular control issues observed in this population.

Various constraints can be employed during static balance training tasks in order to isolate or emphasise a particular component. For example, performing the balance task with eyes closed eliminates visual input. Conversely, tilting or turning the head modifies the challenge with respect to vestibular system input. Finally, performing the balance task without shoes eliminates the stabilisation provided by the athlete's footwear, thereby accentuating proprioceptive afferent input from cutaneous and joint mechanoreceptors. All of these constraints may be manipulated individually or in combination in order to progress the challenge posed by the balance task.

Dynamic balance training

There are essentially two approaches to developing dynamic postural control. The first method is typically performed on a stable supporting surface and the athlete is challenged to maintain equilibrium whilst performing predetermined movements with the other limbs and body segments from a fixed base of support. One example of this form of dynamic balance training task is the star excursion balance test (Bressel *et al*. 2007). This is a single-leg balance task that requires the athlete to reach out with the contralateral (opposite) leg away from the supporting foot in a variety of directions, aiming for maximum distance.

The alternative form of dynamic balance training involves balance tasks performed on unstable supporting surfaces. This form of training employs labile surfaces (for example, foam pads or inflatable cushions) or training devices such as 'wobble-boards' or 'tilt-boards' (DiStefano *et al*. 2009). In contrast to the former approach, this form of dynamic balance training requires the athlete to minimise motion of limbs and body segments whilst balancing on a movable base of support. Training adaptations following dynamic balance training of this type appear to be mediated predominantly by changes in central or 'supra-spinal' neural input (Taube *et al*. 2007).

A variety of training regimens employing unstable training modes have reported improvements in dynamic balance measures with athlete subjects and some carry-over of these training effects to static balance abilities is also evident (DiStefano *et al*. 2009). Progression can be achieved with the particular dynamic balance training device by manipulating the same constraints as described for static balance training. Examples of such progressions include employing head movements, visual tracking tasks and/or introducing an eyes-closed variation of the task.

Finally, the two forms of dynamic balance training can be combined by employing exercises on an unstable surface that require the athlete to maintain equilibrium whilst performing movements with the non-supporting lower limb and/or upper limbs.

Dynamic stabilisation

Feed-forward control of ankle stabilisers during the preparatory phase prior to touch-down is suggested to be the most important factor in improving active stabilisation during landing or stopping movements (Holmes and Delahunt 2009). This is a learned effect and

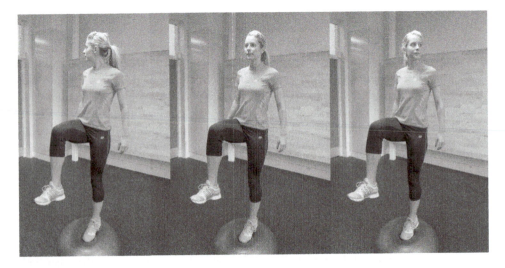

Figure 3.2 Single-leg balance and head turn on domed device

thus amenable to development via repeated exposure to relevant movements in conjunction with appropriate coaching (Zuur *et al.* 2010). A variety of landing tasks can be employed, depending upon what is demanded by the characteristic athletic movements employed in the sport.

Variations of these dynamic stabilisation training tasks can also be performed landing onto an unstable surface by employing labile surfaces and unstable training devices, as described for dynamic balance. Progression can also be achieved by performing dynamic stabilisation tasks under reactive conditions (McKeon *et al.* 2008). Qualitative criteria can be employed in order to assess the quality of each attempt with dynamic stabilisation tasks. Movement 'errors' include touching down with opposite (non-stance) leg, loss of control in trunk posture or motion, and bracing non-stance limb against supporting leg when attempting to balance following landing (McKeon *et al.* 2008).

'Movement skills' neuromuscular training

Corrective neuromuscular training interventions that are reported to be successful in reducing incidence of injury often include some form of movement skills instruction and practice (Hewett *et al.* 2006a). A good example is the *sportsmetrics* training protocol developed at the Cincinnati Sports Medicine Research and Education Foundation, which has been documented to successfully reduce injury incidence among female athletes predisposed to lower limb injury (Hewett *et al.* 1999). A key element of this protocol is instruction and coaching of safe movement mechanics for common athletic movements (for example, jumping and landing).

By happy coincidence 'safe' movement mechanics and postures are often also more efficient and more effective. Adopting 'safe' movement mechanics is frequently shown concurrently to improve performance, particularly when the subjects in these studies exhibit suboptimal neuromuscular control or movement patterns prior to the corrective training intervention.

For example, a neuromuscular training intervention for high school and collegiate female basketball players achieved alterations in movement mechanics during a stop jump movement that resulted in a 50 per cent reduction in measured shear forces at the knee, and players' jump height performance was maintained or improved with the altered technique (Myers and Hawkins 2010). A number of studies have reported improvements in speed and change of direction performance alongside the changes in movement mechanics elicited by this form of training with female athletes (Hewett *et al.* 2006a).

Recently, modified versions of these generic corrective neuromuscular training protocols have been developed which aim to deliver more comprehensive instruction and development of the specific movement skills that feature in a given sport. For example, a protocol has been developed for high school volleyball players which incorporates locomotion and change of direction movements, as well as a variety of jumping and bounding activities (Noyes *et al.* 2011). Preliminary data indicate that this more progressive approach to neuromuscular training confers greater improvements in athletic performance (vertical jump) in comparison to those observed with more established corrective neuromuscular training protocols. This protocol was also similarly effective in eliciting significant improvements in measures of neuromuscular control during a drop jump assessment (Noyes *et al.* 2011). The latter finding is perhaps unsurprising as the training featured in this study included

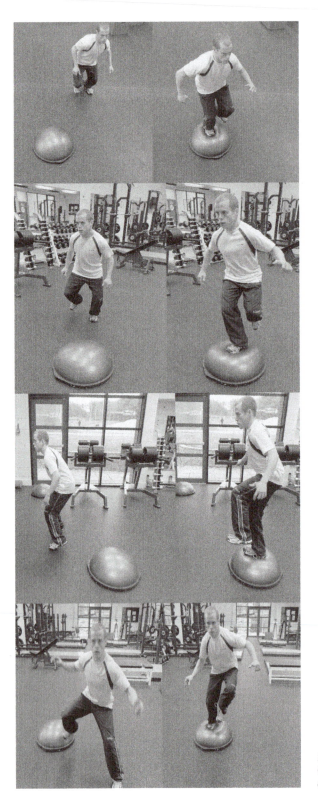

Figure 3.3
Compass bound and stabilise onto domed device

the same exercises that feature in corrective neuromuscular training protocols proven to improve neuromuscular indices and reduce injury incidence, in addition to the novel exercise modes.

The application of neuromuscular training to improve athletic performance is not a new concept. In track athletics the importance of 'neural' training has long been emphasised, and this form of training is commonly applied, particularly with sprinters. It would seem to follow that employing a more progressive approach to neuromuscular training for the locomotion movement skills that feature in other sports, such as team sports and racquet sports, might confer performance benefits as well as addressing injury risk factors (Gamble 2011c). In these more complex sports there is often an assumption that athletes will naturally acquire the requisite athletic movement skill development during the course of their technical and tactical development. This notion may not be valid – anecdotally there are a number of examples in these sports of athletes who have highly developed technical and tactical skills but are lacking in athleticism and movement abilities.

Neuromuscular training in this form can therefore serve dual aims:

• Addressing known biomechanical injury risk factors;
• Enhancing movement efficiency and performance.

Assessing movement skill competencies

As has been described in an earlier section, there are tools available to evaluate neuromuscular function during basic athletic movements, for example single-leg squat and vertical drop jump landing and take-off activities. These forms of assessment offer a valid means to identify gross deficits in neuromuscular function and control. However, qualitative assessment of movement skill competencies during more complex movements is likely to require more subjective assessment using the trained eye of a coach or practitioner. While speculative, it is likely that this type of qualitative assessment is best conducted by observing the athlete in their natural training and competition environment.

Unfortunately, the ability to recognise good versus poor athletic movement is a skill that is rarely taught. Rather this tends to be a skill that comes from a great deal of observation and experience. The ability of a coach or practitioner to be able to correct and develop good movement skills by coaching intervention is rarer still.

Neuromuscular training to develop locomotor abilities

Whilst established neuromuscular training protocols are often reported to be effective in improving landing mechanics as well as favouring vertical jump performance, it has been identified that there may be a lack of transfer to more complex athletic activities with these protocols. For example, DiStefano and colleagues (2011) reported that a standard corrective neuromuscular training protocol failed to produce any improvement in lower limb kinetics assessed during a reactive cut task in a group of prepubescent athletes. These findings might be interpreted with a degree of caution given that studies report that young athletes at this early stage of development appear to be less responsive to neuromuscular training interventions. However, a more progressive neuromuscular training protocol which featured cutting movements under both preplanned and reactive conditions was successful in producing some improvement in lower limb kinematics in the same subject population (DiStefano *et al.* 2011).

It has been identified that 'proximal' neuromuscular control of the lower limb demonstrated by athletes varies in a task-dependent manner (Mendiguchia *et al.* 2011). It is therefore not entirely surprising that changes in neuromuscular function and control developed during particular types of activities (for example, straight-line hopping and bounding tasks) may not carry over to other activities, particularly those which involve different planes of movement. In view of the apparent specificity of neuromuscular training effects, it follows that in order to develop neuromuscular function and control for pivoting and other change of direction tasks (for example, cutting movements) these specific movements must feature in the neuromuscular training intervention.

Furthermore, lower limb neuromuscular control also differs for the same task according to the conditions involved – specifically, whether the movement is executed under pre-planned versus reactive or unanticipated conditions (Besier *et al.* 2001). It therefore follows that not only must the neuromuscular training protocol incorporate the relevant pivoting and change of direction movements for the sport, but the constraints imposed during training must also reflect the unplanned and reactive conditions encountered during competition.

4

METABOLIC CONDITIONING

Introduction

The metabolic conditioning of a team sports player serves a crucial role in defining and ultimately limiting their contribution to the game (Helgerud *et al.* 2001). The effectiveness of players' conditioning and resulting level of fitness is a critical factor that determines their ability to fulfil the specific demands imposed by the playing position.

Specificity in relation to metabolic conditioning involves both energy systems and modes of activity. The bioenergetics of the training activity will determine the impact of training on different aspects of metabolic conditioning – such as aerobic versus anaerobic adaptations. In much the same way, the benefits of metabolic conditioning are reflected principally in the mode(s) of locomotion employed during training. Conditioning responses show a high degree of training mode specificity (Jones and Carter 2000), particularly in trained athletes (Millet *et al.* 2002a).

To satisfy training specificity, it follows that the format of conditioning for team sports should employ the same modes of activity featured in the sport and aim to impose corresponding stresses on metabolic systems to those experienced during match-play. In accordance with this contention, sport-specific conditioning modes that replicate and overload physiological and kinematic conditions encountered during athletic performance are identified as being most effective for preparing players for competition (Deutsch *et al.* 1998).

Applying metabolic specificity thus essentially requires the format of conditioning to reflect the parameters of competition. Practically achieving this for a team sports player poses unique difficulties. Team sports rarely involve continuous locomotion at a consistent intensity. Devising training to exert proportionate stresses upon energy systems for the modes of activity identified for a particular team sport therefore represents a considerable challenge.

Metabolic conditioning and team sports performance

It is reported that measures of fitness for players in sports such as soccer are significantly related to distance covered in a game (Castagna *et al.* 2010; Reilly 1994). Level of fitness also shows significant correlation to the number of high-intensity efforts players attempt (Helgerud *et al.* 2001). Hence, metabolic conditioning influences players' work rate and also their involvement in the game. The relationship between endurance fitness parameters and running performance in matches (total distance covered and high-intensity running bouts completed) are to some extent position-dependent in these team sports (Buchheit *et al.* 2010c). This reflects the influence of playing position, and other aspects of team strategy and tactics on patterns of activity during matches and the associated endurance demands for players in team sports such as soccer.

In general, a player's ability to retain their capacity to perform high-intensity efforts at the key moment is often crucial in the events that ultimately decide matches (Drust *et al.* 1998; Reilly 1997). This can be via a positive influence: making a break or evading a tackle, keeping up with play to be available in support at the critical instant, or being able to chase back in defence to make a crucial intervention. Likewise, it can be telling in a negative sense – such as missing a tackle or interception, failing to support a team-mate in possession of the ball leading to an attack breaking down, or being unable to cover in defence at the critical moment.

Methodological challenges for profiling demands of team sports competition

Attempts to quantify demands of team sports as a basis upon which to model sport-specific conditioning practices have commonly analysed players' movements during match-play. Distance covered during the course of a match is often recorded as a global measure of energy expenditure and physiological demand (Reilly 1994). Previously, time–motion analysis has been employed to document the types of activity players engage in during a match (Duthie *et al.* 2003; McInnes *et al.* 1995). These methods were highly time-consuming. Over recent years, the development of global positioning system (GPS) technology and its increasing use in a professional team sports setting has provided a much faster and easier means to quantify distance covered by players during both competition and training (Aughey 2011). In addition to total distance, this technology also allows distance covered per minute to be evaluated for players wearing a GPS device.

However, intermittent sports have been shown to have energetic demands far in excess of those that would be predicted from covering the same distance continuously (Drust *et al.* 2000). It is notoriously difficult to evaluate physiological stresses associated with intermittent sports by indirect methods, such as time–motion analysis (Gamble 2004a; Reilly 1994, 1997). Similarly, despite the technological advances of GPS, its reliability and validity for quantifying high-intensity efforts is still questionable (Coutts and Duffield 2010). In general GPS devices with higher sampling rates provide more accurate data; however, the greater the velocity of locomotion, the more error is associated with GPS measurement. These factors are compounded by the relatively brief durations of high-velocity bouts during matches, which further decrease the likelihood of accurate measurement of distances for high-intensity running bouts completed by players (Aughey 2011).

The intermittent nature of match-play activity in different team sports is illustrated by studies such as that of McInnes and colleagues (1995), which identified 997±183 movements during the course of a basketball match, with transitions between modes of activity on average every 2 seconds. A study examining rugby union football has similarly reported 560 discrete activities during a 70-minute age-grade match (Deutsch *et al.* 1998). Bangsbo and colleagues (1991) likewise recorded 1,197 changes in activity during a 90-minute professional soccer match. Such intermittent and variable patterns of exertion have major implications for the bioenergetics, and in turn the conditioning demands, of team sports. The frequent changes in direction and velocity of movement require inertia to be repeatedly overcome, and involve accelerations and decelerations which constitute considerable added metabolic and physiological demands (McInnes *et al.* 1995; Wilkins *et al.* 1991).

Without the facility to quantify the player's inertia, and the associated physiological costs of changes in velocity (that is, both speed and direction), the GPS data in isolation will therefore fail to reflect the metabolic demands associated with team sports play. Even when performing straight-line running, the physiological costs of performing intermittent bouts under controlled conditions on a treadmill is associated with greater physiological strain (higher ratings of perceived exertion and ventilatory responses) than exercise of the same average intensity performed continuously (Drust *et al.* 2000). Performing intermittent bouts of shuttle running with 180-degree turns is similarly found to significantly increase physiological and metabolic demands, in comparison to intermittent bouts of straight-line running performed at the same speed for the same duration (Dellal *et al.* 2010). This finding was apparent even in the elite senior team sports players studied, despite their familiarity and skill performing these change of direction movements. The added demands of changes in velocity when performing the intermittent activity required during team sports play are likely to necessitate a greater contribution from anaerobic metabolism, based upon the elevated blood lactate concentrations observed (Dellal *et al.* 2010).

In addition, studies show that unorthodox (sideways and backwards) modes of locomotion feature prominently in team sports, with certain playing positions having a particular emphasis on these modes of locomotion (Duthie *et al.* 2003; McInnes *et al.* 1995; Reilly 1994; Rienzi *et al.* 1999). The metabolic demands of these movements are greater than conventional running in a forwards direction (Reilly 1997), and this added physiological cost rises disproportionately with increases in speed of movement (Reilly 1994). Game-related activities similarly impose considerably higher energy expenditure than running (Reilly 1994, 1997). These factors further compound the underestimation of physiological cost of match-play for team sports from indirect observation such as time–motion analysis or GPS data.

Even when the metabolic cost of these unorthodox forms of locomotion and game-related activities are quantified and taken into account, the transitions between movements are of similar importance to the individual component activities themselves. Estimations based on the individual component activities performed in isolation will therefore underestimate the physiological stresses imposed on players, and can thereby give a false indication of the metabolic pathways implicated in real game situations.

Direct monitoring of physiological indices during matches

It follows that accurate assessment of exertion levels requires players to be directly monitored during competition. The consensus is that assessment of energetic demands in team sports should include sampling of markers of physiological stress under performance conditions (Duthie *et al.* 2003; McInnes *et al.* 1995; Reilly 1994; Reilly 1997). Despite technological advances, gas analysis apparatus will inevitably restrict players' movements and interfere with match-play, and certainly would not be safe for contact sports. In view of this, studies to assess energy expenditure typically use heart rate (HR) or blood lactate (BLa) as the physiological marker (Reilly 1994).

The main argument against BLa as an index of exertion levels during competitive matches is the dynamic nature of lactate as a metabolite (Bangsbo *et al.* 1991). Blood lactate levels are essentially determined by relative rates of production, release, uptake and removal. Consequently, single blood samples merely give a snapshot of the activity performed during the interval immediately prior to when the sample was taken. Concentrations of blood lactate are commonly used to indicate contribution of anaerobic glycolysis to energy production (Coutts *et al.* 2003). However, beyond establishing that anaerobic metabolism plays a role in match-play exertion for a given sport, sporadic determination of BLa is of little value in profiling activity or intensity patterns throughout a match (Impellizzeri *et al.* 2005). Theoretically, serial measurements of BLa may better reflect shifts in intensity of exertion throughout a game, but the frequency of sampling required would be unfeasible during a competitive match.

Assessments of the demands of competitive matches have thus tended to favour HR monitoring as the sole reliable and practical indicator of physiological strain or energy expenditure (Boyle *et al.* 1994). There is some indication that the elevated HR values recorded under competitive conditions will tend to overestimate the actual energy costs of match-play (Hill-Haas *et al.* 2011). That said, the relationship between HR recorded and measured oxygen uptake (VO_2) during match-play activities (5-a-side games) is reported to be robust and comparable to the HR–VO_2 relationship assessed under laboratory conditions (Castagna *et al.* 2004). Combining both HR monitoring and analysis of accompanying GPS data has the potential to offer greater insights into the demands of competition in team sports.

Quantifying physiological demands of match-play in collision sports

The element of violent bodily contact with opposing players and the playing surface has tended to preclude direct measurement of physiological responses during game-play in collision sports (Duthie *et al.* 2003). A consequence of this failure to objectively define the specific demands of match-play is that training specificity has often been neglected in the design of conditioning regimes for players at all levels in these collision sports in past years.

The development of lightweight and miniaturised GPS devices has made this technology more amenable to implementation for contact sports (Aughey 2011). However, given the intermittent nature of activity during matches and issues of quantifying high-intensity activity with GPS described, combined with the non-running physical work undertaken by players in these sports, direct monitoring of physiological parameters such as HR would still be required to augment GPS data. Attempts that have been made to implement HR monitoring during match-play in contact sports such as rugby union and rugby league have typically been limited to youth and semi-professional playing grades (Coutts *et al.* 2003; Deutsch *et al.* 1998). The relevance of these data for senior players at elite level may, however, be questionable.

Sources of variability when evaluating demands of sports performance

The strength and style of play of the opposition will inevitably influence the nature, frequency, duration and density with respect to time of activities players are required to perform (Duthie *et al.* 2003; Woolford and Angove 1991). These aspects will similarly be affected by the officiating styles and environmental conditions (Duthie *et al.* 2003). The referee has a major bearing on the format the game takes in terms of number of stoppages and duration of phases of play, particularly in highly technical sports such as rugby union, ice hockey and American football. Similarly, environmental conditions will influence tactics and the errors committed by both sides, which will in turn influence the pattern and mode of activity players will be engaged in. Thus, there is significant variation not only within a match but also between consecutive games (Duthie *et al.* 2003).

Notwithstanding the difficulties outlined in gathering data pertaining to the global demands of match-play as they relate to a team, individual roles of particular playing positions within a team are also quite diverse (Duthie *et al.* 2003). Precise roles of the respective playing positions therefore vary between teams, depending on their particular structured game plan, and associated demands imposed upon players in different positions. This is reflected in the GPS data derived from matches in team sports such as soccer: total distance covered during matches has been observed to differ significantly between different playing positions (Buchheit *et al.* 2010b).

A significant volume of data would therefore appear to be required to overcome the inherent variability within and between games to establish an accurate assessment of demands during competition that are representative for a particular team. This demand is multiplied several-fold if the aim is to gather a complete picture of the associated demands for individual playing positions within that team.

Physiological and neuromuscular bases of team sports endurance

Based upon the available evidence, a number of different physiological and neuromuscular factors have been identified as critical to meeting the specific endurance demands of team sports competition. Characteristically, physical exertion during team sports is of an intermittent nature, comprising sprints and other modes of high-intensity activity. These bouts of intense activity are interspersed with periods of variable duration engaged in lower intensity locomotion, during which active recovery and removal of lactate can take place (Hoff 2005). Metabolic demands thus alternate between energy provision for bouts of high-intensity work, and replenishing energy sources and restoring homeostasis during the intervals in between (Balsom *et al.* 1992).

A capacity termed 'repeated sprint ability' has therefore been identified as a key determinant of team sports performance (Glaister 2005). Studies indicate that a number of discrete elements are associated with this ability, as will be discussed in the following sections.

Repeated sprint ability

As implied in the title, repeated sprint ability describes the capacity to perform repeated bouts of high-intensity work with short (incomplete) recovery periods between successive efforts. Superior performance on measures of repeated sprint ability differentiates players at elite level from those competing at a lower standard of competition in team sports such as soccer (Impellizzeri *et al.* 2008). Studies also report strong statistical relationships between tests of repeated sprint ability and the number of high-intensity efforts and total distance recorded during matches in team sports (Rampinini *et al.* 2007a). These observations would seem to underline the importance of this capability for team sports players.

What constitutes good repeated sprint ability is the capacity to record high average sprint performance over successive sprint efforts. This requires the player to be (a) fast, in order to record good sprint times for individual bouts, and (b) able to maintain a high level of sprint performance during each successive bout (Bishop *et al.* 2011). Repeated sprint ability is therefore related to neuromuscular aspects associated with speed performance, as well as physiological and metabolic components (Pyne *et al.* 2008). Combating the effects of fatigue in order to maintain performance across successive efforts similarly involves a variety of metabolic, physiological and neuromuscular aspects (Girard *et al.* 2011a).

Anaerobic capacity

Anaerobic capacity represents an athlete's endurance when performing an exhaustive bout of running at supramaximal velocities (that is, above vVO_2max or MAS). This parameter is typically quantified via measures of performance during maximal efforts over longer distances, for example shuttle sprints over 300m (Moore and Murphy 2003), or average work output relative to body mass during a 30-second all-out work bout, such as the Wingate test (Zupan *et al.* 2009).

Anaerobic capacity is dependent upon factors such as the player's muscle fibre profile (type II fibres have higher anaerobic capacity), muscle glycolytic enzyme content and activity, and lactate handling and muscle buffering capacities (Maughan and Gleeson 2004). Despite the apparent relevance of this aspect of conditioning with respect to intermittent exercise performance, it has been highlighted that there is a lack of data pertaining to anaerobic capacity of team sports players, especially those competing at elite level (Duthie *et al.* 2003).

The content and activity of enzymes associated with glycolytic metabolism are responsive to training (Kubukeli *et al.* 2002). However, as alluded to above, the ability to mobilise glycolytic metabolism during repeated sprint bouts is dependent on not only enzyme content but also the ability to offset the inhibition of glycolytic metabolism due to the accumulation of metabolites. Therefore lactate handling and muscle buffering capacity are similarly critical factors.

Muscle buffering capacity

Athletes with a history of repeated sprint training are shown to exhibit an enhanced ability to buffer the hydrogen ion accumulation associated with glycolytic metabolism in order to minimise changes in muscle pH (Edge *et al.* 2006a). Buffering of hydrogen ions is important to counteract the inhibition effects of acidosis and corresponding impairments in repeated sprint performance (Bishop *et al.* 2011). The specific peripheral adaptations observed with improvements in buffering capacity include increased capilliarisation of muscle fibres (Jones and Carter 2000) and improved capacity of buffering agents and up-regulation of lactate/H^+ transporters within the muscle cell (Billat *et al.* 2003). Similarly, appropriate conditioning can improve the capacity for handling and clearance of metabolites from adenosine triphosphate (ATP) breakdown, in particular inorganic phosphate (P_i) which contributes to fatigue when performing repeated sprint activity (Glaister 2005).

Another relevant adaptation concerns the expression and activity of sodium/potassium pumps within the muscle cell. Loss of potassium (K^+) ions from the muscle cell with repeated muscle activation during high-intensity running exercise is identified as a key fatigue mechanism (Iaia and Bangsbo 2010). The action of sodium/potassium pumps works to counteract this loss of K^+ ions.

Lactate handling and metabolism

Oxidative processes within the muscle cell play an important role in handling lactate produced via glycolytic metabolism. Lactate is used directly as a substrate for oxidative metabolism within the mitochondria, and lactate is also the main precursor for *gluconeogenesis* during prolonged exercise, a process that produces glucose for carbohydrate metabolism (Brooks 2009). As this capacity is exceeded during high-intensity exercise, lactate transporters within skeletal muscle also act to remove excess lactate from the muscle cell during exercise, in order to offset the inhibition of glycolysis. In particular, monocarboxylate transporters (MCTs) in the muscle cell membrane are identified as critical to the removal of lactate and H^+ ions, and there is some evidence that the expression of MCTs is responsive to appropriate training (Bishop *et al.* 2011).

There is a large amount of evidence that lactate transported out of the muscle cell can be taken up and metabolised by adjacent muscle fibres as well as other organs, which serves to assist lactate handling (Brooks 2009). This is the central tenet of 'lactate shuttle' theory. It is now well established that a variety of tissues and organs use lactate as a substrate for energy metabolism under both aerobic and anaerobic conditions, and that the contribution of lactate to energy production can be considerable (Brooks 2009). In much the same way as lactate produced via glycolytic metabolism is taken up by the mitochondria within the muscle cell and used for oxidative metabolism, lactate transported out of the muscle cell during high-intensity exercise can be taken up and oxidised by adjacent muscle fibres within the working muscle – particularly those with high mitochondrial capacity (Brooks 2009).

Aerobic capacity

Some authors have inferred that aerobic fitness is of lesser relative importance based upon the comparatively lower values of VO_2max reported for players in some team sports, particularly in rugby union football and basketball (Duthie *et al.* 2003; Hoffman *et al.* 1999). Measures of aerobic capacity have, however, been reported to show significant statistical relationships with repeated sprint ability (Bishop *et al.* 2004). Of the respective measures of aerobic capacity, it has been suggested that vVO_2max or MAS is of more relevance to repeated sprint ability than VO_2max or VO_2peak, which may explain the modest correlation between VO_2max and repeated sprint ability scores reported in some studies (Girard *et al.* 2011a).

Previously it had been suggested that the role of aerobic metabolism during team sports play is limited to rest periods during stoppages between periods of activity (Duthie *et al.* 2003). However, repeated sprint exercise of the type featured during matches in fact involves a significant aerobic contribution to energy production (Bogdanis *et al.* 1996a). Oxidative metabolism contributes a major portion of the energy during successive efforts following the first sprint. A study investigating repeated maximal 30-second bouts reported that the aerobic contribution increased from 31 per cent in the first 30-second sprint in a set to almost 50 per cent in the second, even with four minutes' recovery between sprints (Bogdanis *et al.* 1996a). This increasing contribution from aerobic metabolism serves to offset losses in power output resulting from reduced capacity for anaerobic energy production. More recent investigations reported that peak VO_2 values recorded during successive 30-second all-out efforts are observed to reach close to VO_2max even in trained athletes (Buchheit *et al.* 2012; Girard *et al.* 2011a).

Aside from the direct contribution of oxidative metabolism to energy production during successive sprint efforts, the role of aerobic capacity during rest intervals is another key aspect. Oxygen uptake kinetics measured during recovery periods are identified as a key component of repeated sprint ability (Dupont et al. 2010). This is indicative of the relationship between the oxidative capacity of muscle and the oxygen-dependent processes associated with phosphocreatine (PCr) resynthesis during the recovery intervals between work bouts (Bogdanis et al. 1996a). It is identified that PCr is a particularly important high-rate energy source for repeated sprint exercise, and marked depletion of muscle PCr stores (35–55 per cent) is observed following a 6-second sprint bout (Girard et al. 2011a). Rest intervals between high-intensity efforts in team sports are typically too brief to allow for complete restoration of PCr stores (Spencer et al. 2005), which can take in excess of four minutes (Bogdanis et al. 1996a); therefore, improving the initial fast component of PCr resynthesis is key to supporting repeated sprint ability.

It appears that peripheral components of aerobic capacity, as opposed to cardiopulmonary aspects, are most influential with regards to repeated sprint ability (Bishop et al. 2004). Muscle oxidative capacity and peripheral adaptations resulting in improved muscle reoxygenation during rest intervals are suggested to be most relevant when performing repeated sprint activity (Girard et al. 2011a). An investigation of physiological responses during a maximal intensity interval protocol (30-second all-out cycling bouts interspersed with two minutes' recovery) observed an increasing level of deoxygenation at the muscle fibre during successive efforts, which is offset by corresponding increases in rates of muscle reoxygenation during the rest intervals between each work bout (Buchheit et al. 2012). A highly significant finding is that improvements in repeated sprint ability following high-intensity interval training are also found to be related to increases in muscle reoxygenation rates measured during rest intervals (Buchheit and Ufland 2011).

Another potential adaptation associated with training to develop aerobic capacity is an improved ability to utilise fat stores within the muscle as an energy source during games, which will help to spare players' finite glycogen stores (Hoff 2005). This is significant adaptation in team sports such as soccer where glycogen depletion during the second half of matches results in decreased work capacity, reflected in decreased distances covered and reduced high-intensity activity (Hoff 2005).

Maximum speed capabilities

When undertaking repeated sprint exercise the athlete's sprint performance in the first sprint bout shows strong statistical relationships with both their performance in the final sprint bout, and their overall sprint performance (Girard et al. 2011a). A player's maximum speed per se is therefore strongly related to their repeated sprint ability. In addition to genetically determined anthropometric factors (such as limb length) and muscle fibre profile (proportion of type II fibres), sprinting speed capabilities also involve a variety of strength qualities and neuromuscular attributes, as discussed in Chapter 8.

Running economy and neuromuscular factors

Exercise economy is identified as a key component of cardiorespiratory fitness (Jones and Carter 2000). Movement efficiency and economy during different forms of locomotion are therefore key determinants of endurance during matches. From this point of view, neuro-muscular control and motor patterns featured in training would appear to be a critical factor in terms of the carry-over of metabolic conditioning to performance. In support of this, it has been reported that measures of running economy when performing shuttle runs showed a positive statistical relationship with weekly training and competition volume in the team sports players studied (Buchheit *et al.* 2011b). This would appear to indicate that exposure to training and matches which feature game-specific movement patterns and change of direction activities serves to enhance economy when performing these forms of locomotion.

Relevant neuromuscular adaptations that underpin running economy concern intra-muscular and intermuscular co-ordination (Girard *et al.* 2011a); the ability to maintain these capabilities under fatigue is similarly a trainable quality (Behm 2005). Repeated sprint running is associated with significant reductions in force and power output of lower limb muscles during maximal voluntary contractions and evoked muscle twitch responses, indicative of peripheral fatigue (Perrey *et al.* 2010). Developing neuromuscular capabilities and fatigue resistance may therefore help to reduce the decline in power output and speed during successive sprint efforts.

Intramuscular co-ordination also comprises stiffness regulation of the muscle–tendon complex of locomotor muscles. Alterations in lower limb stiffness and spring properties have been observed during the course of a repeated sprint protocol, which are reflected in progressive reductions in sprint performance (Girard *et al.* 2011b). Another study reported that team sports athletes demonstrated a superior ability to maintain stiffness regulation during successive sprint efforts, which appears to reflect their training history with this form of repeated sprint exercise (Clark 2009).

Factors determining relevant training adaptations

The nature of the conditioning response is dependent upon the work intensity and volume and/or duration of training performed. Some changes, such as growth in the size and capacity of the heart and increases in lung vital capacity, are only apparent in athletes who have completed high volumes of endurance training over a period of years. Other training adaptations are much more responsive to training.

Enzyme adaptation

Increases in content and activity of anaerobic enzymes, specifically those involved in glycogenolysis and glycolysis, have been reported with sprint training (Kubukeli *et al.* 2002). It appears that relatively longer work bouts, which require a greater contribution from glycolytic metabolism, are most effective for eliciting increases in these enzymes, in comparison to repeated sprint exercise involving shorter (≤ 10-second) work bouts (Bishop *et al.* 2011). Conversely, relatively longer rest intervals appear to be beneficial from the point of view of allowing a more complete return to homeostasis, in order to limit the inhibition of glycolysis during successive work bouts. On that basis, the optimal conditioning format for eliciting changes in glycolytic enzymes would feature 30-second all-out work bouts, interspersed with extended rest periods (>4 minutes) (Bishop *et al.* 2011).

A range of high-intensity interval training protocols involving work intensities at or above vVO_2max have reported improvements in enzymes involved in oxidative metabolism. For example, '30-second sprint interval training' protocols involving repeated 30-second all-out efforts, that is, supra-(VO_2) maximal intensity, with rest periods of 4 minutes have consistently shown these changes (Gibala and McGee 2008). This reflects the contribution of aerobic metabolism during successive work bouts with this conditioning format (Bogdanis et al. 1996). High-intensity aerobic interval training involving longer (4-minute) work bouts conducted at close to vVO_2max or MAS intensity interspersed with 2-minute rest periods are also effective in producing changes in oxidative enzymes (Talanian et al. 2007). With these long aerobic interval methods it is recommended that the rest intervals employed should be less than the duration of work bouts in order to maximise the aerobic contribution and resulting adaptations in oxidative enzymes (Bishop et al. 2011).

Energy substrate availability and restoration

High-intensity interval conditioning appears to be a potent training stimulus for eliciting adaptations in muscle oxidative capacity (Gibala and McGee 2008), which supports the oxygen-dependent resynthesis of muscle PCr stores during rest intervals between maximal efforts. Accordingly, preliminary data suggest that high-intensity interval conditioning conducted at VO_2max intensity can elicit significant improvements in the initial rate (that is, the 'fast component') of PCr resythensis observed within the first 60 seconds following high-intensity work bouts (Bishop et al. 2011). Adaptations associated with high-intensity interval conditioning and repeated sprint training that serve to reduce the breakdown and diffusion of substrates for ATP resynthesis are also of relevance to repeated sprint ability (Glaister 2005; Spencer et al. 2004).

Increases in resting muscle glycogen content have also been reported with high-intensity training studies involving short-term 30-second all-out intervals separated by 4-minute recovery periods (Gibala and McGee 2008). There are some data to suggest that aerobic interval training promotes oxidative metabolism of fats, in comparison to the same exercise performed as a continuous bout (Billat 2001a). Relatively longer work bouts ($\approx$4 minutes) at correspondingly lower relative intensity ($\approx$90 per cent vVO_2max) appear to promote these adaptations (Gibala and McGee 2008). The preferential use of fats as an energy substrate and sparing of finite stores of glycogen (carbohydrate) is an important adaptation in terms of prolonging the player's ability to perform at higher work intensities, given the significant depletion in muscle glycogen that is observed towards the end of matches in team sports such as soccer (Hoff 2005).

Capacity to clear and buffer metabolites

Training at moderate exercise intensity does not produce changes in lactate clearance and muscle buffering capabilities (Tabata et al. 1996, 1997). A more recent study reported that when matched for volume, short-term training (5 weeks) at an intensity just above lactate threshold elicits superior improvements in buffering capacity than training at an intensity just below the athletes' measured lactate threshold (Edge et al. 2006a). The efficacy of conditioning in developing anaerobic capacity is therefore intensity-dependent, requiring training at intensities that exceed lactate threshold or 'maximum lactate steady state' intensity. By definition, the conditioning stimulus must elevate lactate above steady state levels in order to stimulate lactate handling and buffering mechanisms (Billat 2001b).

However, recent data indicate that the intensity of work bouts and relative duration of work:rest selected should not elevate H^+ concentrations excessively so that muscle pH falls too far, in order to ensure a favourable adaptive response, in terms of MCT isoform expression (lactate and H^+ transport proteins) and intracellular buffering capacity (Bishop *et al.* 2008). The training history of the athlete and buffering capacities at the start of the training period may be an important factor in terms of what constitutes appropriate training. Conversely, if rest periods between sets are too long and thereby allow lactate and H^+ concentrations to return towards baseline levels, then this is also likely to limit the training stimulus for adaptations associated with buffering capacity (Bishop *et al.* 2011). A range of repeated sprint and high-intensity interval training protocols have reported positive changes in buffering capacity and expression of MCT isoforms in various study populations.

Peripheral adaptations supporting muscle oxygenation

Muscle oxygenation is dependent upon muscle blood flow (and therefore oxygen delivery), and oxygen uptake and consumption at the muscle cell (Buchheit *et al.* 2012). Relevant adaptations therefore include muscle capilliarisation and muscle oxidative capacity (content and capacity of mitochondria, and mitochondrial enzyme activity). Improvements in muscle reoxygenation rates have been observed following a high-intensity aerobic interval training intervention conducted at intensities in the range 90–115 per cent MAS that also reported concurrent improvements in aerobic capacity and repeated sprint ability (Buchheit and Uffland 2011).

Aerobic capacity and maximum aerobic speed

For well-trained athletes it is suggested that training intensities at or above vVO_2max or MAS are likely to be required in order to produce any further improvements in aerobic capacity (Laursen and Jenkins 2002; Midgley *et al.* 2006). High-intensity and low-volume training interventions have been shown to produce comparable improvements in endurance performance (over both short and long distances) and similar changes in measured muscle oxidative capacity in comparison to traditional moderate-intensity high-volume training (Gibala *et al.* 2006). The similar improvements elicited by the high-intensity conditioning group in these studies are particularly notable given both total training time and volume with this approach is only a fraction of that completed by subjects who performed moderate-intensity high-volume training. It is suggested that part of this potency of high-intensity conditioning is due to its recruitment of a larger pool of motor units during the conditioning activity, and the greater use of larger high-threshold type II muscle fibres, compared to submaximal conditioning protocols (Gibala and McGee 2008).

Improvements in measures of aerobic capacity, including muscle oxidative capacity and measures of vVO_2max or MAS, have been recorded with a range of high-intensity training formats. In some studies these improvements have been seen without any measured changes in subjects' VO_2max scores (Gibala and McGee 2008). The standard high-intensity conditioning protocol employed in a number of studies consisted of four to six sets of 30-second all-out efforts with 4 minutes' recovery between sets. However, improvements in aerobic capacity have also been produced with other high-intensity aerobic interval training formats, including a protocol involving long aerobic intervals involving 4-minute work bouts at close to vVO_2max (Talanian et al. 2007, 2010). Similarly, a mixed protocol comprising both short (20–50-second runs) and long (2:30–15-minute) intervals at a range of intensities (85–120 per cent vVO_2max) has also elicited improvements in measures of aerobic capacity, including MAS scores (Buchheit and Ufland 2011).

Neuromuscular adaptations

Unsurprisingly, neuromuscular training responses relating to work economy and movement efficiency are dependent upon the exercise mode used in conditioning (Jones and Carter 2000). For example, the endurance performance of elite triathletes on a given competition element (running, cycling, or swimming) shows no relationship to the training completed by these athletes on other elements (Millet et al. 2002a). In trained non-athletes, cross training (swimming) is similarly shown to be inferior to running training in improving running performance parameters (Foster et al. 1997). Specificity of neuromuscular adaptations associated with running economy is also apparent for running locomotion. For example, the amount of exposure of team sports athletes to shuttle sprints and change of direction movements during training and competition is related to their running economy measured using a shuttle sprint protocol (Buchheit et al. 2011b).

It follows that it is necessary to replicate the type of locomotion and movements encountered during competition when undertaking metabolic conditioning in order to develop economy or efficiency. As such, conditioning modes for team sports should necessarily include the change of direction movements and unorthodox forms of locomotion (sideways, backwards and tracking movements) that feature in matches (Reilly 1994).

Improvements in work economy are also specific to the velocity at which conditioning is performed. For example, in runners the improvements observed in running economy are greatest at the running velocity at which the athlete habitually trains (Jones and Carter 2000). From this it appears that conditioning performed should reflect the movement velocities encountered during match-play in order to develop work economy at these specific velocities.

By extension, improving repeated sprint ability by developing players' maximum speed capabilities will require that their training includes acceleration and sprint bouts performed at maximal velocity (Bishop et al. 2011). When different forms of training are employed in isolation, performing sprinting-based training itself is shown to be the single most effective means to improve sprinting-specific neuromuscular co-ordination aspects and thereby sprint performance (Kristensen et al. 2006). In accordance with this, a short-term training intervention solely comprising speed and acceleration drills reportedly produced improvements in both acceleration and scores on a test of repeated sprint ability in well-trained team sports players (Buchheit et al. 2010b). In this study, equivalent improvements were not seen in another group of players who completed high-intensity running conditioning comprising 30-second shuttle sprint bouts with 2-minute recovery and improved only in a measure of vVO_2max or MAS at the end of the study period.

Strength training also represents means to elicit neuromuscular adaptations in order to improve movement efficiency and endurance performance. Maximal strength training has proved to be effective in reducing oxygen cost at a given workload with endurance athletes (Hoff 2005). It follows that strength training similarly has a role to play for developing running economy for team sports players. Improvements in measures of repeated sprint ability have also been reported with an explosive strength training intervention with young elite soccer players (Buchheit 2010). Exercise selection and the workout format employed are likely to be decisive factors in determining the transfer of strength training to work economy and repeated sprint ability for the particular movements required during a match in a given team sport. The potential for strength training to impact upon endurance performance is discussed in greater detail in Chapter 5.

Training strategies to develop different aspects of metabolic conditioning

High-intensity training methods

It is suggested that well-trained endurance athletes require higher training intensities to produce further gains in performance and enhancement in VO_2max (Midgley *et al.* 2006). The requisite levels of intensity identified are in the range of 95–100 per cent of the velocity attained at VO_2max. By definition, continuous work over an extended period is limited to submaximal work intensities – higher work rates cannot be sustained over these longer periods. Interval conditioning provides a framework to allow higher work intensities to be performed over repeated bouts; this means that the accumulated total time spent at these higher intensities is longer than would be possible if working continuously (Billat 2001a).

By their intermittent nature, team sports would appear to be most amenable to aerobic and anaerobic interval conditioning. Importantly, interval-based conditioning also enables both aerobic and anaerobic capacity to be developed simultaneously (Laursen and Jenkins 2002). This not only represents the more 'sport-specific' approach, but is also more time-efficient – this is an important consideration in view of the volume of technical and tactical practices and other training athletes in these sports are required to perform.

High-intensity interval training is shown to improve cardiorespiratory fitness parameters and measures of performance in team sports athletes (Helgerud *et al.* 2001). A range of conditioning modes have been used successfully, including hill running (Helgerud *et al.* 2001) and high-intensity game-related drills (McMillan *et al.* 2005). One such study reported increases in aerobic power, lactate threshold and running economy observed in junior elite soccer players following training that were also reflected in concurrent improvements in performance measures. Significant increases were observed in distance covered in a match, average work intensity in both halves of play, number of sprints and frequency of involvement in play (Helgerud *et al.* 2001).

High-intensity interval exercise is shown to elicit significant concurrent improvements in both aerobic power (VO_2max) and a selection of anaerobic capacity and intermittent exercise performance measures (Gaiga and Docherty 1995; Tabata *et al.* 1996). If work bouts are conducted at paces that correspond to those occurring during competition, this form of training will also favour improvements in running economy and work efficiency at competition velocities (Jones and Carter 2000).

High-intensity interval running conditioning

Investigations of interval training protocols have found aerobic and anaerobic systems are taxed to a different relative extent depending on the format of training: key factors are the intensity of work bouts and the relative length of work and recovery phases (Tabata *et al*. 1997). For example, what separates aerobic interval training from anaerobic interval training is the intensity and relative duration of work and rest periods, so that either aerobic metabolism or anaerobic metabolism predominates (Billat 2001a). It appears that optimal combinations of high-intensity work bouts and brief rest intervals might also exist that simultaneously tax both aerobic and anaerobic systems almost maximally (Tabata *et al*. 1996, 1997).

Running intervals at individualised maximum aerobic speed intensities

The emergence of a field test that allows an equivalent parameter to vVO_2max or MAS to be accurately evaluated for each player has facilitated the development of a high-intensity interval running conditioning approach involving work bouts conducted at individual-ised running speeds. Each player is required to cover an individualised distance, deter-mined by their MAS score and the specified duration of each work bout. Practically, this is often achieved using running lanes of varying length so that players run together, and the respective distances covered are determined by the player's individual MAS score (and the duration of work bouts employed). The most common work:rest formats featured in the literature are:

• 30 seconds' work : 15 seconds' rest;
• 15 seconds' work : 15 seconds' rest.

A modification to this approach can also allow anaerobic interval training to be performed, by employing velocities above players' measured MAS to provide 'supra-maximal' work intervals. For example, a protocol involving 15-second work bouts at 120 per cent MAS interspersed with 15-second rest intervals has been described for soccer players (Dupont *et al*. 2004). In this study, players recorded significant improvements for both aerobic capacity (vVO_2max) and 40m sprint times when this form of training was performed twice per week during the playing season. Based upon physiological responses observed with different work:rest combinations, it appears that supramaximal work intervals (that is, >100 per cent MAS) may in fact be required when shorter 10- or 15-second work bouts are employed in order to elicit the requisite intensity for trained elite players (Dellal *et al*. 2008).

As described in the previous sections, an alternative approach is to perform 'long' aerobic intervals comprising work bouts typically ranging from 90 seconds to 4 minutes, performed at intensities close to vVO_2max or MAS (Billat 2001a). It is suggested with this approach that the rest bouts should be relatively shorter than the work bouts, in order to maximise the aerobic training stimulus (Bishop *et al*. 2011). For example, a high-intensity aerobic interval training format that has proven to be successful involves repeated 4-minute bouts performed at ≈90 per cent VO_2max intensity, interspersed with 2-minute rest periods (Talanian *et al*. 2007, 2010).

This approach is highly structured and is beneficial in terms of delivery and the ease with which individual players' work rates can be monitored. This is reflected in highly reproducible physiological responses when players perform high-intensity interval running at individualised MAS intensities (Dellal *et al.* 2008). As a result, it is relatively easy to ensure consistent levels of work intensity between sets and sessions.

On the other hand, the exclusive use of this approach for players' metabolic conditioning could conceivably affect motivation and compliance over time due to the monotony of this form of training. In addition, the lack of sports skill element and the fact that it features only straight-line running in a forwards direction means that training of this type is highly unlikely to confer any improvements in economy for other forms of game-related locomotion and the various change of direction movements that feature in matches.

Repeated sprint conditioning

When interval training features maximal work intensities, this form of training is more accurately defined as repeated sprint training (Billat 2001b). It has been suggested that for clarity this term should only be used for protocols employing maximal sprints of relatively short duration (that is, ≤10 seconds) that involve minimal deterioration of work output within each sprint bout, as opposed to longer, all-out efforts of 30 seconds or more, which would fall under the bracket of the supramaximal interval training described above (Girard *et al.* 2011a).

Relatively longer recovery durations are often employed with this form of training, in order to allow more complete restoration of PCr stores within the muscle (Billat 2001b). Protocols in the literature have employed recovery intervals as long as 4 minutes between work bouts (Bodganis *et al.* 1996). Depending on conditions, such as work intensity and nature of recovery employed, rest intervals of this length allow almost complete restoration of PCr stores within the muscle; this enables the contribution of the phosphagen system to energy production to be maintained over consecutive sprints (Billat 2001b). The contribution of oxidative metabolism also increases with each work bout, despite the near maximal work intensities and extended recovery periods used in these protocols (Bodganis *et al.* 1996).

Some authors have suggested that repeated sprint conditioning over short distances using work:rest ratios recommended to optimise PCr resynthesis may be a suitable approach for developing the capacities required by team sports players (Little and Williams 2007). Proponents of this approach have suggested that the sprint distances and work:rest ratios recommended also correspond quite closely to those reported for various field team sports.

A study has investigated a range of repeated sprint protocols with reference to the physiological responses of soccer (Little and Williams 2007). Variations of two protocols were used: 15 sets of 40m sprints with either 1:4 or 1:6 work:rest ratio; and 40 sets of 15m sprints, again with either 1:4 or 1:6 work:rest. Based upon physiological responses recorded the authors of the study suggested that the 40x15m sprints with 1:6 work:rest ratio would be most applicable to soccer (Little and Williams 2007). With both 15m and 40m sprint distances the decrement in sprint times when 1:4 work:rest ratios were employed was concluded to be too great for use with soccer players. However the authors did also suggest that the 15x40m sprints with 1:4 work:rest might have application as an overload training stimulus for soccer players (Little and Williams 2007).

Performing maximal shuttle sprints has been investigated as an alternative approach to repeated sprint training (Buchheit *et al.* 2010a). This involves maximal efforts covering the same total distance but incorporating one or more 180-degree turns; each bout is performed against the clock in the same way as for the straight-line repeated sprint protocol. Due to the shorter distances to attain top speed, and the need to decelerate to stop and turn, sprinting speed is markedly lower when performing shuttle sprints compared to straight-line sprints over the same total distance. Sprint times were reportedly around 30 per cent worse (that is, higher) when performing 2 × 12.5m shuttle sprints (one 180-degree turn) compared to 25m straight-line sprints in a sample of senior team sports athletes (Buchheit *et al.* 2010a). In the same study a variety of physiological indices were also higher under the shuttle sprint protocol, indicating that repeated shuttle sprint conditioning is also associated with greater physiological load.

Tactical metabolic training approach

The 'special endurance' approach to conditioning models training intensities upon the workloads and the 'effort distribution' observed during competition (Plisk 2000). In the case of sports featuring intermittent activity, a key parameter for structuring conditioning is the work:rest ratios observed from competition (Plisk 2000). The process of identifying relevant parameters from competitive match-play in order to apply this data to players' metabolic conditioning has been termed 'tactical modelling' (Plisk and Gambetta 1997). The tactical metabolic training (TMT) approach to conditioning is essentially an extension of the high-intensity intervals and repeated sprint conditioning approaches – the difference being that the intensity of work intervals and work:rest ratios employed are directly based upon those observed during competitive matches.

Such an approach gives recognition to the interrelationship between energy systems during competition, as energy systems are trained in combination in a way that aims to reflect the bioenergetics of competition (Plisk and Gambetta 1997; Plisk 2000). Proposed advantages of TMT include greater time efficiency, as skill elements can be incorporated into metabolic conditioning (Plisk and Gambetta 1997). This is favourable from a coaching viewpoint as it allows technical and tactical elements to be executed in simulated game conditions, and would likely also be advantageous in that it would engender greater motivation and enhanced training compliance among athletes (Plisk and Gambetta 1997).

The 'special conditioning' TMT approach for team sports was originally developed in American football. This sport is highly structured with the ball only being live for brief periods until the player in possession of the ball is tackled or the ball goes out of play, at which time there are extended stoppages until play restarts. As described in an earlier section, the majority of team sports are less structured and feature highly variable patterns of activity, which poses greater challenges to application of this approach. Objectively quantifying competition demands tends to demand extensive analysis of physiological and time–motion or GPS data, and this would also need to reflect the respective demands placed on each playing position.

If these data are available for the sport in question, the application of the TMT approach might be possible by structuring conditioning drills based upon relevant data, such as work:rest ratios (Plisk 2000; Plisk and Gambetta 1997). Application of the TMT approach based upon work:rest ratios published in the literature has previously been described for collegiate basketball (Taylor 2004); however, in general this approach is not widely employed as a consequence of the logistical difficulties described.

Skill-based conditioning drills

As outlined there are significant methodological issues that compound the inherent difficulty in collecting data to quantify demands associated with team sports in general, and particularly collision sports. The complexities and inherent variability of team sports renders efforts to design conditioning drills to simulate match conditions all the more difficult (Gabbett 2002). Furthermore, strength and conditioning specialists seek to not merely simulate typical match-play demands, but rather impose overload in terms of the intensity, frequency, duration and density of specific activities demanded in match-play (Gamble 2007).

An alternative approach to provide appropriate overload is to employ skill-based conditioning drills that require the player to operate at the extremes of frequency, duration and intensity of activity levels that they could expect to experience during a competitive match.

Small-sided conditioning games

This approach to metabolic conditioning comprises purpose-designed games involving reduced numbers of players on each team and featuring modified playing areas and rules, which allows training intensity to be manipulated (Hoff et al. 2002; Hill-Haas et al. 2011). The application of small-sided games as a metabolic conditioning modality has been described for various team sports, including soccer (Dellal et al. 2008), rugby union (Gamble 2004), rugby league (Gabbett 2006), basketball (Castagna et al. 2011), handball (Buchheit et al. 2009) and volleyball (Gabbett 2008). A variety of small-sided conditioning games with different rules can be adapted from other ball games, while still using the same regulation ball and similar skill set to that featured in the sport for which the athlete is training (Gamble 2007b).

Depending on the choice of conditioning game and other related parameters, it is possible to elicit different levels of training intensity. Factors identified as influencing training intensity with conditioning games include pitch dimensions, players per side and presence of coaching and/or instruction (Rampinini et al. 2007b). Typically, the highest training intensities are produced with small-sided games on a relatively larger playing surface (Hill-Haas et al. 2011). However, there does tend to be an optimal size of playing area, in relation to numbers of players on each side, which requires greatest exertion without allowing the player in possession too much time and space (Jeffreys 2004). In general, lower player numbers are associated with the greatest work intensity, with most studies reporting that the 2-versus-2 format elicits the highest physiological responses (Castagna et al. 2011). Manipulating player numbers so that there are uneven numbers on each team, for example implementing a floating player who joins whichever team is in possession, is another option for altering work intensity (Hill-Haas et al. 2011). Other rule modifications that can influence demands placed on players include restricting the time the ball is out of play (Hoff et al. 2002; Rampini et al. 2007b).

Hoff and colleagues (Hoff et al. 2002) concluded that small-sided games fulfilled the necessary criteria to be an effective means of interval training for soccer players, on the basis of HR and respiratory responses recorded during training. A study of junior elite volleyball players likewise showed that the skill-based conditioning game studied involved comparable time in specified intensity zones (defined ranges of players' percentage HRmax) as those recorded when the players were engaged in competitive matches (Gabbett 2008). In support of this, a training study employing small-sided conditioning games with young elite handball players reported significant improvements in various measures of repeated sprint ability and aerobic capacity following training (Buchheit et al. 2009). The application of small-sided conditioning games during pre-season training for rugby league football players similarly produced equivalent gains on measures of aerobic fitness to a control group that performed interval running conditioning (Gabbett 2006). Similarly, in rugby union football, a pre-season conditioning programme exclusively employing conditioning games was shown to produce significant improvements in cardiorespiratory responses to a standardised shuttle test with elite-level senior players (Gamble 2004b).

Small-sided conditioning games are suggested to be a superior method for metabolic conditioning based upon the specificity of this training mode (Buchheit et al. 2009). For example, small-sided games require decision-making under fatigue and simulated game conditions, encompassing both movement and context specificity (Gamble 2004b; Jeffreys 2004). This would appear also to be a highly time-efficient and integrated approach, as small-sided games not only incorporate relevant sport skills and modes of locomotion, but these skills and movement responses are also executed in reaction to game-related cues, thereby providing concurrent development of technical and tactical elements (Hill-Haas et al. 2011). The skill and competition elements that are the key features of skill-based conditioning games are suggested to promote enhanced effort despite the apparently lower perceived exertion ratings by participating players (Gabbett 2006). As such the skill-based conditioning games approach is likely to engender greater compliance, making this form of conditioning amenable to continued use over an extended period (Gamble 2007b; Jeffreys 2004).

The skill element that is a feature of conditioning games has been suggested to offer concurrent sports skills development as it requires relevant sport skills to be executed under game conditions and while fatigued (Gabbett 2006; Gamble 2007b). A study of elite junior volleyball players reported that skill-based conditioning games conferred some improvement in scores for certain sport skill measures, albeit they did not produce the degree of improvement on the same range of measures as a training group that engaged in specific skill practices (Gabbett 2008). Accordingly, this form of conditioning should complement players' skill work, but should not replace dedicated skill practice.

There is also some indication that this approach to conditioning is associated with lower injury rates, in comparison to other forms of training (Gabbett 2002). Gabbett (2002) reported reduced rates of injury when rugby league players were engaged in skill-based conditioning games, in contrast to the far higher incidence of injury reported when performing traditional conditioning (without any skill element) reported in this study. It is conceivable that enhanced motor control when performing game-related movements may be one factor responsible for the apparent decreases in injury rates, in comparison to traditional running conditioning (Gamble 2004b).

One caveat with this approach is that a greater level of variability in players' physiological responses is reported with small-sided games, in comparison to more structured conditioning such as high-intensity running intervals (Dellal et al. 2008; Hill-Haas et al.

2011). Physiological responses and movement patterns also appear to be influenced by the skill level and technical abilities of the players performing this form of conditioning (Dellal *et al.* 2011). There is also some suggestion that individuals with higher endurance capacities may not receive the same training stimulus as other players within the team when partici-pating in small-sided games conditioning (Hill-Haas *et al.* 2011).

The manner of delivery when conducting metabolic conditioning with small-sided games, and the way in which players are monitored during these sessions, would appear to be critical in terms of minimising variability in players' physiological responses both within and between training sessions. Small-sided games with fewer players on each side appear to produce more consistent work rates (Hill-Haas *et al.* 2008). If larger player numbers are used it is recommended that the conditioning game is played on a correspondingly larger pitch, so that the relative playing area per player is equivalent (Hill-Haas *et al.* 2011). It would also appear to be important that the teams for small-sided conditioning games are selected carefully so that opposing teams are well matched in terms of both playing ability and aerobic capacity. The presence of the sports coach to provide verbal encouragement and instruction when conditioning games are being conducted also appears to enhance the consistency of players' work rates over time (Rampinini *et al.* 2007b).

Training using such an inherently unstructured format as conditioning games requires some objective marker to evaluate the work rates of individual players (Gamble 2007). Heart rate (HR) monitoring is extensively used as the most effective and practical means to objectively monitor intensity during a training session (Potteiger and Evans 1995), and quantify training loads in the athlete's weekly training log (Gilman and Wells 1993). The use of HR to monitor exercise intensity has also been validated against direct measure-ment of ventilatory responses during small-sided conditioning games in soccer players (Hoff *et al.* 2002). Monitoring of players' HR therefore would appear a crucial adjunct to the skill-based conditioning games approach, in order to quantify training intensity in the conditioning game setting (Gamble 2007b). It has also been suggested that the HR data recorded should be expressed as percentages of players' individual $HR_{Reserve}$, in order to reflect both maximum and resting heart rate values for each player (Dellal *et al.* 2008). Providing timely and appropriate feedback to players, ideally following each set or after the training session, and based upon objective data, provides a means to increase levels of compliance and ensure players work consistently at the desired level of intensity.

Conclusions and training recommendations

High-intensity interval training and repeated sprint conditioning appear to be the training approaches best suited for concurrent development of the physiological and metabolic capacities required to prepare players for the intermittent exertion that is characteristic of team sports. It is likely that a blend of both these forms of training represents the best approach in order to elicit adaptations across the full spectrum of factors that have been identified as contributing to repeated sprint performance. Given the complex nature of the metabolic requirements of team sports play, and the host of physiological and neuromus-cular factors described, it is perhaps unsurprising that there is no single training approach that is optimal, and a mixed approach is likely to be most effective (Bishop *et al.* 2011).

A range of different conditioning modes may be employed to provide high-intensity interval training and repeated sprint conditioning. For example, high-intensity interval conditioning may be undertaken using conventional running conditioning, small-sided conditioning games, or any combination of these two methods. Small-sided conditioning games might be viewed as equivalent to 'long' aerobic interval training (set durations are typically in the range of 2–8 minutes), whereas high-intensity running conditioning might be employed for short intervals (for example, 30–15 second or 15–15 second work:rest intervals). Likewise, repeated sprint training might feature a selection of conventional sprints, shuttle sprints and maximal-intensity conditioning drills featuring game-related movements. Finally, these metabolic conditioning modes should be complemented with appropriate speed development, strength and speed-strength training, in order to provide concurrent development of speed and neuromuscular qualities (Bishop *et al.* 2011).

Each of these training modes has various strengths and limitations in terms of specificity, practicality, physiological responses and issues of motivation and compliance over time. A blend of these different approaches, implemented strategically throughout the training year, would again seem to be the best approach. Similarly, the selection of conditioning approaches and prescription of intensity, volume and work:rest parameters should follow a coherent progression, according to the periodised plan for the sport season and the individual athlete.

5

STRENGTH TRAINING

Introduction

Specificity is manifested in both the ability of the athlete to express their strength in a particular athletic movement and the nature of the training response to a particular strength training intervention (Carroll *et al.* 2001). Fundamentally, a player's strength capabilities when lifting in the weights room is of less relevance than their ability to express that strength when executing athletic and skilled movements on the field of play. How training effects ultimately transfer to sports performance therefore represents a primary consideration when designing a strength training programme.

The obvious application of specificity with regard to the outcomes of strength training is exercise selection. Particular modes of strength training have greater transfer of training effect in terms of what performance effects are manifested, based upon the mechanics and kinetics of the training exercise (Stone *et al.* 2000a). Strength training outcomes are also dictated by the particular combination of strength training variables employed. Training intensity, repetition scheme and volume all interact to determine the specific strength training response (Baechle *et al.* 2000). These factors in turn influence the nature of the training response elicited with respect to different strength qualities – for example, maximum strength versus strength-endurance (Young 2006).

In turn, the requirement for a particular strength quality for a team sports player will depend on the typical demands placed upon them during competition. It follows that sport-specific and position-specific considerations should be addressed in the design of strength training, in order to develop the required combination of strength qualities for the sport and playing position. The final consideration for strength and conditioning specialists is that strength training design should also be specific to the needs of the player. From this viewpoint a starting point in attempts to tailor a programme for a player might include musculoskeletal and movement profiling, in combination with a battery of performance tests to identify any areas in need of particular attention.

Requirements and relevant strength qualities for team sports

There is currently a lack of contemporary strength testing data published from professional team sports players; the studies that have been published mainly concern contact team sports. Scores on strength and power measures are shown to distinguish elite professional players in collision sports from those at lesser levels (Baker 2001b, 2001d). This asserts the importance of developing strength properties for contact sports such as rugby football – in fact it appears to be a prerequisite for participation at the highest level (Baker 2002).

There is a significant progression reported in these strength qualities at each stage from high-school level, through college age, to senior professional level (Baker 2002). Independent of any difference in lean body mass, elite professional rugby league players are able to express greater upper-body strength and power than semi-professional and college-aged players (Baker 2001b, 2001d). Upper- and lower-body power measures of elite rugby league players are shown to be heavily dependent on their levels of strength (Baker and Nance 1999a). Given the observed importance of strength and lean body mass, it is thus crucial to maximise the effectiveness of the strength training players are able to perform within the constraints of other training and team practices.

In collision sports such as American football and rugby football, physical size and muscularity confer an advantage to the player during contact situations. Accordingly, body mass and size of players in these sports have risen disproportionately in recent times. It is reported that over a 25-year period the body mass and levels of mesomorphy of top-level rugby union players has shown consistent increases at five times the rate of that seen for the general population in the same period (Olds 2001). Individual players are similarly predisposed to, and selected for, particular playing positions on the basis of their anthropometric characteristics and strength capabilities (Quarrie et al. 1995; Quarrie and Wilson 2000; Duthie et al. 2003). Site-specific hypertrophy is also important in contact sports such as American football and rugby football (Kraemer 1997). The shoulders are a key area for development as this is frequently the point of impact when tackling opponents.

Based upon what data exist in the literature, there appear to be significant differences in strength demands between playing positions in the sports studied. For example, it has been identified that different playing position groupings in professional rugby league vary in their performance on various strength, speed and endurance measures (Meir et al. 2001). Specifically, rugby league forwards exhibit greater upper-body strength than backs. Conversely, outside backs in rugby league are faster over 15m than forwards – and faster than all other positional sub-groups over 40m (Meir et al. 2001). All playing positions, irrespective of differences in body mass and positional demands, require high levels of dynamic muscular strength relative to body mass in order to contend with the physical aspects of the sport (Baker 2001b; Meir et al. 2001).

When athletes are required to perform movements repeatedly, other capabilities are implicated that relate to the strength qualities described. Strength-endurance, speed-endurance, and power-endurance are identified as discrete elements and should be considered independently, as opposed to merely derivatives of strength, speed and power (Yessis 1994). The capacity to activate musculature under conditions of fatigue has been identified as a trainable quality (Behm 1995). Under conditions of fatigue, trained individuals appear to have superior ability to fully activate the musculature (Behm 1995). Two key adaptations identified as underlying strength-endurance are acid–base buffering (Kraemer 1997) and neural mechanisms (intramuscular co-ordination) that make the athlete better able to more fully activate fatigued motor units (Behm 1995).

Sport-specific strength

Strength training has become established as a key component in a programme of physical preparation for the majority of sports. However, the diverse physical demands involved in team sports pose unique demands for strength training design. For the majority of sports it is suggested that athletes require *optimal* levels of strength as opposed to *maximal* levels in order to successfully compete in their sport (Murray and Brown 2006). It is therefore important to recognise that 'optimal strength' may be a more important training goal than maximal strength for these athletes. The design of strength training should therefore reflect the specific demands of the particular sport – and in the case of team sports, the playing position.

What defines 'sport-specific' strength capabilities is the ability of the player to express their strength qualities during the execution of game-related activities or sport skills in the context of a match situation (Smith 2003). Anecdotally, many coaches will be familiar with the scenario that their top performing players are not necessarily those that have the best strength test scores or lift the heaviest weights in the weights room (McGill 2006d). One aspect of this is that team sports performance requires more than just strength performance. However, another implication is that the strength and speed-strength capabilities expressed in the context of team sports are somewhat different to the classical weights room definition of strength performance.

Fundamentally, strength and conditioning specialists cannot lose sight of the fact that they are preparing the athlete to perform on the field – not to increase the athlete's strength test results for their own sake. Strength tests may show some correlation to performance, playing level or selection in certain sports. However, the focus should remain on building athleticism to allow the athlete to compete in their sport, not to convert the athlete into a powerlifter. Strength test scores may well improve – preferably in those tests that resemble the demands of the sport – but this is secondary to improving athleticism and the athlete's ability to express functional or sport-specific strength. The ultimate measure of the success of the athlete's programme is the extent to which it improves their performance in the field of play, not in the weights room. Transfer of training effects is a crucial factor: one of the key criteria when judging the efficacy of a strength training programme is the degree of performance improvement relative to the training time invested (Young 2006).

Associated benefits of strength training for team sports players

Reducing risk of injury

Sport-specific physical conditioning can favourably influence injury risk when playing team sports. One general protective effect is that appropriately conditioned athletes are more resistant to neuromuscular fatigue, which renders athletes susceptible to injury (Hawkins *et al.* 2001; Murphy *et al.* 2003; Verrall *et al.* 2005). This is illustrated in the common trend observed in many team sports for higher injury rates in the latter stages of matches when players are fatigued (Best *et al.* 2005; Brooks *et al.* 2005a; Hawkins and Fuller 1999; Hawkins *et al.* 2001). Strength training also serves a general protective effect in making the musculoskeletal system stronger and thereby more resistant to the stresses incurred during games (Kraemer and Fleck 2005). The addition of strength training to the physical preparation of male collegiate soccer players was followed by an almost 50 per cent reduction in injury rates during subsequent playing seasons (Lehnhard *et al.* 1996). One aspect of this is that trained muscle is more resistant to the microtrauma caused by strenuous physical exertion and also recovers faster (Takarada 2003).

In addition to the general benefits of strength training and metabolic conditioning, targeted interventions have the potential to specifically guard against certain injuries to which athletes may be exposed. Injury prevention-oriented strength training employs particular exercises specifically designed to address certain risk factors and injury mechanisms associated with a particular type of injury in the sport. This application of specific training interventions, of which strength training is a key component, is discussed at length in Chapters 9 and 10.

Strength training to improve endurance performance

Neuromuscular aspects that can influence players' endurance performance can be developed via appropriate strength training. Neuromuscular factors that contribute to endurance performance include neural and elastic components of stretch-shortening cycle capabilities, intermuscular co-ordination influencing running mechanics and movement economy, and also the strength qualities of locomotor and postural muscles (Paavolainen *et al.* 1999). Improving these aspects independently of any changes in aerobic or anaerobic endurance parameters has the potential to improve endurance performance (Mikkola *et al.* 2007, Millet *et al.* 2002b, Paavolainen *et al.* 1999).

Such beneficial effects of strength training on parameters of endurance performance have been demonstrated in athletes in various sports. A number of studies of endurance athletes report that time trial performance is improved by the addition of strength training to their physical preparation, and these improvements occur independently of any changes in physiological parameters such as VO_2max scores (Mikkola *et al.* 2007, Millet *et al.* 2002b, Paavolainen *et al.* 1999). Accordingly, a recent study showed that strength training intervention was effective in producing improvements in measures of endurance and repeated sprint ability with team sports players (Buchheit *et al.* 2010d).

The force-generating capacity of the locomotor muscles and the ability to maximally recruit these muscles during conditions of fatigue are important factors when engaged in endurance activities (Paavolainen *et al.* 1999). It follows that improving strength, speed-strength and strength-endurance should positively influence economy and performance when engaged in endurance activities. In addition, neuromuscular control and co-ordination aspects influence the stiffness and elasticity of the muscle–tendon complex during foot strike when running (Paavolainen *et al.* 1999). For example, increases in measures of lower limb muscle stiffness were shown following a period of strength training in elite triathletes (Millet *et al.* 2002b). Improving such capacities via appropriate strength and speed-strength training can increase the non-contractile contribution to work output during locomotion. Reducing energy cost of locomotion in this way will improve movement economy and thereby improve endurance capacity (Millet *et al.* 2002b). Given that team sports feature a variety of modes of locomotion in multiple directions, it follows that selection of strength-training exercises should reflect this in order to confer such improvements in movement-specific work economy.

Approaching strength training for team sports players

A number of the practices and conventions observed in athletic preparation – in particular with regard to strength training – have evolved from competitive powerlifting, weightlifting and bodybuilding (Fleck and Kraemer 1997). This should be recognised when evaluating and designing strength training programmes for team sports. It is important that strength and conditioning specialists are able to discern between practices, even at the level of exercise selection, that are based predominantly on convention as opposed to those that serve a specific purpose with regard to players' physical preparation for the sport.

A survey investigating the practices of strength and conditioning coaches in US Division One collegiate competition revealed that what most influenced their training design and prescription was the input and practices employed by their peers (that is, other collegiate strength coaches) (Durell et al. 2003). In contrast, only 9 per cent of these collegiate strength and conditioning coaches ranked journals or books as their primary information source when designing programmes. Similar surveys of professional North American team sports did not include this question. However, responses of strength and conditioning coaches in National Football League, National Hockey League, Major League Baseball and National Basketball Association indicated similar reliance on convention and non-scientific sources with respect to different aspects of training programme design and implementation rather than evidence-based practice (Ebben and Blackard 2001; Ebben et al. 2004, 2005; Simenz et al. 2005).

All team sports feature common fundamental movement abilities to some degree: these include gait and locomotion (for example, running), squatting and/or lifting, pushing and/or pulling, lunging, twisting and maintaining balance (McGill 2006c). A logical starting point for a strength training programme is to address any deficiencies or areas of weakness that restrict the player's ability to efficiently execute these fundamental athletic movements. From a performance viewpoint, a player can be deemed to be only as strong as the weakest link in the kinetic chain from the supporting lower limb to the limb which is executing the movement. This kinetic chain may extend from the supporting foot to the upper limb, for example when executing a throwing or striking movement. Lack of mobility and deficits in strength or function at any one of the integrated system of joints in the kinetic chain will ultimately limit performance, as well as potentially causing pain and injury.

Traditional approaches to training can serve to strengthen areas where the athlete is already strong without addressing the weak links that will ultimately limit performance. Without corrective training, this has the potential to make the athlete more imbalanced and place tissues around any weak links under further strain. The approach and the strength training modes that are most appropriate will therefore depend upon the constraints of the individual. For example, the barbell back squat is an exercise that is employed year-round as the cornerstone of the strength programme for some sports. Based upon electromyographic (EMG) data recorded from muscles during the classical barbell back squat, this lift can be categorised as primarily an exercise for the quadriceps muscles – at least for the majority of the exercise range of motion (McGill 2006b). The back squat is a good option if the aim is improving general strength of the knee extensors. However, an emphasis on the back squat in the training for an athlete who already exhibits quadriceps dominance and weak gluteal muscles might in fact exacerbate this dysfunction and further predispose the athlete to injury and impaired performance.

Similarly, selection of exercises should reflect the programme goal for the training phase. Consideration should be given to specificity with respect to transfer of training effects, as well as the capabilities of the athlete. For example, if the primary aim of the strength-training programme is producing gains in speed capabilities in the short term, bilateral strength training modes such the back squat would not represent the best option for a player who already exhibits adequate maximum strength levels (Young 2006). For example, an 8-week strength training intervention with the back squat exercise reported this training mode to be highly effective in improving back squat 1-RM strength (21 per cent gain) and vertical jump performance (21 per cent); however, very limited improvement (2.3 per cent) was seen in sprinting speed (Wilson *et al.* 1996).

A recent trend in the strength and conditioning industry and the field of athletic preparation has been the growth of 'functional training' approaches, which are often employed to the exclusion of conventional heavy resistance training methods. This approach ignores the longer-term implications of training adaptation and the size principle of motor unit recruitment, and is therefore very unlikely to produce consistent gains in performance. The paradox of specificity and transfer of training effects was discussed in Chapter 1. Whilst highly task-specific modes offer a high degree of dynamic correspondence, by their nature these training modes are unable to provide the levels of force required to elicit the requisite adaptations that will ultimately optimise performance (Bondarchuk 2007). For example, the maximal loading the standing cable press is able to provide is reportedly only 40.8 per cent of the athlete's body mass (Santana *et al.* 2007). The loading provided by common functional training exercises and sport-specific training modes is therefore typically insufficient to recruit high-threshold motor units and elicit the gains in strength and produce the morphological adaptations that are the prerequisites for the development of athletic performance.

Conversely, heavy resistance training modes impose the loading conditions required for mechanical and morphological adaptations that underpin strength and power performance. However, as illustrated in the previous study investigating the transfer of heavy resistance training modes to speed performance (Wilson *et al.* 1996), employing these methods in isolation will also not confer the desired improvements in athletic performance. It follows that the optimal approach to strength training is likely to feature a blend of training modes that span a continuum, ranging from heavy resistance training modes to highly sport-specific training.

Specificity of dose–response relationships with strength training experience

Training experience is a key consideration for strength-training prescription: there is an obvious need to progress intensity, volume and frequency of training, as the neuromuscular system grows more accustomed to strength training with increased exposure (Rhea *et al.* 2003). Exercise prescription guidelines accordingly make a distinction in terms of resistance training experience and feature separate recommendations for untrained, recreationally trained and advanced lifters (Kraemer *et al.* 2002). Meta-analysis of the strength-training literature demonstrates that training responses vary depending on subjects' training status (Rhea *et al.* 2003). Thus the levels of intensity, volume and training frequency shown to maximise gains differ based upon the training experience of the subject population (Peterson *et al.* 2004). It appears logical that individuals with different training experience will require different 'doses' of training parameters in order to elicit a maximal training response, in terms of strength gains.

Such dose–response relationships with regard to optimal resistance load, volume and frequency of strength training have previously not been identified in competitive athletes. There is a paucity of data from elite team sports athletes in particular – for example, the absence of contemporary data concerning strength levels of elite players in rugby union football has been highlighted (Duthie *et al.* 2003). However, one study has undertaken a meta-analysis of 37 studies in the strength training literature that directly examined athlete subjects (Peterson *et al.* 2004). Summarising the findings of these studies, the authors found that the training parameters that optimise training effects (measured strength gains) in competitive athletes differ from those based on similar studies employing strength-trained non-athletes. Training volume (sets per muscle group), training frequency (days per week for each muscle group) and training intensity (resistance load) found to be most effective in the studies examined differed markedly from those for non-athletes – even non-athlete subjects experienced in strength training (Peterson *et al.* 2004).

Hence, competitive athletes show different dose–response relationships with regard to strength training in comparison even to strength-trained non-athletes (Peterson *et al.* 2004). From these studies it appears that a continuum exists in terms of optimal training variables for maximal strength gains, which is dependent on the training status and training experience of the individual (Rhea *et al.* 2003) – and that elite athletes appear to sit further along this dose–response continuum (Peterson *et al.* 2004). As such, elite team sports players are shown to require considerably different intensity, frequency and volume of strength training to maximise strength gains (Peterson *et al.* 2004).

This consideration raises questions regarding the relevance of findings in the strength-training literature based on investigations involving non-athletic populations, even using subjects with strength training experience (Peterson *et al.* 2004). The lack of studies denies any opportunity for comparison of the current findings to existing data. There remains a critical need to gather data pertaining specifically to athletes, in particular those engaged in team sports. Obtaining access to elite athletes is likely to require some compromise in terms of study design (Millet *et al.* 2002a). However, only in this way will it be possible to provide an objective alternative to the ongoing tendency of strength and conditioning coaches working in many team sports to rely upon their own observations and personal experience as the primary basis for selection of training modes and methods (Kraemer 1997).

Strength training prescription for elite athletes

The specific needs of competitive athletes are vastly different from those of recreationally trained individuals: it is logical that by extension the optimal training for athletes will likewise be different. On this basis, elite performers should be treated as a special population (Cronin *et al.* 2001b). Maximal strength gains are demonstrated in untrained individuals training at an average intensity of 60 per cent 1-RM (repetition maximum), whereas individuals experienced with strength training exhibit maximum gains with 80 per cent 1-RM resistance; competitive athletes appear to exist further still along this continuum. From what data are available, some suggestions for training prescription applicable to team sports players can be made: a mean training intensity of 85 per cent 1-RM has been found to have greatest effect in competitive athletes from the majority of relevant studies (Peterson *et al.* 2004). This equates to an average intensity of 6-RM (that is, the greatest weight that can be lifted for six repetitions with proper form).

This is in general agreement with the finding that loads greater than 80 per cent 1-RM were necessary to maintain or improve strength throughout the playing season in college American football players (Hoffman and Kang 2003). Observation of elite weightlifters likewise noted a significant decrease in EMG recorded during the phase of the training year when training intensity dropped below 80 per cent 1-RM, which recovered once training intensity was increased above 80 per cent in the subsequent training period (Hakkinen *et al.* 1987). This requirement for greater average intensity appears to be a common theme for athletes as a special population. Of all training variables, training intensity was the only significant predictor of strength changes during an in-season period in college American football players (Hoffman and Kang 2003). Training studies featuring protocols in which the athlete subject group lifted to failure report greater average strength gains (Peterson *et al.* 2004). Therefore, it appears there is a need for strength training regimes to stipulate the athlete must exert maximal effort at the specified load, as training at lesser intensities appears to elicit minimal improvements in competitive athletes (Hoffman and Kang 2003).

In terms of frequency of strength training, recommendations are based on the number of times per week individual muscle groups should be trained. From data examining athletes, training a particular muscle group two or three days per week was observed to be similarly effective (Peterson *et al.* 2004). How many strength training sessions this equates to will depend on the layout of the workout. It could be two workouts per week in the case that both days are whole-body sessions. On the other hand, if a 'split routine' format is being used (for example separating upper- and lower-body workouts), this may comprise four or more strength-training sessions per week. There is some evidence that a 5-day programme incorporating split routine loading may offer greater strength and muscle mass gains (Hoffman *et al.* 1990). However, given the time constraints imposed in many team sports, the former 2- or 3-day whole body format may be more time-efficient during the majority of the season.

Recommendations for volume of strength training for competitive athletes are similarly made in terms of individual muscle groups. A mean number of eight sets per muscle group per week appears to maximise strength gains in groups of athletes (Peterson *et al.* 2004). This represents double the equivalent volume recommendations based on studies for non-athletes: the majority of studies employing non-athletes found four sets per muscle group per week to be effective in evoking maximal strength gains (Rhea *et al.* 2003). Competitive athletes thus appear to require a much greater volume of strength training to provide an effective training stimulus for gains in strength. Similarly, players in contact sports for whom hypertrophy is a programme goal require greater training frequencies to elicit the necessary gains. It has been identified that quite extreme training frequencies (four and five days per week) are required to elicit body mass gains in college-aged American football players experienced in strength training (Hoffman *et al.* 1990; Kraemer 1997). These distinct differences in optimal training volumes again reinforce the specific needs of competitive athletes as a special population.

Strength and conditioning specialists must, however, be careful with what constitutes an 'advanced athlete' with respect to strength training. Most players will have strength training experience to the extent that they have been engaged in some form of resistance training for a period of time. However, despite – or potentially as a result of – having been resistance trained for a number of years, an individual player may still exhibit deficits in mobility, stability and/or imbalances in strength that impair their ability to perform fundamental athletic movements. Following a neuromuscular skill-based approach to strength training, training status and therefore the starting point for the individual player's strength training programme will depend upon an assessment of their functional move-ment abilities alongside their scores on strength, power and performance tests. Similar ongoing qualitative assessment of the player's neuromuscular skill and movement abili-ties can likewise be used to help govern the rate of progression in their strength training programme.

Format of strength training

Another application of specificity, which is typically not fully accounted for, is the format in which strength training workouts are performed. Team sports involve a wide array of movements in multiple directions executed repeatedly in an unspecified order with high force. Contact field sports feature the added element of movements executed against resistance, often with the upper body as the point of contact. For team sports players, the optimal training format has yet to be adequately investigated. Anecdotally, some strength and conditioning specialists working with professional team sports players attempt to address this by incorporating the use of 'compound sets' – that is, alternately performing sets of one exercise (for example, a pushing lift) with another exercise (such as a pulling lift).

Taking this approach further, a circuit format might be considered for the entire workout. This should not be mistaken for traditional circuit training which features submaximal loads and relatively high repetitions; the same loads are used: it is solely the format of the workout that is altered. The circuit format would also appear to have the advantage of reducing workout time (as players will move onto the next lift in the interval during which they would normally be resting) and potentially stimulating improvements in strength-endurance. A study investigating this approach termed this method 'heavy resistance circuit training' and found that subjects were able to lift the same load and volume with no alternation in bar kinematics compared to the traditional sequential format, and that it also elicited a greater cardiovascular response (Alcaraz et al. 2008). The authors concluded this approach to strength training could be expected to elicit similar strength improvements with additional cardiovascular benefits.

A subsequent study has confirmed the efficacy of strength training performed in a 'heavy-resistance' circuit format. An 8-week training intervention with resistance-trained subjects produced similar improvements in strength (bench press and squat 1-RM) and bench throw power output scores, and gains in lean mass to subjects who trained with the traditional strength format (Alcaraz et al. 2011). The session duration for the high resist-ance circuit format was significantly shorter, and there were also additional improvements in body composition that were not observed with the traditional strength-training group (Alcaraz et al. 2011). The latter finding corresponds to the greater cardiovascular response previously reported with this training format (Alcaraz et al. 2008). An earlier study by Kraemer (1997) reported improvements in strength-endurance (number of repetitions the subject was able to complete at 80 or 85 per cent 1-RM) with American football players following a multi-set strength training at 8–12RM, performed in a circuit fashion. This was attributed in part to improvements in lactate buffering and whole body acid–base balance associated with the circuit format (Kraemer 1997).

It has been shown that with adequate rest (3 minutes) between sets, RM loads can be lifted repeatedly (Kraemer 1997). The crucial factor influencing capacity to repeatedly perform sets at RM load was identified as rest period between sets. When rest is reduced, ability to perform the prescribed number of repetitions at the RM load may be compromised (Kraemer 1997). The sequential approach of lifting the prescribed sets for one lift before moving on to the next exercise may lead to insufficient rest between sets to successfully complete the stipulated repetitions with the RM load. Players typically self-select rest between sets and may rush through the sets in an effort to perform all the exercises within the limited time allotted for the workout. The circuit format described avoids this, as the muscle groups involved in a particular lift are allowed to rest while the player completes the intervening exercises in the circuit prior to performing next set.

Strength-training methods and modes

The particular constraints of a given training mode serve to determine the stimulus provided to the neuromuscular system in terms of intra- and inter-muscular co-ordination (Carroll *et al.* 2001). In this way, biomechanical aspects that include the kinematic and kinetic profile of a particular strength-training exercise will influence the degree to which there is any direct transfer of training effects to a given aspect of neuromuscular performance in the short term (Newton *et al.* 1999). This concept has been termed *dynamic correspondence*.

The method employed for applying resistance during strength training is accordingly a key factor that influences the neuromuscular stimulus provided. For the majority of multi-joint training movements, free weight application of resistance has generally been considered to be more functional as the lifter is required to stabilise their own body and the external resistance, while simultaneously controlling and directing the movement (Kraemer *et al.* 2002; Stone *et al.* 2000b). For example, free weights exercises develop intra- and inter-muscular co-ordination to a greater degree than training with conventional weight-stack resistance machines. This is reflected in greater strength gains and superior transfer to athletic and ergonomic performance measures in comparison to machine-based resistance training (Stone *et al.* 2000b).

A number of other methods for applying resistance and novel strength training practices have emerged with the growth of the strength and conditioning industry. The strength and conditioning specialist is therefore faced with a variety of options, depending on access to the appropriate equipment. These options range from suspension training methods whereby the player's own body weight provides the resistance, to highly specialised devices including variable resistance machines and pneumatic resistance training modes. In addition, bands, ropes and chains have been employed to provide variable resistance when performing conventional free weights training exercises.

There is currently very little data to support manufacturers' claims regarding the superiority of these devices and equipment for athletic development. In general, most devices restrict the motion and in turn the degrees of freedom of the strength-training exercise; the mechanical and associated neural stimulus provided therefore does not correspond to the conditions encountered during normal activities (Frost *et al.* 2010). It has similarly been suggested that manipulating the resistance provided at different points in the exercise range of motion with the use of bands or chains alters the kinetic and kinematic profile of the strength-training mode in an artificial manner that may not produce appropriate adaptation in neural co-ordination when related movements are performed under 'real-world' conditions during competition (Frost *et al.* 2010).

Conversely, cable pulley devices employing either weight-stack or pneumatic resistance offer a means to provide resistance in a variety of directions. One limitation with isoinertial free weights exercises is that by definition the forces applied are dictated by the acceleration due to gravity, which acts only in a downward vertical direction.

The majority of game-related movements in team sports are executed partly or fully from a single-leg base of support. It follows that unilateral support exercises should necessarily comprise a significant portion of the team sport athlete's training (McCurdy and Conner 2003). Unilateral strength training was reported to be similarly effective in producing improvements in strength and vertical jump performance in comparison to bilateral strength training in a study of untrained subjects (McCurdy *et al.* 2005). Unilateral support exercises also do not allow the athlete to favour their dominant limb during the movement as can occur with bilateral lifts (Newton *et al.* 2006). For example, differences in force production have been observed between dominant and non-dominant legs in collegiate female softball players when performing the bilateral barbell back squat exercise (Newton *et al.* 2006). The number of sets and/or repetitions can also be manipulated to increase the training stimulus provided to the weaker side. Unilateral support exercises offer a means to address such imbalances in strength between limbs. This is important both in terms of function and performance, but also from an injury prevention perspective in view of the reported association between strength and flexibility imbalances with injury incidence (Knapik *et al.* 1991).

Similarly, upper-body movements in team sports are typically unilateral. It follows that training to develop players' upper-body strength and power should feature an appropriate emphasis on alternate arm and single arm lifts. Such exercises also require greater stabilisation of the trunk, as the unilateral resistance results in destabilising torques that must be compensated for by the trunk muscles on the opposite (contralateral) side (Behm *et al.* 2005). This stabilising challenge corresponds to what occurs during match-play, hence can be viewed as beneficial in terms of transfer of training effects.

The quantity of muscle mass involved in the training exercise, as well as frequency and volume load (repetitions multiplied by mass lifted) of training will influence adaptations in body composition (Stone *et al.* 2000a). Free weight exercises that recruit a large amount of muscle mass have greater metabolic demand and hormonal responses, which tends to favour alterations in body composition. This is important for contact team sports in which developing high levels of lean muscle mass are a key programme goal. Similar considerations underpin recommendations for multiple-joint free weights exercises recruiting large muscle mass to develop local muscular endurance and strength-endurance (Kraemer *et al.* 2002).

Progression of strength training variables

There is a need for progressive increases in training stress applied as training advances to achieve continued adaptation. Even the best designed programme will not produce significant gains over time without continuing to take the neuromuscular system beyond what it is accustomed to. Progressions in training intensity may be achieved by increasing force demands, either by increasing mass lifted or increasing the acceleration at which the movement is executed (or any combination of these two variables). Progression can likewise be achieved by manipulating volume load via repetitions performed, training volume (number of sets and exercises in the workout) and/or training frequency (weekly number of sessions per muscle group) (Kraemer *et al.* 2002). Finally, the neural stimulus with respect to intra- and inter-muscular co-ordination requirements provided by the strength-training intervention represents another option for achieving progression. With increasing training experience and as training status advances, more challenging training regimes and more sophisticated manipulation of training parameters are required to elicit a training response (Newton and Kraemer 1994; Kraemer *et al.* 2002).

Progression of strength training modes: the specificity continuum

Manipulating exercise selection to progress the neuromuscular and motor control demand, in a systematic and sequential manner over time, provides not only progression but also facilitates transfer of training effects from preceding training phases. It is important not to ignore the role of training adaptations elicited by preceding training cycles, in terms of building the athlete's capabilities for the training scheduled in successive training cycles, as this will also ultimately determine the longer-term training effects observed at the culmination of the training macrocycle (Bondarchuk 2007). When taking account of specificity and transfer of training effects, consideration must therefore be given not only to the direct effects observed in the short term, but also to the indirect long-term effects on the player's capabilities that will ultimately be reflected in performance improvements if progression is used appropriately. This principle is the central tenet of the study of the transfer of training effects and the staged model described by Bondarchuk (2007).

For example, strength training implemented early in the training year might feature heavy resistance training modes designed to maximise increases in force-generating capacity and produce adaptation in both contractile elements and connective tissues. Once this foundation development has been completed early in the training year, successive training cycles might then see a shift towards more technically demanding lifts and those that require greater balance and stabilisation. This sequential progression in exercise selection might then culminate with the most specific training modes which show a high degree of dynamic correspondence to the movements performed in the sport being employed towards the end of the competition season, in order to facilitate the greatest short-term transfer of training effects.

Manipulating neuromuscular demands in this way as a means to achieve progression is in keeping with the alternative approach to strength training for team sports characterised by a neuromuscular emphasis that was described previously. Given that it is motor control rather than gross strength capabilities that commonly separates the best performers in many team sports (McGill 2006d), it follows that the means for achieving progression when designing players' strength training should reflect this.

General strength development

As discussed in a previous section, traditional heavy resistance training modes provide the most potent means to elicit mechanical and morphological adaptation that are the prerequisites for optimal development of strength and power. As such, exercise selection during the general strength development phase will feature conventional 'powerlifting' training modes, for example barbell squat and deadlift. However, alternative training modes that demand greater co-ordination and provide additional development of postural strength will also have a role during this phase. For example, the front racked variation of the barbell squat exercise is shown to elicit comparable levels of muscle recruitment to the conventional back squat, with lesser compressive loads, which may be important for those players with a history of lower limb injury (Gullet *et al.* 2009).

The front squat also has apparent benefits in terms of developing sound technique: essentially it is very difficult to perform this lift without maintaining proper technique simply due to the constraints of the exercise. Specifically, the fact that the barbell rests on the front of the shoulders means that in order to execute this lift the athlete must control their posture and maintain form through the full range of motion, otherwise they risk losing the bar. Equally, once sound technique has been developed, the conventional back squat should not be neglected during this phase, as it allows greater loads to be handled and has proven efficacy in terms of developing strength (Wilson *et al.* 1996).

In addition to bilateral heavy training modes, exercise selection should also comprise unilateral heavy resistance training modes. Issues of dynamic correspondence remain a consideration even during the general development stage, which favours the use of training modes that feature a unilateral base of support for team sports players' strength development. Crucially, a study that compared muscle activity and hormonal responses during unilateral versus bilateral strength-training modes reported that a version of a free weight resisted single-leg squat (termed a 'pitcher squat' in that study) produced similar values for muscle activation and post-exercise testosterone concentrations in trained college-level athletes (Jones *et al.* 2012). These findings support the use of unilateral barbell exercises for heavy resistance training.

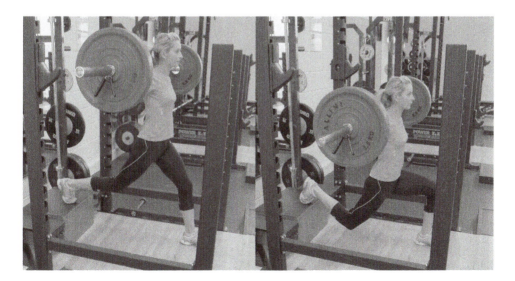

Figure 5.1 Barbell single-leg squat

One unilateral strength training mode that would appear to have a particularly important role in the strength training of team sports players is the barbell step up exercise. This training mode has been identified as eliciting marked activation of the hip musculature during both concentric and eccentric phases of the exercise (Simenz *et al.* 2012). For example, the levels of activation of gluteus maximus during a 6-RM step up onto an 18-inch (45.75cm) box are considerable during both eccentric and concentric phases, and markedly greater than the values reported for the squat exercise. From a biomechanical viewpoint, this exercise also represents a closed kinetic chain movement that comprises simultaneous hip and knee extension executed from a unilateral base of support, which is reflective of jumping and locomotion movements that feature during competition.

Transition strength training modes

Often there is a dichotomy in the training modes employed with athletes: general or 'nonspecific' heavy resistance training modes are often combined or immediately followed with highly specific training modes and 'functional training' practices. In order to achieve a coherent and stepwise progression in terms of exercise selection, there is a clear need to consider the intermediate training modes that exist between these two extremes of the specificity continuum. It follows that 'transition' strength training modes should therefore be implemented during the training blocks that follow the general preparation phase and precede the highly specific training employed during the middle and latter stages of the playing season. This approach is analogous to the *specialised preparatory* and *specialised developmental* cycles described in the staged model described by Bondarchuk (2007).

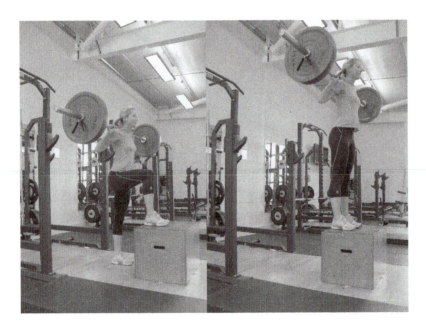

Figure 5.2 Barbell step up

The transition training modes implemented to fill this void will essentially be variations and progressions of conventional strength training modes. There will be an increasing emphasis on specificity and dynamic correspondence with respect to the exercise modes employed in each successive training block. From this viewpoint, there will be an increased emphasis on unilateral modes for lower limb strength training. Likewise, exercise selection should feature a progression in terms of the neuromuscular co-ordination and postural stability challenge imposed. To this end, front racked variations of barbell resisted unilateral support strength-training exercises might be considered, in a similar way as described in the previous section with the bilateral barbell squat exercise.

Another key factor with respect to exercise selection will be the direction of force application. Whereas the bilateral and unilateral lower limb strength-training modes featured in the general strength development block comprised the application of vertical ground reaction forces, exercise selection during this phase should also account for the horizontal ground reaction forces that are a feature of locomotion activities. Similarly, there will necessarily be a shift from predominantly sagittal plane movements to training modes that feature movements in a variety of directions. For example lateral, diagonal and crossover variations of the lunge and step up exercise have been described in the literature. An investigation of the loaded step up exercise performed on an 18-inch (45.75cm) box that employed lateral, diagonal, and cross-over versions of this exercise reported that the respective variations produced different levels of activation of the hip muscles studied, which included gluteus maximus and medius, biceps femoris and semitendinosis, and rectus femoris, vastus medius and vastus lateralis (Simenz *et al.* 2012). Each of these variations and progressions would appear to merit consideration during this phase.

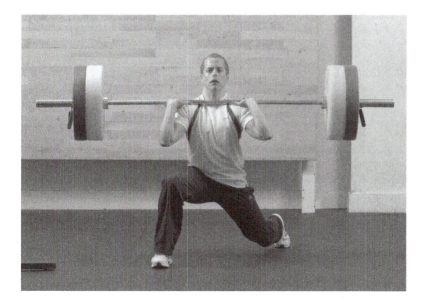

Figure 5.3 Front racked barbell diagonal lunge

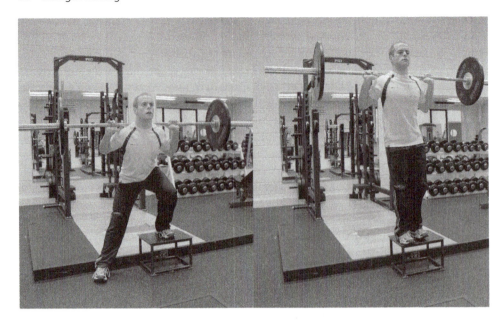

Figure 5.4 Barbell lateral step up

Exercise selection for upper limb strength development during this phase will similarly feature variations of conventional strength training modes. For example, alternate arm variations of standard upper-body strength training exercises with dumbbells provide a strength training stimulus that is combined with a stabilisation challenge for the lumbopelvic region and shoulder girdle. It has previously been reported that single limb versions of resisted upper limb strength training exercises with dumbbells (Behm *et al.* 2005) and cable resistance (Tarnanen *et al.* 2012) elicit significant activation of various stabiliser muscles of the trunk.

'Transfer' strength training

As implied, exercise selection during this phase places the greatest emphasis on dynamic correspondence. Hence there will be a further progression in terms of the specificity continuum, and the training modes selected will favour the greatest immediate transfer to movements in the sport. Accordingly, the strength training exercises employed in this phase will be the most challenging in terms of co-ordination and stabilisation demands. The versions of conventional lower limb strength training modes that feature will thus comprise the most challenging overhead variations (Figure 5.6), and exercises involving movements in multiple directions (Figure 5.7).

Similarly, strength training modes for the upper limbs will feature exercises performed in a weight-bearing stance. Single-arm variations of resisted upper limb movements in various directions will likewise feature. As such, upper limb strength training modes selected will recruit muscles of the upper and lower limbs, as well as comprising considerable activation of the trunk musculature to resist destabilising torques and maintain 'postural integrity' (Fenwick *et al.* 2009; Santana *et al.* 2007).

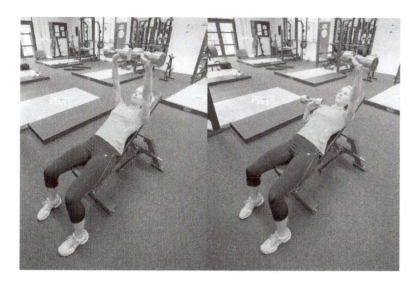

Figure 5.5 Alternate arm incline dumbbell bench press

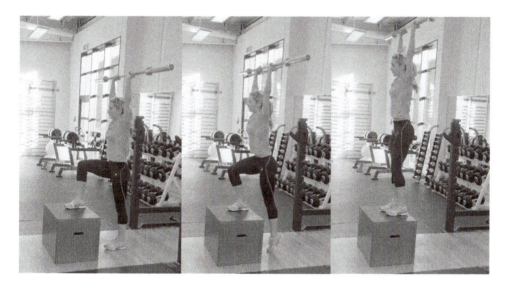

Figure 5.6 Barbell overhead step up

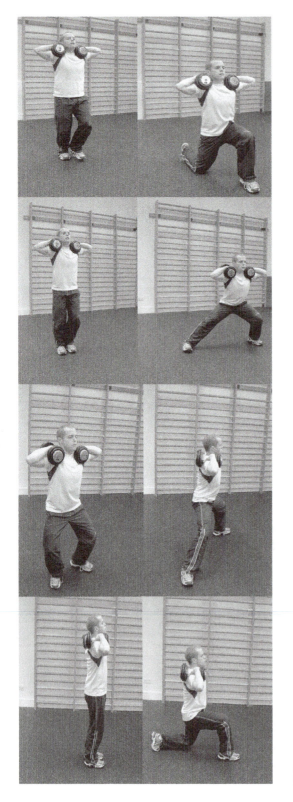

Figure 5.7
Dumbbell clockwork lunge

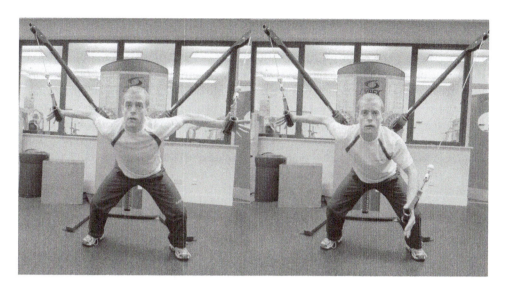

Figure 5.8 Alternate arm cable fly

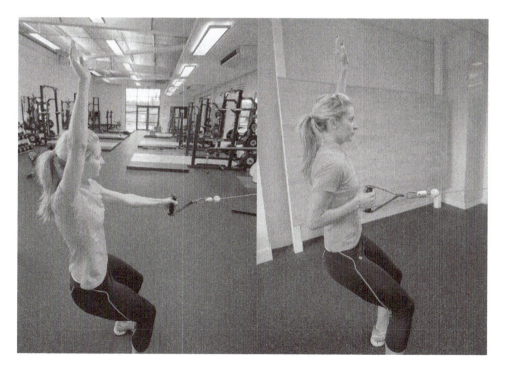

Figure 5.9 Single-arm cable row

Conclusions and training recommendations

Given the time constraints imposed by extended playing seasons and high volumes of concurrent training and team practices common to all team sports at elite level, the efficiency and effectiveness of physical preparation is paramount (Peterson *et al.* 2004). One of the key criteria when evaluating a strength training programme for a team sports player is the degree of improvement in the player's capacity to perform and remain fit to participate in matches and team practices versus the training time invested (Young 2006). This need to optimise any strength training performed is particularly important given the potential for interference effects from concurrent metabolic conditioning (Leveritt and Abernethy 1999) – and in the case of contact sports particularly, the disruption due to the physical stresses of bodily contact during practices and matches (Hoffman and Kang 2003). Such complications place even greater emphasis upon the effectiveness and efficiency of strength training for team sports players.

In this chapter a neuromuscular emphasis has been described for approaching strength training for team sports. Whatever the sport or training history of the player, the initial programme goal suggested is addressing any deficits in mobility and stability that have been identified that impair the player's ability to effectively perform fundamental athletic movements. Once this foundation is established, exercise selection should progress towards integrated multi-joint movements, which are specific to movements that are characteristic of the sport (Baechle *et al.* 2000; Stone *et al.* 2000a). Accounting for specificity in this way will benefit gross motor activation or intramuscular co-ordination as well as enhancing inter-muscular co-ordination and local neural control at in a way that facilitates transfer to performance (Sheppard 2003; Young 2006).

Progression of exercise selection within the strength training macrocycle might feature a gradual introduction of unilateral support lifts, as well as alternating upper limb and single limb variations of strength training exercises – in order to increase balance, stabilisation and neuromuscular control demands. Similarly, speed-strength and plyometric exercises that involve similar progressions can be introduced into players' preparation, particularly as they approach key phases in the playing season. In this way, acceleration can be manipulated as a way of progressing intensity in the players' programme. From a specificity viewpoint, it follows that these speed-strength exercises should also be executed in a manner that corresponds to the rate of force development associated with competition (Sheppard 2003) and features inter-muscular co-ordination demands appropriate to the sport (Young 2006).

In terms of the format of strength training for team sports players, strength and conditioning specialists might consider experimenting with the structure of the workout. Manipulations to the traditional set configuration for Olympic lifts (adopting short rest intervals between consecutive repetitions) have proven to reduce impairments in lifting kinematics in successive repetitions in a set, by reducing residual fatigue (Haff *et al.* 2003). It is possible that the circuit format may allow similar enhanced lifting kinematics by offsetting fatigue between consecutive sets of a particular exercise. There is also early evidence that such an approach might increase cardiovascular responses (Alcaraz *et al.* 2008) and confer similar benefits in terms of strength-endurance (Kraemer 1997), as well as reducing the time required to complete the workout.

In general the strength and conditioning specialist should adopt a neuromuscular training emphasis with respect to maintaining the focus on the quality of movement during strength training rather than solely load lifted. Such a neuromuscular skill-focused approach would appear to make sense given that it is commonly motor control rather than gross measures of strength or power that distinguishes the best athletes from their peers (McGill 2006d); and this is the case particularly in team sports. In this sense, rather than coaching by numbers and focusing on improving loads lifted, the players should be instilled with the principle that if they are unable to lift a given load with perfect form then they cannot lift it. In keeping with this approach, measures to facilitate maintaining posture and form, and offset the effects of acute fatigue, should be considered – for example breaking a set up into smaller chunks (particularly during the initial stages after load has been increased). This is analogous to the use of cluster sets – a practice employed by Olympic weightlifters and which has been suggested to have applications for other athletes (Haff *et al.* 2003, 2008).

6

TRAINING FOR POWER

Introduction

Expression of power is determined by the constraints of the task and phenomena characteristic of the neuromuscular system, such as the force–velocity curve and muscle length–tension relationship (Cormie *et al.* 2011a). Several discrete aspects of the neuromuscular system that influence power output have been isolated (Newton and Kraemer 1994; Newton and Dugan 2002). These individual neuromuscular components involved in expression of explosive power can be considered trainable; developing each of these components either in isolation or in combination can favourably impact upon expression of power (Newton and Kraemer 1994). Developing each of these neuromuscular factors that contribute to explosive power expression in turn requires an appropriate training stimulus specific to the respective component.

Training specificity is evident when training to develop 'explosive power' or speed-strength. It has been identified that the neuromuscular firing patterns observed during strength-oriented and explosive movements are grossly different (Ives and Shelley 2003). Neuromuscular firing patterns and intra-muscular co-ordination demands are accordingly key factors which differentiate training methods which are effective for developing explosive power from other forms of strength training (Young 2006).

Speed-strength training comprises a special category of training modes that fulfil the requisite conditions to develop explosive power production. Speed-strength training modes have a demonstrated capacity to impact specifically upon explosive performance (for example, jump-and-reach height) independently of any changes in other strength properties such as maximum strength (Newton *et al.* 1999; Winchester *et al.* 2008).

Aside from considerations regarding neuromuscular firing patterns and intra-muscular co-ordination, in much the same way as strength training exercises, transfer of speed-strength training methods to sports performance is also determined by the dynamic correspondence of the training mode to the sports movement. Speed-strength training therefore must likewise satisfy kinetic, kinematic and biomechanical criteria related to the athletic or sport skill movement in order to be most effective.

Approaching training for power or 'speed-strength'

There have historically been differing schools of thought regarding the best training approach for developing explosive muscular power. It has been suggested by some that it is sufficient to solely develop force-development capabilities (that is, strength) and then transfer the gains in strength by subsequent practice with the particular athletic activity (Kraemer 1997). Such an approach essentially accounts for the force element in the force × velocity equation for power. However, explosive power is a learned motor skill of the neuromuscular system and is identified as a capacity that is distinct from maximal force production (Ives and Shelley 2003). Although maximal power output is dependent upon strength to a varying extent depending on the resistance involved (Stone *et al.* 2003a), expression of sport-specific power has elements that are independent of the basic force-generating capacity of the musculature. This is illustrated by the dissociation of maximum (1-RM) strength and explosive power scores in elite athletes (McBride *et al.* 1999; Delecluse *et al.* 1995).

The efficacy of specific training to develop power is demonstrated by the observed improvements in measures of explosive power performance with short-term speed-strength training interventions in the absence of any maximal strength gains (Newton *et al.* 1999; Winchester *et al.* 2008). Likewise, Olympic lifts have been found to increase concentric power (squat jump height) in elite strength athletes (champion weightlifters) (Hakkinen *et al.* 1987). This is similarly significant, as traditional heavy resistance training modes are relatively ineffective in developing lower-body power (vertical jump height) in trained power athletes, despite significant concurrent gains in 1-RM strength (Baker 1996).

Such considerations led to the genesis of a multidimensional construct for explosive muscular power. Several discrete elements of the neuromuscular system have been isolated, all of which influence power output (Newton and Kraemer 1994; Newton and Dugan 2002). Each of these individual components of the neuromuscular system that contribute to expression of power can be considered trainable. 'Mixed methods' training strategies propose employing a range of training modalities to specifically train each neuromuscular capacity implicated in the expression of explosive power (Newton and Kraemer 1994). These factors, targeted via appropriate training, have the potential to individually contribute to the development of explosive power capabilities. Developing these components in combination can further have a cumulative impact upon the athlete's ability to develop explosive power.

Evidence as to the efficacy of mixed methods training is seen by the superior results elicited by combination training in comparison to either high-force or high power training (Harris *et al.* 2000). Greater gains are reported with strength-trained team sports players (collegiate American football players) on a wider range of performance measures following a combination of both high-force and high-velocity 'power' training. Performed individually, high-force training effects are limited to gains in maximal strength (1-RM) and heavy load speed-strength (hang pull 1-RM) measures, with no impact on dynamic athletic measures. Conversely, the high-velocity 'power' training resulted in gains in dynamic measures, with no change in heavy load capabilities (Harris *et al.* 2000). Interestingly, combination training not only yielded the benefits associated with both single training modes, but also produced gains on measures (10-yard shuttle agility run and average vertical jump power) not seen with either high-force or high-velocity training alone (Harris *et al.* 2000). Adaptation to high-force or high-velocity training performed in isolation by strength-trained athletes are restricted to the region of the force–velocity curve that characterised the training. Furthermore, combined methods are observed to be most effective in developing vertical jump height (the standard measure of lower-body power production) (Baker 1996). Superior performance effects on a broader spectrum of the force–velocity curve with combined training were attributed to exploiting different avenues of explosive performance development simultaneously (Harris *et al.* 2000).

Factors in the expression of explosive muscular power

The individual elements that have been implicated in the expression of explosive muscular power will be discussed in turn.

Maximum dynamic strength

In accordance with the force–velocity curve, maximum strength is developed at slow movement velocity. This strength quality is nevertheless required at the initiation of any explosive movement to overcome inertia when system velocity is zero or slow (Stone 1993). Maximum strength therefore has a major influence on the initial rate at which force is developed early in the movement (Stone *et al.* 2003a). For locomotion and jumping movements in particular, even in the absence of external resistance, there is a significant inertia component due to the athlete's own body mass. This inertia component is particularly significant if there is any change of direction involved, as the athlete's own momentum in the original direction of movement must first be halted and overcome in order to generate movement in a new direction.

Accordingly, maximum strength relative to body mass is a key element in expression of power for gross motor actions involved in a variety of athletic movements (Peterson *et al.* 2006). High correlations are observed between 1-RM strength and power output even for unloaded jumps. Furthermore, slow velocity strength development influences the mechanical power output a player is able to generate in higher resistance regions of the load/power curve (Stone *et al.* 2003a). For players in contact sports in particular, the ability to generate power against external resistance is an important factor, which similarly relies heavily upon high levels of force output and therefore maximum strength.

Rate of force development

Rate of force development (RFD) describes the ability to develop force within a limited timeframe. This component represents the slope of the force–time curve for a muscular action (Newton and Dugan 2002). The time interval for force development in many athletic movements is very brief – typically within 300ms (Newton and Kraemer 1994). On this basis some authors identify RFD as possibly the most important capacity influencing athletic performance (Wilson *et al.* 1995). Accordingly, RFD is associated with the ability to achieve rapid acceleration for a given movement (Stone 1993).

Rate coding is identified as a major factor influencing RFD; specifically the maximal firing rates of motor units within the window for force development allowed by the movement (Behm 1995). Motor unit recruitment is another critical factor: the ability rapidly to recruit high-threshold motor units associated with the highest force-generating capacity and power output is directly related to maximal power development. For rapid contractions that occur during ballistic activities, the threshold of motor unit activation is relatively lower than for slow graded contractions (Cormie *et al.* 2011a). It follows that training modes which feature ballistic contractions will be favourable for developing this capacity.

It also follows that the duration of the concentric portion of the training exercise must be similarly brief to train the neuromuscular system to develop maximal force across the shorter timeframes permitted by rapid athletic and sports skill movements. In support of this it is reported that the closer the time interval of a given strength measure to the contact time observed for athletic movements, the greater the correlation to performance (Young et al. 1995). Similarly, on this basis traditional heavy strength training would appear to be suboptimal for developing this RFD component. For example, a heavy barbell squat can take around 1.5–2 seconds to complete (Baker 2001b). Conversely, motor unit firing rates are appreciably higher during the short window for force development associated with maximal ballistic concentric actions (Hedrick 1993; Behm 1995). Under certain conditions improvements in isometric RFD have been noted following isometric training in non-athlete subjects (Behm and Sale 1993); however, the relevance to athletic performance of both isometric training (Morrissey et al. 1995) and isometric measures of RFD (Wilson et al. 1995) has been questioned.

High-velocity strength

High-velocity strength represents the ability to exert force at high contraction velocities. Increasing maximum strength at slow movement velocity is of limited relevance if the athlete is unable to express this greater force-generating capacity at the movement velocities encountered during athletic and sports skill movements (Hedrick 1993). This ability is in part determined by anatomical and mechanical factors associated with muscle fascicle length. In particular, more sarcomeres in series will serve to share the overall muscle fibre shortening between a greater number of subunits, so that the rate of shortening at the level of the individual sarcomere will be less for a longer muscle fascicle (Cormie et al. 2011a). In turn, this reduced shortening velocity at sarcomere level will allow more force to be developed. Muscle fascicle length is determined to a large degree by genetic factors. However, there may be scope for chronic adaptive responses to training that may include increases in muscle fascicle length and/or the addition of more sarcomeres in series (Cormie et al. 2011a).

The neural basis for improvements in force development at higher velocity regions of the force–velocity curve include adaptations relating to the capacity of motor units to fire rapidly for short intervals (Hedrick 1993) and may also include the preferential recruitment of high-threshold motor units (Stone 1993; Cronin et al. 2001a). Such adaptations in intra-muscular co-ordination appear to result in specific improvements at the higher movement velocity region of the force–velocity curve (Stone 1993). Improvements in high-velocity strength may also include changes at the level of the muscle fibre. Adaptations in the contractile properties of muscle fibres that lead to increased maximal shortening velocity and peak power have been shown to be elicited by appropriate training (Malisoux et al. 2006).

Stretch-shortening cycle capabilities

The majority of movements in sport involve some kind of pre-stretch or countermovement which serves to increase force and power output for the concentric portion of the movement (Cormie et al. 2011a). This increase in power output originates from the interaction between muscle and tendon structures during the transition between eccentric and concentric action, referred to as the *stretch-shortening cycle*. The stretch-shortening cycle (SSC) comprises not only mechanical aspects associated with the contractile (muscle) and connective tissue structures, but also neural aspects including reflexes at local spinal level.

Authors increasingly distinguish between 'fast SSC' (100–200ms) and 'slow SSC' (300–500ms) movements based upon the duration of ground contact or force application. Changes in SSC performance are found to be relatively independent of maximal muscle strength in highly trained athletes (Plisk 2000). The contribution of SSC to concentric power output in part depends on the capacity of the musculoskeletal complex to store and use elastic tension (Yessis 1994; Newton *et al.* 1997). As such, mechanical adaptations that alter the compliance of these structures may contribute to improved concentric power output (Cormie *et al.* 2011a).

In addition to mechanical adaptations that alter the passive properties of connective tissue structures, changes in active stiffness are also apparent following exposure to SSC movements due to changes in muscle activation which modify the interaction between muscle and tendon during these activities. In the case of bounding movements, the 'fast SSC' contribution to concentric power output can also be modified via changes in neural input in the interval prior to and during ground contact. Such modification in descending neural input to the muscles from higher motor centres is responsible in part for the improvement in fast-SSC performance following appropriate training (such as plyometrics).

Another component of the underlying neural mechanisms that may contribute to augmenting concentric power output immediately following pre-stretch is associated with the 'stretch reflex'. This is a peripheral reflex at local spinal level that acts to stimulate the stretched muscle to contract, in an attempt to return the muscle to its previous length (Potach and Chu 2000). This stretch reflex-mediated neural drive is superimposed upon voluntary drive to the agonist muscles, which leads to augmentation of power output in the subsequent concentric phase (Newton *et al.* 1997).

Neuromuscular skill and co-ordination

The final component of explosive power is neuromuscular skill. In much the same way as sport-specific strength, a player's effectiveness is limited to the extent that they are able to express the elements of explosive power described above during the execution of game-related activities and sport skills at the decisive time in match situations (Smith 2003). This encompasses both inter-muscular and intra-muscular co-ordination (Newton and Kraemer 1994).

Broadly, intra-muscular co-ordination comprises the recruitment and firing of motor units of muscle groups involved in the movement. Intra-muscular co-ordination thus encompasses descending neural drive from the motor cortex and excitatory and inhibitory inputs originating from local spinal level (Cronin *et al.* 2001b). Increasing motor unit recruitment, descending neural drive and net excitatory input to the motor units involved in an athletic or sports skill movement will have a favourable effect on force and power output. The constraints of the task will largely dictate what is required in terms of intra-muscular co-ordination. For example, a key aspect of intra-muscular co-ordination in the context of power expression is the ability to develop force within the time window allowed by the athletic or sports skill movement (Cormie *et al.* 2011a).

Inter-muscular co-ordination concerns the co-ordinated action of muscles that are involved in producing athletic or sports skill movements (Young 2006). The interaction between agonist, synergist and antagonist muscle groups employed during a particular movement is highly complex and entails both the magnitude and timing of activation (Cormie *et al.* 2011a). Increasing force or power output of a single muscle group in isolation could conceivably impair athletic performance if the increased single muscle function is not achieved in co-ordination with other muscle groups acting on the kinetic chain of joints involved in a movement. Inter-muscular co-ordination therefore comprises both the timing of activation and also relaxation of muscles involved in producing movement in order to allow fluid and rapid motion (Cormie *et al.* 2011a). For example, one important adaptation in inter-muscular co-ordination is reduced co-contraction of agonist and antagonist muscle groups, which allows for greater angular velocity and torque development (Newton and Kraemer 1994).

Inter-muscular co-ordination is a critical factor for the relatively 'gross' motor skills involved in athletic movements. In the case of fine motor skills involved with sports skill movements, such as throwing and striking, the ability to co-ordinate motion between joints and limbs of the kinetic chain involved in the activity assumes even greater importance with respect to movement velocity and power output. For example, the one-handed overarm throwing skill that features in sports such as baseball, cricket and netball is described in terms of multiple linked segments operating in series, comprising lower limbs, pelvis, trunk, shoulder and upper limb, with motion ultimately translated to the finger tips and imparted upon the ball. The degree and relative timing of the sequential motion of these segments is identified as critical to torque generation and efficient throwing mechanics (Aguinaldo *et al.* 2007).

Inter-muscular co-ordination does not only concern the limbs generating force and producing the movement. A characteristic double peak pattern associated with activation of the trunk musculature is observed during striking and kicking movements (McGill *et al.* 2010). The contract-relax-contract sequence includes a preparatory pulse to stiffen the core to provide a strong base from which to accelerate the limbs to initiate the striking action, followed by a relaxation phase to allow fluid and rapid whole-body motion, prior to a second 'pulse' timed to stiffen the body again as the limb strikes the target. It follows that adaptations in inter-muscular co-ordination will be closely related and highly specific to the particular movement(s) featured in training (Young 2006).

Speed-strength training modes for development of explosive muscular power

Conventional strength training provides a means to develop maximum strength and provide the requisite foundation development that will ultimately confer the ability to express explosive muscular power with the aid of subsequent specific training. Strength training therefore serves a critical role in the long-term development of power capabilities. Without this baseline development of force-generating capacities, as well as the morphological and neural adaptations that are produced by heavy resistance training, the athlete will not be able to generate high levels of muscular power. Athletes therefore require optimal levels of strength – developed via appropriate heavy resistance training – as a precursor to training to specifically develop power. The specific approach that may be taken to strength training has been covered in a previous chapter. In support of this, there is evidence that improvements in power output following *speed-strength* training (ballistic resistance training) are greater in stronger subjects (Cormie *et al.* 2010a). That said, it should be noted that the 'weaker' subjects in this training study did also respond positively to the speed-strength training intervention.

Following this initial foundation development there remains a need for specific speed-strength training in order to develop the specific ability to express explosive muscular power. Accordingly, the addition of speed-strength training has been shown to produce gains beyond those elicited by heavy resistance training alone (Newton *et al.* 1999; Baker 1996; Delecluse *et al.* 1995). Speed-strength training modes have been identified as the optimal means to develop a number of the qualities identified that underpin explosive power expression. As implied by their title, speed-strength exercises combine both high force (the product of mass and acceleration) and high velocity (Hydock 2001). Speed-strength exercises are characterised by maximal rates of force development (Hedrick 1993) throughout the movement range of motion (Stone 1993). These power development-oriented exercises have thus been termed 'full acceleration' exercises by some authors (Baker 2003).

Potential adaptations to speed-strength training include improvements in contractile elements – such as increased maximum shortening velocity and power output of muscle fibres (Malisoux *et al.* 2006). Speed-strength training is also associated with preferential hypertrophy of high-threshold type II muscle fibres (Stone 1993). Intent is key to the neural adaptations associated with speed-strength training (Behm and Sale 1993). Due to their explosive nature, speed-strength exercises are more suited to evoke explosive intent. In the case of conventional strength training lifts such as the bench press, aside from mechanical considerations, athletes also must be coached to make a conscious effort to lift with explosive intent to optimise training responses on explosive power scores (Jones *et al.* 1999). Velocity gains following training are reportedly reduced by half when subjects are left to self-select lifting speed (Jones *et al.* 1999).

Olympic weightlifting training modes

Olympic lifts are classified as speed-strength exercises (Stone 1993), on the basis that they feature both a force (strength) and speed component (Hydock 2001). These lifts are unique in that the resistance is accelerated up the natural line of the body and gravity acts to decelerate the load, which means the neuromuscular system does not have to intervene to brake the motion of the barbell (Kraemer 1997). Elevating the athlete's own centre of mass represents a significant component of the work done when performing Olympic lifts (Garhammer 1993). In contrast to ballistic resistance training modes in which the load is released at the end of the movement, with Olympic weightlifting movements the external load (typically a barbell) is held throughout: in the event that the barbell is still travelling upwards at the termination of the concentric phase, the lifter's feet merely come off the floor.

Applications

Average mechanical power output values reported for the Olympic lifts are 3,000W for the barbell snatch and 2,950W for the clean, which are nearly three times greater than for back squat or deadlift (approximately 1,100W) (Stone 1993; Garhammer 1993). Peak power output recorded during the 'second pull' phase can be five times greater (5,500W) (Stone 1993). Peak propulsion forces for these lifts are similarly comparable to those during jumping movements (Stone 1993).

The unique nature of Olympic lifts allows heavy loads to be handled in an explosive fashion (McBride *et al.* 1999). This enables high-force 'speed-strength' and rate of force development (RFD) elements to be developed simultaneously. Olympic weightlifters exhibit equivalent strength scores and superior dynamic power scores to powerlifters, which reflects the combination of heavy loads and high velocity of movement featured in Olympic lift training (McBride *et al.* 1999). That said, Olympic weightlifters do also perform classic strength-oriented lifts in their training, which contributes to their strength development. Olympic lifters are reported to generate greater velocity and power than powerlifters when performing countermovement jumps with or without added loading (McBride *et al.* 1999).

Similarly, Olympic lifters exhibit superior strength (1-RM squat) in comparison to sprinters (McBride *et al.* 1999). From these data it could be inferred that Olympic lift training is similarly effective to sprint training and more effective than powerlifting training in developing dynamic power, and more effective than sprint training in developing maximal strength. Similarly, of particular relevance to contact team sports is the observation that Olympic lifters perform better than sprinters in dynamic movements against resistance (McBride *et al.* 1999). The superior performance exhibited by Olympic lifters in this capacity suggests that the heavy load speed-strength training provided by Olympic lifting has the potential to develop this ability to generate power against resistance. Such observations point to the potential benefits of heavy load speed-strength training, and specifically the use of Olympic lifts for rugby football and other contact sports. However, controlled prospective studies are required to draw definitive conclusions.

The kinetic and kinematic specificity of Olympic lifts with regard to the vertical jump movement are suggested to develop speed-strength in a way that transfers more readily to jumping performance (Baker 1996). A study of semi-professional rugby league football players also reported that players' scores on hang power clean relative to body mass discriminated between those who showed superior performance on vertical jump and 20m sprint, as well as speed-strength measures with a loaded jump squat (Hori *et al.* 2008). A previous study with similar subjects reported hang power clean scores relative to body mass to be significant predictors of acceleration (10m) and short distance (40m) sprint scores in rugby league players (Baker and Nance 1999b). In accordance with this a study using non-athlete subjects reported that short-term (8 weeks) training using Olympic lifts in combination with heavy resistance training improved both squat jump and countermovement jump, and 10m sprint scores – although 30m performance was unchanged (Tricoli *et al.* 2005).

The relative load used is shown to influence the power output with which a lift is executed. Taking the hang power clean as an example, peak and average power output varied with loads from 50 per cent to 90 per cent of subjects' recorded 1-RM for the hang power clean (Kawamori *et al.* 2005). One characteristic that makes Olympic weightlifting movements unique is that the relative loading at which mechanical power is optimised is relatively higher than for other strength and speed-strength training exercises, including ballistic resistance training modes. This may be favourable from the viewpoint

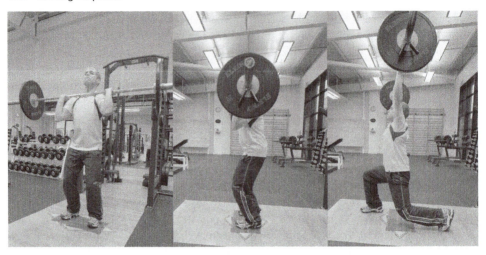

Figure 6.1 Barbell split jerk

of activating high-threshold motor units, in accordance with the size principle of motor unit recruitment (Cormie *et al.* 2011b). Peak and average power output were reported to be maximised at the 70 per cent 1-RM load for the hang power clean, albeit peak power output values did not vary dramatically across a range of loads in this study (Kawamori *et al.* 2005). A more recent study that measured peak power for both the barbell and athlete's body mass identified that peak power for the body + barbell 'system' is maximised at 80 per cent of squat 1-RM for the power clean (McBride *et al.* 2011).

Selection of training loads will also depend in part upon the team sport in question. For example, relatively lighter loads may be appropriate for sports such as volleyball and basketball. Conversely, relatively higher loading towards the 90 per cent 1-RM value might be preferred for collision sports, such as rugby football and American football, given the need to overcome external resistance provided by opposing players in these sports (Cormie *et al.* 2011b). In either case, a range of loads may be used during the course of periodised strength and speed-strength-oriented training cycles.

Olympic lifts combine strength, power and neuromuscular co-ordination elements in a way that favours transfer to athletic activities, such as vertical jump performance (Kraemer *et al.* 2002). Peak propulsion forces relative to body mass generated during the power clean lift are shown to be similar to those exerted during jumping movements (Stone 1993). Likewise, Olympic lifting movements involve a comparable time interval for force production, typically between 100–200 milliseconds for the second pull phase (Garhammer 1993). On the basis of their biomechanical similarity and comparable timeframes for concentric force production, Olympic lifts are routinely used in athletes' physical preparation as a means to replicate sport-specific movements (Souza *et al.* 2002).

Mechanisms

The majority of the Olympic weightlifting exercises feature predominantly concentric force and power production. During rapid concentric actions such as those occurring during Olympic weightlifting movements, the muscle shortens throughout the concentric phase, so that the majority of the shortening of the musculo-tendinous unit occurs at the muscle fascicle rather than the tendon (Kawakami *et al.* 2002). Underlying mechanisms for the gains in concentric power output are generally ascribed to improvements in rate of force development (RFD) and high-velocity strength (Stone 1993; Garhammer 1993; McBride *et al.* 1999; Souza 2002). Increased peak RFD has been reported with concurrent gains in Olympic lift (snatch) 1-RM and performance test (shot put distance) scores (Stone *et al.* 2003b). Both inter-muscular and intra-muscular co-ordination elements are implicated in the training responses observed (Newton and Kraemer 1994; Hedrick 1993). Potential adaptations in inter-muscular co-ordination include improved recruitment of high-threshold (high-force) motor units, enhanced co-ordination of synergist muscle activation and reduced co-contraction of antagonist muscles.

Developments in intra-muscular co-ordination are manifested in both recruitment of high-threshold motor units and enhanced capability of individual motor units to fire rapidly for short intervals (Hedrick 1993). Other aspects of adaptation in intra-muscular co-ordination are neuromuscular learning effects associated with rapid muscular contractions (Morrissey *et al.* 1995). Such learned 'neural strategies' include over-riding inhibitory input and an anticipatory priming of agonist motor units during the interval immediately prior to initiating the movement (Baker *et al.* 2001d).

Limitations

Most Olympic lifts – particularly the pulling lifts – develop concentric power output (Hakkinen *et al.* 1987), as opposed to stretch-shortening cycle (SCC) components. Observations of a year's weightlifting training in elite weightlifters registered significant improvements in unloaded and loaded squat jump height in the absence of any significant change in countermovement jump height (indicative of 'slow SSC' performance) with equivalent loads (Hakkinen *et al.* 1987). Similarly, these athletes also exhibit very small differences between squat jump and countermovement jump scores, indicating limited SSC augmentation of jumping performance (Baker 1996).

Although Olympic weightlifting training is consistently shown to improve vertical jump performance, there is some uncertainty as to whether bilateral speed-strength training of this type will transfer to sprinting performance (Young 2006). A number of studies have failed to show improvements in sprint scores even when improvements in jump height and performance on other tests were seen (Harris *et al.* 2000). A training study with collegiate football players that included derivatives of the Olympic lifts (mid-thigh pull and push press) failed to show improvements in 30-metre sprint scores – although improvements in jump height and performance on a stair climb power test were seen (Harris *et al.* 2000). A more recent study, also examining collegiate football players, compared Olympic lift training to powerlifting training and likewise showed no changes in 40-yard sprint or T-test change of direction performance in either group (Hoffman *et al.* 2004).

Change of direction performance also appears to be both independent of hang power clean test scores (Hori *et al.* 2008) and similarly unresponsive to training involving standard weightlifting movements (Hoffman *et al.* 2004; Tricoli *et al.* 2005). This may be a consequence of the bilateral nature and predominantly vertical force production that is characteristic of the classical weightlifting movements. That said, single-leg and split variations of the Olympic lift movements do exist that may transfer more readily to a broader range of athletic and sports skill movements.

Limitations imposed by technique flaws in the catch phase when employing the classical Olympic lifts can potentially restrict the load players are able to handle (Hydock 2001). The pull variations of the Olympic lifts allow higher loads (≈110–120 per cent) to be handled relative to the classical clean and snatch lifts, which tend to be more limited by deficiencies in lifting technique (Hydock 2001). The clean pull variation has the same biomechanical characteristics of the power clean lift (minus the catch phase) and comprises the maximal power second pull portion of the lift (Souza *et al.* 2002). Likewise, the snatch pull also features the second pull phase, and power outputs during the second pull for the snatch and clean are found to be very similar (Garhammer 1993). Purely in terms of concentric power production, the 'catch' phases that characterise the classical Olympic snatch and clean lifts are of little consequence (Hydock 2001).

The pull variations of these lifts are a good option for introducing Olympic lifts into players' training for speed-strength development and to allow technique for the key 'second pull' phase to be developed. Furthermore, these lifts will allow relatively higher loads to be handled than would be the case for the full clean or snatch lifts, particularly for those players who are less technically proficient. For both these reasons it is suggested that the pull variations of the Olympic lifts might be the best option when the player initially moves into speed-strength-oriented training phases in their training macrocycle.

Ballistic resistance training

Ballistic resistance exercises represent one of the other major speed-strength training modalities for developing concentric power capabilities. This form of training is unique in that the load is released or projected into free space at the end of the movement. It is this characteristic that makes ballistic resistance training superior to conventional strength-training exercises in developing elements of explosive muscular power (Cronin *et al.* 2003). Specifically, ballistic resistance exercises allow power to be generated throughout the full range of motion, as there is no requirement to brake the motion of the load to bring it to a halt at the end of the movement. As the acceleration phase is not terminated before the

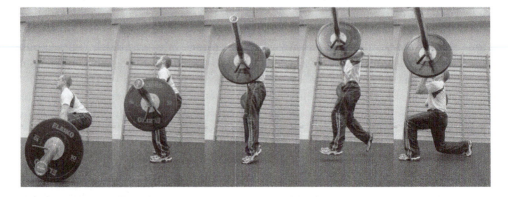

Figure 6.2 Barbell split clean

end of the range of motion (ROM) for the exercise, this in turn allows higher velocities to be produced with the result that a higher peak velocity (hence peak power) can be attained later in the movement (Newton *et al.* 1996). Accordingly, Cronin and colleagues identified projection (that is, release) of the load as the most crucial factor influencing expression of peak power (Cronin *et al.* 2003, 2001a). This is reflected in greater average and peak velocities observed with upper body movements for a range of loads (30–60 per cent 1-RM) under conditions where the load is projected into free space (Cronin *et al.* 2003).

Conventional strength training modes are unsuitable for speed-strength training. Attempting to use traditional strength training exercises in an explosive fashion (lifting the load as rapidly as possible, keeping hold of the barbell at the termination of the movement) has been shown to be counterproductive (Newton *et al.* 1996). Lifting lighter 'maximal power' loads (45 per cent 1-RM) in this manner results in a significant deceleration component, which can be up to 40 per cent of the range of motion (Newton *et al.* 1996). As a result, in the case of the bench press, beyond the initial 10 per cent of the range of motion at the initiation of the concentric movement, both force and velocity are less than the corresponding values for the ballistic bench throw at equivalent loads (Newton *et al.* 1996). This is accompanied by a loss of motor activity in agonist muscles, reflected in reduced EMG recorded for the bench press versus bench throw movement at these loads (Newton *et al.* 1996).

Antagonist co-contraction is likewise increased when explosively performing the bench press exercise, particularly with light loads (Cronin *et al.* 2001a). As a result, the training stimulus is compromised for the affected portion of the movement (Cronin *et al.* 2001a). Furthermore, efforts to lift a submaximal resistance with maximal acceleration results in the barbell gathering considerable kinetic energy, which will ultimately have to be absorbed by the muscles and joints at the end of its range of motion (Newton and Kraemer 1994). Attempting to use conventional strength training exercises in this manner therefore engenders the risk of injury.

Applications

Jump squats have been identified as an effective training modality for developing measures of lower-body explosive power (vertical jump height) in elite power athletes (Newton *et al.* 1999; Wilson *et al.* 1993; Baker 1996). Short-term (5 weeks) jump squat training was also reported to produce significant improvements in high-force speed-strength measures (power clean 1-RM) in collegiate American football players (Hoffman *et al.* 2005). Such changes in speed-strength and vertical jump performance appear to be relatively independent of changes in 1-RM strength and peak force measures or changes in muscle morphology. A recent study examining performance effects and underlying mechanisms for training adaptations with jump squat training in recreational athletes reported significant gains in peak power, rate of force development and peak velocity (Winchester *et al.* 2008). However, there were no significant changes in peak force, 1-RM squat or muscle fibre type expression accompanying these improvements in speed-strength measures.

The obvious upper-body equivalent to the jump squat is the bench throw. Accordingly, this mode of training has been shown to elicit significant upper-body power gains (Lyttle *et al.* 1996). It is suggested the greater velocity and movement pattern specificity of ballistic training is more likely to stimulate functional high-velocity adaptations (Cronin *et al.*

2003) than traditional resistance training. Accordingly, bench throw training is shown to elicit significant improvements in functional performance in elite baseball players (McEvoy and Newton 1998). A practical consideration with this ballistic training mode is that it requires costly apparatus to safely restrict the barbell to vertical-only movement and to brake the descent of the bar once it is released. One alternative is to substitute the ballistic push-up exercise; this circumvents the need for expensive specialised equipment to catch an external load as the athlete's own body mass is the load that is projected into free space. When compared to standard modified push ups (supported on the knees), ballistic modified push-up training (hands leaving the floor at the top of the movement) is reported to elicit significantly greater improvement in ballistic power, as assessed by medicine ball throw distance, and similar gains in strength (chest press 1-RM) scores in female subjects (Vossen *et al.* 2000).

Mechanisms

The majority of ballistic resistance training exercises are preceded by an eccentric action or countermovement. As such, the interaction between muscle and tendon during these training modes differs to that seen with concentric training modes such as Olympic weightlifting exercises. Specifically, the majority of the shortening during the concentric portion of the movements occurs at the tendon, with limited change observed in muscle fascicle length (Kawakami *et al.* 2002). Essentially, the muscle contracts in a quasi-isometric fashion in order to add tension to the tendon 'spring'. The significance of the eccentric action is evident in that the majority of the improvement in (concentric) power output following ballistic resistance training (jump squats) is attributed to adaptations associated with the eccentric phase (Cormie *et al.* 2010b). These adaptations may include changes in the mechanical properties of the muscle–tendon unit, as is observed following plyometric training (Foure *et al.* 2010).

Intra-muscular co-ordination aspects include improved recruitment and firing of high-threshold motor units at the high contraction velocities associated with the ballistic training movement (Stone 1993; Hedrick 1993). Maximal ballistic muscle actions involve appreci-ably higher motor unit firing rates than those observed with conventional strength training (Behm 1995; Hedrick 1993). Ballistic contractions appear to be part pre-programmed by higher motor centres in anticipation of how the ballistic action is expected to occur, with some modification of motor unit activation based upon sensory feedback during the movement (Behm 1995). It follows that repeated exposure will result in a learning effect, resulting in an enhanced ability for motor units to fire rapidly during the short interval for force development allowed by the ballistic action (Ives and Shelley 2003). In support of this, training adaptations reported following ballistic training include an increase in peak firing frequency, and this higher rate of firing also appears to be maintained throughout an extended portion of the concentric movement (Cormie *et al.* 2011a).

Inter-muscular co-ordination and antagonist co-contraction is likewise largely pre-programmed, and is believed to be a protective mechanism acting to maintain joint integ-rity in anticipation of the forces and limb accelerations during the ballistic action (Behm 1995). Fine-tuning of antagonist input with repeated exposure to the ballistic training movement may occur to reduce co-contraction to increase net concentric force output. The acceleration–deceleration profiles associated with bench throw training have been suggested to more closely resemble sporting activities (Cronin *et al.* 2003). This being the case, similar advantages in terms of improving performance via enhanced inter-muscular co-ordination may be conferred by ballistic training.

Controversy regarding maximal power 'P_{max}' training approach

It has been contended that ballistic training with 'P_{max}' loads that maximise mechanical power output is the optimal means of developing explosive muscular power (Wilson *et al.* 1993; Baker *et al.* 2001a, 2001b). These methods have proven effective in developing power output and scores for dynamic athletic performance (Wilson *et al.* 1993). However, from a methodological point of view, attempts to identify players' individual P_{max} loads often produced variable results. Values for P_{max} derived by many earlier studies appear to be affected by numerous factors including the constraints of the training activity and the relative strength and strength-training history of subjects tested (Baker 2001c; Harris *et al.* 2007).

Similarly, the practical significance of this P_{max} load has been called into question by a number of authors. In view of the multidimensional nature of explosive muscular power developed discussed earlier in the chapter, it seems counterintuitive that training a single percentage 1-RM load would be the optimal way to develop speed-strength capabilities (Cronin and Sleivert 2005). Data from elite senior team sports athletes (rugby union players) also show that power output at different loads either side of the P_{max} load value in fact differs very little for a given training movement (machine jump squats) (Harris *et al.* 2007).

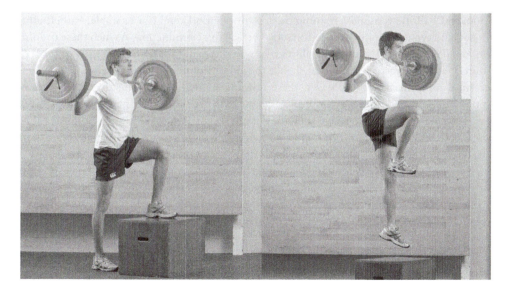

Figure 6.3 Barbell bound step up

More recent studies have highlighted flaws in the methodology and calculation methods used to derive P_{max} values (Cormie *et al.* 2007a). For instance, it has been identified that measured peak power differs for the barbell versus the athlete's own body, and peak *barbell* power values are maximised at a considerably different external load (80 per cent of squat 1-RM for the barbell jump squat) than the peak power measured for the athlete's body (0 per cent of squat 1-RM) (McBride *et al.* 2011). When calculated correctly, the actual external load that maximises mechanical power output for the body + barbell 'system' for the jump squat ballistic training exercise has been repeatedly shown to equate to zero – i.e. body mass resistance (Cormie *et al.* 2007b; Dayne *et al.* 2011; McBride *et al.* 2011).

Whatever the P_{max} load identified, employing this training approach in isolation tends to neglect the principles of specificity. Although a particular training load may be optimal for developing mechanical power output for a given movement, if the loading bears no relation to the resistances the athlete faces during competition then the degree of transfer to performance appears questionable. Training at a single relative load is similarly unlikely to elicit improvements in other regions of the force–velocity curve. Employing a variety of loads would therefore appear the best approach (Cronin and Sleivert 2005).

The contribution of the player's own body mass should be considered when selecting the external load for ballistic resistance exercises such as jump squat and ballistic push up which involve the body being projected into free space (Cronin and Sleivert 2005). Practically, there will also tend to be a trade-off between the degree of external loading used versus lifting form and the explosiveness with which the player is able to execute the movement. Qualitative assessment of posture and lifting technique as well as velocity and height achieved should therefore also be used to guide loading when players perform ballistic resistance exercises.

Limitations

Standard ballistic resistance training modes are often bilateral (for example, barbell jump squat) and typically feature predominantly vertical force production. As such these training modes develop speed-strength qualities in a way that will transfer most readily to bilateral movements in a vertical direction – hence the efficacy of jump squat training in improving vertical jump measures. However, these training modes are less effective in developing power expression during cyclic unilateral movements in a horizontal direction – such as sprinting. A 10-week study employing jump squats improved jump height measures, isokinetic knee extension scores and 6-second cycle performance without any significant improvement in 30m sprint (Wilson *et al.* 1993).

Variations of ballistic resistance training modes performed in a split stance or from a unilateral base of support could be employed, which could conceivably offer greater transfer to unilateral movements. One such example is the bound (barbell) step up exercise (Figure 6.3). Other examples include concentric only versions of training exercises commonly used for plyometrics. These exercises typically use only body weight resistance, but potentially added resistance in the form of a barbell or dumbbells could be applied. To date, very little attention has been given to such exercises in the literature – further study would be required in order to establish if these training modes might be effective and identify what degree of external resistance would be appropriate.

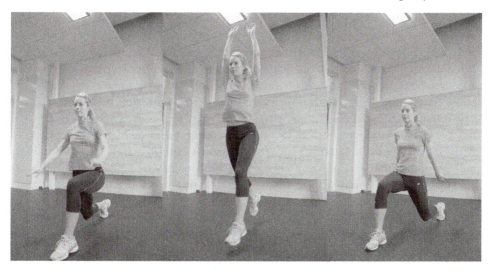

Figure 6.4 Alternate leg split bounds

Plyometric training

Applications

Plyometrics are a special class of speed-strength training exercises that emphasise the coupling of eccentric and concentric actions and the development of SSC capabilities (Matavulj *et al.* 2001). There are essentially two categories of plyometric training modes. Slow SSC plyometric exercises are characterised by a preparatory eccentric phase but are performed from a fixed base of support, for example, the countermovement jump. Fast SSC plyometric training modes essentially feature a preceding flight phase, so that the duration of ground contact is very brief. One example is the drop jump exercise; however, fast SSC plyometrics also include repeated jump movements and cyclic bounding activities.

The major benefit associated with plyometric training is developing the athlete's capacity to harness SSC augmentation of concentric power output. For example, athletes who participate in sports such as long jump and triple jump which have a significant SSC component exhibit increased lower limb active musculo-tendinous stiffness when performing SSC tasks such as hopping (Rabita *et al.* 2008). Accordingly, the addition of plyometric training to the physical preparation of trained elite junior athletes is shown to elicit significant improvements in vertical jump performance in these athletes (Matavulj *et al.* 2001). A meta-analysis of the research literature has reported that both slow SSC (countermovement jump) and fast SSC (drop jump) plyometric training modes produce significant improvement in vertical jump performance (Markovic 2007).

A similar review of the literature on the effects of plyometric training interventions on sprinting performance also reported favourable results (Saez de Villarreal *et al.* 2012). This is a particularly significant finding as other speed-strength training modes often exhibit very limited transfer to measures of running speed. This study also identified factors relating to the design of the plyometric interventions that were associated with superior training outcomes with respect to sprint performance. For example, employing different modes of plyometric training in combination, and the inclusion of plyometric exercises that feature horizontal propulsion, appears to maximise gains in speed performance (Saez de Villarreal *et al.* 2012). From a specificity viewpoint, cyclic unilateral horizontal bounding and jumping plyometric exercises (in a horizontal direction) would appear the most appropriate training modes to develop sprint capabilities (Young 2006). Bounding in particular features comparable horizontal propulsion forces, foot contact position and contact times, and muscle activation to those recorded during sprinting (Mero and Komi 1994). Accordingly, an early study that employed plyometric training which included unilateral jumping and bounding exercises in a horizontal direction reported improvements in acceleration (10m sprint time) and overall 100m sprint scores (Delecluse *et al.* 1995).

It has similarly been identified that the kinematics of the eccentric phase differ markedly for a variety of unilateral countermovement jump movements performed in different directions (Meylan *et al.* 2010). Peak velocity achieved during the eccentric phase showed a positive statistical relationship to horizontal jump distance for both forwards and lateral variations of the unilateral horizontal countermovement jump in this study, whereas no such relationship was seen for jump height achieved in the unilateral vertical countermovement jump test. The necessity for both slow and fast SSC plyometric exercises to reflect the multidirectional activities performed in the sport therefore not only concerns developing horizontal propulsion in the relevant directions, but also exposing the player to the specific eccentric actions involved in these movements in order to confer the specific neuromuscular adaptations required.

Mechanisms

The SSC training stimulus provided by plyometric training has shown to elicit improvements in shortening velocity and peak power output of single type II muscle fibres (Malisoux *et al.* 2006). Plyometric training is also associated with structural adaptations to tendon structures (Fouré *et al.* 2010). Although tendon cross-sectional area appears unchanged following a short-term plyometric intervention, qualitative changes in tendon structure have been observed. These adaptations alter the mechanical properties of the tendon, including changes to both stiffness and energy dissipation (Fouré *et al.* 2010).

In addition to such mechanical adaptations to contractile and connective tissues, the mechanisms for the improved SSC performance with repeated exposure to plyometric training are also of neural origin. Alterations in intra-muscular co-ordination include changes to descending neural input from higher motor control centres. One aspect of the neural activation response to plyometric exercise is the pre-activation of agonist muscles during preparatory and eccentric phases of both slow SSC (for example, countermovement jump) and fast SSC (for example, drop jump) movements (McBride *et al.* 2008). This pre-activation of agonist muscles increases the active stiffness of the muscle–tendon complex. Specifically, activating the muscle in the interval before touchdown means that the tendon is placed under tension prior to ground contact. An associated effect of this is that there is minimal change in muscle fascicle length during ground contact so that the majority of the change in length occurs at the tendon, which is further stretched during the eccentric phase and then rapidly shortens due to elastic recoil during the concentric phase prior to take-off. This serves to enhance the storage and return of elastic energy during eccentric and concentric phases, respectively.

Another postulated effect of this descending input is to modulate locally mediated inhibition of stretch reflex neural pathways (via Golgi tendon organ) immediately prior to and during the pre-stretch phase (Taube *et al.* 2008). Plyometric training is thus suggested to result in 'disinhibition' of stretch reflex-mediated neural drive during the countermovement, which acts to augment power output in the subsequent concentric phase (Newton and Kraemer 1994).

The described adaptations elicited by lower-body plyometric exercises are manifested in enhanced concentric power and rate of force development (RFD) of the lower limb extensor muscles (Matavulj *et al.* 2001). Plyometric training in the form of depth jumps is reported to elicit improvements in eccentric RFD with short-term progressive training at increasing drop heights (Wilson *et al.* 1996). This improvement in rate of eccentric force production is suggested to enhance storage of elastic energy in the musculo-tendinous unit, which underpins observed improvements in SSC performance in response to progressive plyometric training (Wilson *et al.* 1996).

Limitations

Despite the extensive use of plyometric training in particular for lower-body dominated athletic training, there is a lack of systematic investigation to determine the optimal load for plyometric exercises (Wilson *et al.* 1993). Standard methods for upper- and lower-body plyometric training are likewise yet to be established empirically (Vossen *et al.* 2000). In the absence of such data, body weight is typically used as resistance due to convenience; this factor may contribute to the lesser improvements in power output during concentric movements compared to other speed-strength training modes (Wilson *et al.* 1993). However, it may conversely be that it is counterproductive to add loading to plyometric movements on the basis that this may lead to a protective inhibitory effect upon neural activation – as has been noted with depth jumps when added load is applied. In support of this contention, a meta-analysis of studies relating to plyometric training and sprint performance reported that the addition of external resistance produced no further benefit (Saez de Villarreal *et al.* 2012).

Decisions regarding exercise selection and progression when designing plyometric training interventions are complicated by uncertainty regarding the efficacy of published guidelines pertaining to the relative intensity of various plyometric training modes. Recent investigations have reported that muscle activity (EMG) and ground reaction forces measured during a variety of plyometric exercises in some cases bear little resemblance to intensity guidelines published for these exercises (Ebben *et al.* 2008, Wallace *et al.* 2010). Similarly, volume guidelines are often based upon arbitrary limits for the number of 'foot contacts' during a session. In contrast a recent meta-analysis noted greater effects on sprint performance when volume per session exceeded 80 jumps (Saez de Villarreal *et al.* 2012).

Whether the augmented neural activation to agonist muscles during plyometric exercise translates into increased jump height or distance depends on the net balance between the augmented concentric energy production versus the amount of energy absorbed during the eccentric phase (McBride *et al.* 2008). For example, drop jump height may or may not be greater than countermovement jump height, depending on the reactive speed-strength and fast SSC capabilities of the player. A player's performance when undertaking high-intensity plyometric training will therefore depend upon their training history, including maximum strength capabilities and also prior exposure to eccentric loading and SSC movements. Plotting players' jump height for squat jump, countermovement jump, and drop jumps executed from a range of drop heights offers a means to profile their SSC abilities. Above a certain ideal drop height for the player there is a withdrawal of neural pre-activation, which is reflected in a steep decline in jump height achieved when this critical drop height is exceeded. This appears to be a protective response which is modifiable with training.

Drop jumps would appear to be a poor choice for improving sprinting speed, given that they are typically performed bilaterally and feature force production in a vertical direction (Young 2006). Accordingly, a 10-week training period using drop jumps produced no significant gains in 30m sprint scores despite significant improvements in countermovement jump (Wilson et al. 1993). Similarly, the interval for force production during sprinting (dictated by foot contact time) is less than half that for vertical jumping, and much shorter than that allowed by speed-strength training modes (Mero and Komi 1994). This may be a factor in the frequent failure of speed-strength training studies to produce significant effects in sprint performance over longer distances (30–40m), despite concurrent improvements in vertical power measures and acceleration (10m sprint) parameters (Wilson et al. 1993; Lyttle et al. 1996; Harris et al. 2000).

It has been noted previously that specific upper-body power training is underprescribed by strength coaches (Baker and Nance 1999a). The majority of plyometric exercises featured in training and research are typically lower-body intensive (McEvoy and Newton 1998), with training to develop SSC capabilities in upper-body movements receiving little attention in the literature (Newton et al. 1997). The few upper-body-targeted plyometric exercises that are implemented typically employ weighted medicine balls to provide resistance. The training stimulus provided by such weighted implements represents a far smaller external loading compared to the corresponding lower-body plyometric exercises. Practically, to project a medicine ball or other weighted implement heavy enough to provide the requisite external loading (46–63 per cent 1-RM) from a supine position is not feasible without the use of specialised equipment. Accordingly, drop medicine ball throws failed to produce the enhancement in rate of eccentric force development conferred by lower-body plyometric depth jump training (Wilson et al. 1996).

Variations of a ballistic push up show potential use as equivalent upper-body plyometric training modes. For example, a ballistic push up executed with countermovement might be used to develop slow SSC capabilities, whereas a drop ballistic push up initiated from raised blocks could serve as fast SSC plyometric training. The latter training mode is equivalent to the plyometric push up test described in the study by Jones and colleagues (1999).

Complex training

Applications

Complex training, or contrast loading, is a method often used in conjunction with ballistic or plyometric exercises. Contrast loading incorporates a heavier load strength-oriented exercise prior to performing a full acceleration (typically ballistic) exercise (Young et al. 1998; Baker 2003). This approach attempts to harness transient mechanical and neural effects of the preceding heavy load to augment power output when the speed-strength exercise is subsequently performed (Baker 2003). This phenomenon is termed post-activation potentiation (Chiu *et al.* 2003).

Essentially, a preceding muscle contraction has two residual effects which affect twitch contraction force in the interval that follows. One effect is fatigue; the other is post-activation potentiation (Kilduff *et al.* 2007). It is the net effect of these two opposing effects that determine the acute performance response at a given time point following the initial activity. Attempts to manipulate these transient effects therefore aim to minimise fatigue whilst harnessing potentiation effects (Kilduff *et al.* 2007).

The key aspects of optimising performance enhancement and minimising detrimental fatigue effects are the load and volume used with the preceding primer set and the rest interval employed between primer set and the target activity (Kilduff *et al.* 2007). Both isometric (Paasuke *et al.* 2007) and dynamic heavy resistance modes have been successfully employed to produce post-activation potentiation effects – typically studies have used the back squat exercise with near maximal resistance (Chiu *et al.* 2003). However, short-term performance enhancement has also been reported with an intervening set at a heavier resistance with the same ballistic exercise (jump squats) (Baker 2001d). Theoretically employing a speed-strength exercise as the preload set should be beneficial from the point of view of minimising residual fatigue effects. Studies examining rest intervals have typically employed heavy load barbell squat and bench press as the preceding resistance exercises for lower-body and upper-body movement respectively. It has been reported that recovery time in the range of 8–12 minutes appears optimal for observing performance enhancement (Kilduff *et al.* 2007). However, this may vary according to both the contraction mode featured in the preload set and the training history of the individual player (Paasuke *et al.* 2007).

Mechanisms

Tension-sensitive contractile and neural mechanisms have been identified as underlying the acute performance effects observed with contrast loading (Baker 2003, Chiu *et al.* 2003). Mechanical factors are suggested to involve transient changes in stiffness of series elastic components within the musculo-tendinous unit. One of the biochemical changes identified as underlying such contractile effects is phosphorylation of regulatory myosin light chains initiated by calcium release during the initial muscle action (Chiu *et al.* 2003). This process renders the actin–myosin complex more sensitive to further calcium release during subsequent muscle contraction – hence its proposed role in post-activation potentiation (Paasuke *et al.* 2007).

The various postulated neural mechanisms principally involve acute changes in autogenic regulatory inputs to motor units involved in the movement (Kilduff *et al.* 2007). Part of the modification of peripheral pathways involved is likely to originate from descending input from higher motor centres. The probable mediating factors at the level of the motor unit are the Golgi tendon organ (GTO) and Renshaw cell. The net peripheral effects are suggested to comprise reduced inhibitory input to the agonist muscles and increased reciprocal inhibition of antagonist motor units (Baker 2003). These mechanical and neural effects are transient and are reported to dissipate approximately 20 minutes after performing the initial high-intensity preload set (Kilduff *et al.* 2007).

Limitations

Due to the paucity of data regarding contrast loading, chronic effects associated with the use of complex training have to date received little research attention (Paasuke *et al.* 2007). As a result, possible mechanisms for any performance improvement elicited by the long-term use of complex training are yet to be determined. The application of these methods also appears dependent upon the training status of the individual. Significant positive correlation is reported between lower-body strength and the degree of potentiation, which suggests that the mechanisms underlying acute performance augmentation play an increasing role with advances in training status (Young *et al.* 1998). In accordance with this, it was reported that performance enhancement consistent with post-activation potentiation was observed in athlete subjects whereas the recreationally trained subjects studied did not show such a response (Chiu *et al.* 2003). Another study identified that power athletes appear to exhibit differing responses to endurance athletes with respect to post-activation potentiation (Paasuke *et al.* 2007). Both the magnitude and the time course of post-activation potentiation may therefore differ according to players' training background.

To date, acute contrast loading effects have been most widely documented with lower-body exercises, typically with jump squats as the target ballistic activity. Acute potentiation of dynamic lower-body performance has been observed with standing long jump, vertical jump and jump squat scores when performed immediately following a heavy load set with a strength-oriented lower-body exercise (Young *et al.* 1998; Baker 2003). Data for upper-body complex training has been more equivocal. It has recently been elucidated that a lesser load (≈65 per cent bench press 1-RM) for the primer exercise set appears to be more effective in producing enhanced power output in the subsequent target upper body power activity (Baker 2003). This was identified as the reason why previous studies featuring heavier upper-body contrast loads (85–90 per cent bench press 1-RM) did not observe any acute performance augmentation effect (Baker 2003). However, a recent study featuring professional rugby union players did report significant, albeit modest, increases in peak power output for ballistic bench throws at different time points following a bench press 3-RM 'preload' set (Kilduff *et al.* 2007).

Co-ordination training

Applications

In the case of fine motor skills, the training stimulus must feature a high degree of specificity with respect to the movement patterns and velocity encountered in competition in order for improvements in power output to transfer to the particular sports skill movement (Kraemer *et al.* 2002). This is likely to be particularly evident with experienced athletes (Newton and Kraemer 1994). Key factors are intra-muscular and inter-muscular co-ordination, and in particular the degree and timing of agonist, synergist and antagonist muscle activation. The concept of co-ordination training has been introduced to describe training modes that satisfy these criteria (Newton and Kraemer 1994).

The term 'co-ordination training' thus describes training modes that feature co-ordination of agonist, synergist and antagonist muscle groups in a way that closely replicates the movement patterns and velocity of an athletic activity (Newton and Kraemer 1994). Many sports skill activities, such as throwing and striking movements, involve motion in the transverse plane and generation of rotational torques and transfer of angular momentum throughout the kinetic chain via sequential motion of multiple segments (Aguinaldo *et al.* 2007). Conversely, the different training modes described in the previous sections predominantly involve linear acceleration movements. Accordingly, successful co-ordination training modes typically apply resistance directly to the specific skill movement (Escamilla *et al.* 2000; van den Tillar 2004). For example, pulley devices have been used for developing power for the overarm throwing movement (Ettema *et al.* 2008).

A number of studies have investigated co-ordination training interventions to develop power output for the (one-handed) overhead throwing movement. The rationale behind the use of weighted implements when carrying out ballistic sports skills is that resistance is provided during the actual target movement. It therefore follows that the training implement employed for ballistic resistance training should be of the same dimensions as that used in the particular sport. A variety of underweight and overweight balls have been employed as a means to provide overload in the form of velocity and force, respectively (van den Tillar 2004). The benefits of underweight ball training interventions have been reported previously by a number of studies examining overarm throwing sports (van den Tillar 2004). Likewise, combination training, featuring both overweight and underweight balls, has reported to be successful in improving overarm throwing velocity with regulation balls (DeRenne *et al.* 1994, 1990). However, results of studies featuring overweight ball training interventions in overarm throwing sports players have been more variable (Escamilla *et al.* 2000; van den Tillar 2004). Crucially, throwing accuracy also appears to be maintained at the enhanced throwing velocities post-training (Escamilla *et al.* 2000).

Previously, the data of DeRenne *et al.* (1994) indicated that a load variation of ±20 per cent regulation weight was successful for under- and over-weight training interventions, which is consistent with previous data for athletic throwing events (Escamilla *et al.* 2000). Other overarm throwing studies have reported success with balls that are 100 per cent overweight (van den Tillar 2004). The overarm warm-up study by van Huss *et al.* (Van Huss *et al.* 1962), that successfully showed acute enhancement of throwing velocity, employed 11oz balls, which were 120 per cent heavier than regulation ball weight. However, overarm training studies employing overweight balls of this degree of difference (>100 per cent regulation weight) have typically not reported improvements in throwing velocity (van den Tillar 2004).

A more recent study has investigated co-ordination training on the two-handed overhead throwing movement performed in team sports such as soccer, basketball and netball (van den Tillar and Marques 2011). It was suggested that the loading employed with the weighted ball training intervention is likely to be a critical factor. In this investigation, significant increases in overhead throwing velocity were reported following a 6-week training period with a 3kg medicine ball; this is over six times heavier than a regulation soccer ball (van den Tillar and Marques 2011). A similar finding was noted in an investigation of weighted ball training intervention for the two-handed spin pass with a rugby ball (Gamble 2005). These findings suggest that the magnitude of loading for two-handed throwing movements in team sports may exceed what has been reported to be optimal for one-handed overarm throwing.

Mechanisms

The precise mechanisms for increases in throwing velocity with modified (heavy and light) ball training are yet to be elucidated. The increases in velocity for the passing skill observed in the current study are likely to be mediated by neural factors, on the basis that the relative loading offered by the heavy ball is probably insufficient to elicit morphological changes. These underlying neural factors likely include improvements in rate of force development (RFD). This RFD parameter is dependent on the rate at which the musculature is activated (Stone *et al.* 2003b), and increases can be attributed primarily to enhanced motor firing in the brief time interval for force production allowed by the sports skill (Behm 1995). Gains in high-velocity strength in the specific musculature involved in the passing movement may also have been a factor. Authors of a previous overarm throwing study hypothesised that improvements in the ability to selectively recruit high-threshold motor units may play a role (DeRenne *et al.* 1994). It is likewise possible that improved inter-muscular co-ordination of agonist, synergist and antagonist muscle firing may also contribute to gains in throwing velocity.

Limitations

A very high degree of specificity of loading does appear to be necessary in order for speed strength modes to transfer to sports skill performance. This is perhaps unsurprising given the very high degree of co-ordination in the magnitude and timing of sequential motion between multiple segments in series that feature in skilled movements such as throwing (Aguinaldo *et al.* 2007). For example, the divergence in motor patterns involved with two-handed over-head and chest pass medicine ball throws are apparently too great to stimulate a training effect for baseball throwing velocity, even in junior players with no resistance training experience (Newton and McEvoy 1994). Similarly, despite the greater similarity noted for the force–time curve for the bench throw movement, bench throw training was not found to offer any advantage to conventional bench press training in developing netball pass velocity in female players (Cronin *et al.* 2001b). The authors concluded that the movement velocity involved in the bench throw was too dissimilar to the netball chest pass movement to evoke superior gains in chest pass velocity in relation to conventional bench press training.

In the case of fine motor skills, it has been proposed that if the contrast in load is too great then disruption of the precise motor patterns of the sports skill would occur, thereby nullifying any benefits of training (Baker 2001d). Skilled movements such as one-handed overarm throw are reliant upon precise control of the degree and sequential timing of rotational motion of a series of segments in order to translate angular momentum from the hips to the throwing arm (Aguinaldo *et al.* 2007). In this case, if the overweight ball was too heavy, the player will have to adjust their throwing mechanics to compensate, at the risk of causing disruption to this highly co-ordinated sequential motion. For example, in the one-handed overarm throwing study by Straub (1968), subjects threw balls that were progressively increased in weight each week, culminating with 17oz balls (240 per cent heavier than regulation) in the final week of the study, and no improvement in throwing velocity with the regulation ball was derived.

It is also noteworthy that increases in performance reported by co-ordination training interventions that employ weighted implements are often no different from the improvements elicited by performing repetitions without any added load. For example, in the two-handed overhead throwing study, the improvement in throwing velocity following the 6-week training period did not differ for subjects in the group who trained only with a standard ball, in comparison to the medicine ball training group or combination (medicine ball and standard ball) training group (van den Tillar and Marques 2011). Similar findings have been noted previously in a study of sprint training methods, which reported that a training group performing only standard sprint training showed superior improvements to groups that employed either resisted sprinting or assisted sprinting training interventions (Kristensen *et al.* 2006).

Co-ordination training modes that employ heavier or lighter sports skill implements appear most appropriate for ballistic sports skills – such as throwing – where the implement can be released at the end of the movement. It is more problematic to employ this form of training with other sports that involve an implement such as a racquet or a bat which is held throughout. For example, if swinging a heavier version of a racquet, at the termination of the swing the momentum of the heavier implement has to be absorbed by the limbs and joints. This carries obvious risks of injury, particularly if performed repetitively. For these striking sports, resistance in the form of a cable pulley system may offer a safer and more viable alternative for co-ordination training. In particular, cable machines with pneumatic resistance may provide a means to allow ballistic-type striking movements to be performed with lighter loads without the issues of causing damage to the apparatus that can occur with weight stack loaded cable machines. However, studies to date have only investigated the use of pulley devices to develop throwing velocity; there are currently no data to validate the application of this approach for striking movements.

Conclusions and training recommendations

Power is clearly multidimensional, and developing this capacity is dependent upon a range of morphological, mechanical and neuromuscular adaptations (Cormie *et al.* 2011a). It follows that achieving optimal development of power will require a variety of training approaches in order to account for each of the different factors that contribute to the ability to express explosive muscular power. The selection of training modes will depend upon the athletic or sports skill movement in question (Baker and Newton 2005). The optimal approach will to some extent also depend upon the profile and training history of the individual player. The degree to which a particular mode of training is effective in developing explosive power capabilities will be influenced by the amount of adaptation that has already taken place in the corresponding factor underpinning power expression.

For example, a key consideration is the strength base of the individual and their window for adaptation (Baker and Newton 2005). In the case of players with low to moderate strength-training experience, and corresponding maximum strength levels, appropriate strength training is likely to confer improvements in both strength and power (Cronin *et al.* 2001b; Newton and McEvoy 1994). For those with a greater strength-training base, diminishing returns are observed so that only modest improvements in power will be observed despite gains in strength. The emphasis for these players must therefore shift to greater use of specific speed-strength training modes in order to produce any significant increase in power (Cormie *et al.* 2011b).

In general, employing a combination of speed-strength training modes during the course of the training macrocycle is likely to offer superior improvements in power over time (Cormie *et al.* 2011b). Olympic weightlifting training modes confer improvements in concentric power development and maximise power expression against greater external resistance. Ballistic resistance training offers a means to elicit gains in concentric power output due in part to improvements in the eccentric phase; peak power measured for both the athlete's body and body + mass 'system' during the barbell jump squat are also significantly higher than values achieved during the power clean at a range of barbell loads from 0–80 per cent of squat 1-RM (McBride *et al.* 2011). Plyometric training provides improvements in both slow SSC and fast SSC properties, and a high degree of movement specificity is possible with plyometrics, which favours transfer to horizontal propulsion and multidirectional movement. Finally, co-ordination training modes represent a means to develop specific power capabilities for sports skills, such as throwing and striking movements.

Planned variation has been identified as an important factor in optimising gains in explosive power performance over time (Winchester *et al.* 2008). This pertains to both the training modes employed and intensity prescribed for speed-strength training. Superior gains in power are generally achieved when a range of loads are employed in the course of a training intervention (Cormie *et al.* 2011b). An undulating periodisation format, featuring alterations in training intensity both between workouts and successive training weeks, has been employed successfully in short-term (8 week) speed-strength training studies (Winchester *et al.* 2008).

The session format will also have a bearing on the training stimulus and force and velocity parameters during successive sets and repetitions. The amount of rest employed between sets when performing Olympic weightlifting training (three sets of six repetitions of the power clean with 80 per cent 1-RM resistance) was reported to significantly influence the decrement in peak power, force and velocity measures in sets two and three (Hardee *et al.* 2012). Similarly, the format of each set can be manipulated when performing speed-strength training to provide variation and enhance the quality of each repetition (Haff *et al.* 2008). One such approach involves the use of 'cluster' or 'rest-pause' sets: this format incorporates a brief rest period between individual repetitions within the set. Lifting velocity was reported to be better maintained for consecutive repetitions of an Olympic weightlifting exercise (barbell clean pull) when sets were performed in a cluster set format (Haff *et al.* 2003). Similar findings were observed with respect to power output and velocity when repetitions of a ballistic resistance exercise (barbell jump squat) were performed in clusters of one, two or three repetitions with rest intervals between, in comparison to the traditional format of performing six repetitions consecutively (Hansen *et al.* 2011). These findings are particularly noteworthy as the latter study employed professional and semi-professional team sports players with extensive training experience. Implementing this approach is therefore suggested to optimise the mechanical stimulus provided (Hansen *et al.* 2011), and is likewise beneficial in terms of neural co-ordination aspects (Haff *et al.* 2008). Varying the set format at different times in the training cycle according to the goals of the training phase (for example, power versus power-endurance) is another tool strength and conditioning specialists may use when periodising players' speed-strength training.

7

SPORTS SPEED AND AGILITY DEVELOPMENT

Introduction

It is acknowledged that speed and agility in team sports represent complex psychomotor skills (Verkhoshansky 1996). Training to develop speed and agility would therefore appear to demand a high degree of neuromuscular specificity. There are likewise issues of biomechanical specificity that must be considered when designing speed and agility training for a particular team sport. Perceptual components that underpin sports speed and agility must also be accounted for when developing these qualities, which include anticipation and decision-making; these constraints will be specific to the sport and playing position.

Developing speed capabilities necessarily comprises a variety of elements. For example, strength qualities are implicated in the need for the athlete to overcome their own inertia, such as during initial acceleration. Speed-strength and stretch-shortening cycle abilities are likewise required every time the foot touches down to propel the body forwards. In addition to physical capabilities, speed expression is highly dependent upon neuromuscular co-ordination and technique aspects. All of these components must be trained in a way that is specific to the form of locomotion (such as running or skating), and movement velocities that feature in the sport, in order to ultimately transfer to sports performance.

Change of direction performance is relatively independent of straight-line speed performance (Little and Williams 2005; Young *et al.* 2001a). The multidirectional acceleration and deceleration involved in change of direction movements, which in turn underpin agility performance, are therefore specific qualities and should be trained as such (Jeffreys 2006). Team sports agility comprises not only these change of direction abilities, but also the capability to anticipate, read and react to game-specific cues in the environment (Sheppard and Young 2006; Young and Farrow 2006).

Due to the variable nature of match-play, high-velocity movements may be initiated from a variety of starting conditions. Similarly, exhibition of both speed and agility in team sports occurs in response to game situations (Young *et al.* 2001a). It follows that perception–action coupling and decision-making are critical elements in terms of developing the ability to express speed and agility capabilities under match conditions.

Trainability of speed and agility capabilities

Traditionally there has been some debate among coaches about whether speed capabilities are trainable. To some extent there has been a shift in opinion over recent years and coaches increasingly acknowledge that while genetic aspects do exert major influence there is growing acceptance that an athlete's speed capabilities can be developed via appropriate training interventions. In the case of agility development this debate is to some extent ongoing (Gamble 2011a).

There is an increasing body of data that support the efficacy of training interventions to develop both change of direction abilities (Brughelli *et al.* 2008) and the perceptual and decision-making aspects of agility (Serpell *et al.* 2011). It is also clear that dedicated training will be required in order to elicit such improvements; speed training alone will not be reflected in improved change of direction performance (Young *et al.* 2001a), or in turn agility expression in the sport.

Specificity of speed versus agility development

Players' straight-line sprinting scores and measures of change of direction performance that are indicative of agility typically show only limited statistical relationship. In a study of professional soccer players' scores on acceleration, maximum speed and change of direction tests showed low coefficients of determination (Little and Williams 2005). The authors concluded that speed and agility are distinct abilities that are relatively independent of each other. Furthermore, correlations between measures of these abilities reportedly decrease markedly when any sport skill component is incorporated in the agility tests (Young *et al.* 2001a).

These findings reflect the dissimilarity of movement mechanics between straight-line running and the locomotion employed during change of direction tasks (Sheppard and Young 2006; Young *et al.* 2001a). Major differences include stride mechanics and the requirement for deceleration and lateral acceleration, and the fact that change of direction movements involve considerable hip abduction and generation of medial–lateral ground reaction forces (McLean *et al.* 2004).

The specificity of training effects is reinforced by the very limited transfer to change of direction performance reported following a six-week period of straight-line sprint training (Young *et al.* 2001a). In this study, as the complexity of the agility test increased (greater number of changes in direction and more acute angles of cutting), the degree of improvement following the straight-line sprint training became less. The converse also appears to be true of agility training. Following six weeks' agility training, performance was improved in a selection of tests with varying numbers of changes in direction – however, no improvement was seen on a straight-line test (Young *et al.* 2001a). Again, the greatest carry-over was observed on the tests with similar change of direction complexity and angles of cutting to that featured in the agility training employed (Young *et al.* 2001a). As these change of direction abilities which underpin agility performance would appear to be independent of straight-line sprinting ability, it follows that they must be developed via specific training (Jeffreys 2006).

Mechanics of sprint running

Foot strike during sprinting

The duration of ground contact when sprinting is very brief and represents the interval during which the athlete has the opportunity to propel themselves forwards (Weyand *et al.*

2010). For these reasons various aspects relating to the foot strike exert considerable influence, in terms of maximising propulsion and minimising braking forces (Gamble 2011b). One example is the placement of the foot with respect to the athlete's centre of mass at initial contact. When the athlete is in motion, it is critical that the foot is not placed so far in front of the body that excessive braking forces result. During high-speed running the optimal position for initial foot strike is just in front of the centre of mass in order to maximise the effective interval of ground contact (Nummela *et al.* 2007).

Similarly, the orientation of the foot and lower limb, and the relative motion of the foot when it connects with the ground, will also determine relative braking versus propulsion forces. If the foot is moving forwards at initial contact braking forces will result; the aim therefore is that the foot is moving in a rearwards direction so that braking forces are minimised and propulsion maximised (Nummela *et al.* 2007). The region of the foot that makes contact with the ground is also a key factor. If the athlete strikes the ground with their heel a dual spike of ground reaction forces results; this not only increases impact forces but also increases braking forces (Divert *et al.* 2005). Better sprinters are therefore observed to make initial contact with the ground with their midfoot or forefoot (Lieberman *et al.* 2010). In addition to reducing braking and impact forces, this foot strike strategy also allows for improved elastic storage and return of elastic energy (Jungers 2010).

The importance of arm action to stride mechanics

Although not widely identified in the literature, expert sprint coaches frequently cite the importance of arm action to sound sprinting mechanics. During initial acceleration athletes employ a combination of a rapid arm drive in a rearward direction with the ipsilateral (same side) upper limb to the forwards moving leg, and a powerful upwards and forwards arm drive with the contralateral (opposite side) upper limb. The ipsilateral arm drive is a feature of all phases of the sprint; essentially the counter-rotation of the shoulders and arm drive in a rearwards direction facilitates hip rotation and leg drive in a forwards direction. The importance of arm action to running mechanics is illustrated when arm movement is forcibly restricted (Fujii *et al.* 2010). Under these constraints athletes must employ much shorter strides, for which they attempt to compensate by increasing stride frequency.

The forwards and upwards contralateral arm swing serves a specific role during the acceleration phase. This action is analogous to the arm swing (in a forwards direction) that athletes perform during the propulsion phase of the vertical jump. During the jumping action this helps to stiffen the trunk region as the lower limb extensors propel the athlete upwards, as well as helping to generate momentum in an upwards direction, ultimately increasing torque generation and allowing greater jump height to be attained (Feltner *et al.* 1999). During the initial acceleration phase, the forwards arm drive can be seen to serve much the same function (that is, stiffening the torso and augmenting torque generation) for the supporting lower limb that is extending to propel the athlete forwards as the opposite leg is being swung forwards for the first stride.

Team sports players must also accommodate the ball or implement of the sport (for example, hockey stick) when running. Holding or dribbling the ball will require the player to adapt their posture and running technique, and places constraints on arm action when running. These technique modifications represent a specific ability that differentiates elite players from those at lower levels. For example, skilled basketball players are observed to increase shoulder rotation when dribbling the ball in order to maintain normal hip and lower limb mechanics (Fujii *et al.* 2010). It follows that these running technique modifications should be accounted for during speed and agility development.

Running mechanics for different phases of sprint running

The gait cycle when sprinting can be divided into two distinct parts:

- the *contact* or *stance phase*, which begins at initial foot strike and ends when the foot leaves the ground – that is, 'toe-off' – the stance phase can be subdivided into a braking or 'weight-acceptance' phase, and a propulsion phase;
- the *flight* or *swing phase*, consisting of the initial recovery during which the initial rearward motion of the lower limb is first slowed then reversed as the leg is brought forwards to pass under the athlete's centre of mass and then swung forwards before positioning of the foot and lower limb for the next foot strike.

There are marked differences between running mechanics during the initial acceleration phase versus running at maximal speed. One difference is the respective duration of the stance and swing phases. During initial acceleration the period of ground contact is much longer; the duration of foot contacts when running at maximal speed is necessarily very brief. Other key differences include posture and the positioning of initial foot strike. Specifically, during acceleration there is a pronounced forwards lean, whereas at top speed athletes adopt an upright stance (Weyand *et al.* 2010). The position of initial contact during foot strike is to the rear of the athlete's centre of mass during the acceleration phase in order to maximise forwards propulsion (Kugler and Janshen 2010); at maximum speed foot strike is marginally in front of the athlete's centre of mass.

Expression of speed in sports

Sprinting technique of team sports players appears to differ from that of track athletes (Young *et al.* 1995). It is also suggested that the acceleration phase for team sports athletes may be shorter so that they acquire top speed within a shorter distance in relation to track sprinters (Baker and Nance 1999). Studies of both track and field athletes and team sports players report that measures of acceleration performance are not closely correlated to maximum sprinting speed (Young *et al.* 1995; Cronin and Hansen 2005). This is a reflection of the fact that these abilities involve different patterns of muscle recruitment and motor firing.

In the context of some team sports, acceleration and short-distance speed may be of more relevance than top speed attained over longer distances (Cronin and Hansen 2005). The distances covered at high-velocity locomotion are typically short and this generally coincides with direct involvement in attacking or defensive play. Team sports played on a restricted playing area (basketball, volleyball) and some playing positions within other field team sports will rarely engage in high-velocity locomotion over distances sufficient to attain maximum speed (McInnes *et al.* 1995). Hence, training for maximum speed would appear to be a secondary priority for these players given that they will rarely express these capabilities on the field of play (Young *et al.* 2001a). Conversely, the larger playing field in team sports (rugby, soccer) combined with the fact that players may already be in motion when they start sprinting can allow certain playing positions to attain near maximal speeds in some instances (Little and Williams 2005). For these players developing maximal speed capabilities over longer distances remains a key training goal.

Aspects of agility expression in team sports

A categorical definition of agility has recently been offered: 'rapid whole-body movement with change of velocity or direction in response to a stimulus' (Sheppard and Young 2006). In the context of team sports, agility therefore comprises not only change of direction movement capabilities but also perception and decision-making.

Change of direction movement mechanics

Much the same mechanical principles as those described for straight-line running govern propulsion during the acceleration phase of change of direction movements (Gamble 2011c). For example, body lean angle in the intended direction of movement and the positioning of the foot relative to the athlete's centre of mass will serve to determine the vertical and horizontal component of ground reaction forces; and hence the net propulsion in a horizontal direction (Kugler and Janshen 2010). However, by definition change of direction movement requires generation of medial-lateral ground reaction forces that are not evident during straight-line running (McLean *et al.* 2004). As a result there are corresponding differences in muscle recruitment, in particular there is greater adductor and abductor muscle involvement, and there is a direct contribution from different muscles of the hip girdle to producing movement.

Depending on the athlete's initial velocity and degree of deviation from their original path, change of direction movements will often comprise a 'weight-acceptance' phase during which the athlete must decelerate their momentum, closely followed by a propulsion phase to move in the new direction (Brughelli *et al.* 2008). The deceleration component of such change of direction activities requires generation of braking forces. These deceleration movements demand postural adjustments, in order to reposition the player's centre of mass and help slow their momentum, and considerably different foot placement and ground contact from that described for straight-line running. Deceleration movements are therefore described as a specific ability (Griffiths 2005; Lakomy and Haydon 2004). Furthermore, the transition between deceleration and acceleration phases during change of direction activities comprises additional aspects associated with the coupling of eccentric and concentric actions (Gamble 2011c).

Sensorimotor, perceptual and decision-making aspects of agility

Change of direction movements impose greater demands in terms of balance abilities, particularly dynamic stabilisation, and lower limb neuromuscular control. Performing change of direction movements under reactive conditions in turn imposes considerably different sensorimotor control challenges (Gamble 2011c). The greater complexity of the neuromuscular control challenge when the same change of direction task is performed under reactive conditions is reflected in measurably different movement kinetics and kinematics (Besier *et al.* 2001).

In addition to the sensory and cognitive abilities involved in reacting to a stimulus and initiating the movement response, the constraints of the agility task may also demand elements of anticipation and decision-making. For example, when intercepting a ball it is demonstrated that skilled performers often employ a predictive movement strategy which is initiated in advance based on the anticipated trajectory of the ball (Gillet *et al.* 2010). Players at elite level are observed to possess a superior ability to detect, select and process 'task relevant' cues that are available in the competition environment (Holmberg 2009). Following the anticipatory movement response, players will also modify and refine their movement based on the actual observed trajectory of the ball, and these adjustments comprise further visuo-motor abilities which similarly differentiate performers at elite level (Gillet *et al.* 2010). The coupling of perception and action during agility movements is therefore highly refined in elite players, and also highly specific to the constraints of the given situation faced by the player in a match context (Gamble 2011c).

Elements of speed development

A number of different elements contribute to speed performance during competition. Each component can be viewed as an avenue for development through which overall speed expression may be improved. It follows that each element should be addressed via dedicated training in order to maximise overall speed development. A multidimensional approach to developing sports speed therefore appears the most appropriate – in much the same way as the 'mixed methods' approach for developing power (Newton and Kraemer 1994) described in Chapter 6.

Technical and kinematic aspects of speed expression over the first few steps differ from what is observed with maximum speed sprinting over longer distances (Delecluse 1997). First-step quickness (0–5m split sprint time) and acceleration (10m speed) have been identified as distinct capabilities to 30m speed in sports players (Cronin and Hansen 2005). Whilst first-step quickness and acceleration measures correlate closely to each other (r=0.92) in team sports players (professional and semi-professional rugby league players), the relationship with maximal speed scores was much weaker in these players (Cronin and Hansen 2005). It follows that these capabilities must not only be assessed independently but also that developing each of these qualities will require a different training stimulus to speed over longer distances (Cronin and Hansen 2005). Given the importance of speed over short distances in team sports, it follows that dedicated training to develop the technical and neuromuscular aspects that underpin players' acceleration capabilities is warranted (Cronin and Hansen 2006).

Strength and speed-strength training modes

Maximum strength and speed-strength ('explosive power') are key factors from the point of view of overcoming the player's own inertia particularly when initiating high-velocity movements. By increasing the force-generating capacity of the muscles involved, it is possible to improve players' acceleration and speed when engaging in high-velocity locomotion during a game (Cronin and Hansen 2006; Hoff 2005). One aspect of achieving this is through the use of appropriate strength training incorporating specific movements (Verkhoshansky 1996).

Different strength qualities appear to predominate in different phases of a sprint (Young *et al.* 1995). Maximum strength, relative to body mass, is suggested to be relatively more important for the initial acceleration phase (Young *et al.* 2001a). Concentric speed-strength capabilities appear to be important for both initial acceleration (Young *et al.* 1995) and speed over longer distances (Young *et al.* 2001a). As the player attains higher velocity and foot contact time becomes shorter, reactive strength has an increasing role (Young *et al.* 2001a). Fast stretch-shortening cycle abilities are similarly critical during maximal sprinting.

Correlation studies report that measures of speed-strength are closely related to speed capabilities of team sports players. In one study of semi- and full-time professional rugby league players, only scores on loaded jump squat and vertical jump (squat jump and countermovement jump) differentiated between 'fast' and 'slow' groups within the players studied (Cronin and Hansen 2005). In another study of professional rugby league, higher force speed-strength measures (higher load jump squats and 3-RM hang clean) showed strongest relationships to speed performance in the players studied (Baker and Nance 1999). A more recent study reported that players' scores on hang power clean successfully differentiated between those with differing sprinting ability (fast versus slow groups) in a sample of professional Australian rules football players (Hori *et al.* 2008).

The muscles that extend the hip and knee and plantarflex the ankle are a common focus for strength training to improve speed performance due to their involvement in propulsion during sprinting (Deane *et al.* 2005; Delecluse 1997). Olympic weightlifting exercises and ballistic exercises such as jump squat are suggested to favour lower limb speed-strength gains at appropriate hip and knee angles for running (Cronin and Hansen 2006). Short-term training employing Olympic-style lifts was shown to elicit improvement in 10m speed with physically active male college students with strength-training experience (Tricoli *et al.* 2005). This is supported by the correlations between hang clean and jump squat 3-RM with 10m and 40m sprint scores of rugby league players (Baker and Nance 1999).

However, despite the importance of speed-strength of the locomotor muscles inferred from the correlation studies mentioned previously, very few strength and speed-strength training studies consistently report such gains in speed measures. One reason suggested for this finding is that speed-strength training studies use ballistic exercises and/or Olympic-style lifts that are typically bilateral and involve predominantly vertical force production (Young 2006). This raises obvious questions concerning biomechanical and kinematic specificity, given that sprinting involves cyclic unilateral motion and features primarily horizontal force production. Based upon this contention two suggestions can be made: the first is that progression to unilateral and split variations of the Olympic-style lifts and ballistic speed-strength exercises may be necessary to translate gains in speed-strength to sprinting performance. The second is that horizontal speed-strength and plyometric movements – such as unilateral bounding exercises – may develop speed-strength and reactive strength in a way that offers greater transfer to speed performance (Young 2006).

Sprinting-specific plyometrics

Different phases of a sprint rely on slow (300–500ms) and fast (100–200ms) stretch-shortening cycle (SSC) properties to different degrees, depending on duration of foot contact. Slow SSC performance will be required during the longer foot contacts featured during acceleration. Fast SSC then predominates as foot contacts become shorter as the player attains higher velocities. Measures of fast SSC performance are significantly related to sprint performance over 30m, and over longer distances (100m and beyond) in trained athletes (Hennessy and Kilty 2001). In fact, drop jump for height was shown to be the single biggest predictor of sprint performance in the elite female sprint athletes studied.

Specific sprint drills and bounding exercises are the tools typically employed to develop stretch-shortening cycle performance. To account for specificity in order to improve transfer of training, it is important that the force–time characteristics of exercises used reflect those experienced during high-velocity actions on the field of play (Mero and Komi 1994). Particularly important when developing stretch-shortening cycle performance is the ground contact time involved with particular exercises. Excessive braking forces and a compromised propulsion phase occur in particular with stepping and hopping bounding exercises, which reduces the stretch-shortening cycle training stimulus and limits their effectiveness in evoking neuromuscular adaptations (Mero and Komi 1994).

A factor in this is that stepping and hopping bounding exercises involve initial contact with the heel, rather than midfoot as occurs in maximal running – which is again unfavourable from a biomechanical specificity viewpoint. Maximal bounding that features initial contact at the midfoot and shortened ground contact times avoids these problems and so is likely to favour stretch-shortening cycle and neuromuscular adaptations (Mero and Komi 1994). In support of this contention, short-term plyometric training that featured unilateral and horizontal bounding exercises was reported to be successful in improving 10m (acceleration) and 100m (maximum speed) sprint times, albeit in non–athlete subjects (Delecluse et al. 1995).

Resisted co-ordination training modes

One approach employed to specifically develop acceleration involves the use of resisted sprinting methods (Cronin and Hansen 2006). This may be achieved simply by using an inclined surface. The kinematic changes associated with uphill sprinting – including greater trunk flexion and reduced distance between centre of gravity and foot strike – serve to lengthen the propulsive phase during foot contact (Paradisis and Cooke 2001). Such changes would appear to replicate the specific mechanics associated with the acceleration phase (Cronin and Hansen 2006), including pronounced forward lean and greater knee extensor involvement (Delecluse 1997).

Towing weighted sleds or tyres can similarly be used to provide resistance for short-distance straight-line sprinting. Applying resistance in this way demands greater stabilisation of the trunk and pelvis, and should therefore promote development of lumbopelvic stability during the sprinting action (Cronin and Hansen 2006). Towing tends to produce similar kinematic changes to those described with uphill sprinting (greater trunk lean, hip flexion and ground contact time) (Lockie et al. 2003), which may be beneficial to developing acceleration. Heavier towing loads appear to interfere with sprinting mechanics to a greater degree (Lockie et al. 2003). For this reason, lighter loads (approx 10 per cent body mass) are typically recommended – however, the friction provided by the running surface is another contributing factor that is harder to quantify (Cronin and Hansen 2006). An alternative and possibly more practical approach is to assess the degree to which a given load impacts upon performance (sprint times). The guideline suggested is that if sprint times are affected by more than 10 per cent the loading is too great and should be adjusted (Cronin and Hansen 2006).

Adding weight to the athlete is another means by which coaches have increased resistance during speed training (Cronin and Hansen 2006). Weighted vests provide a different form of overload by imposing greater vertical (rather than horizontal) forces. Although step length and step frequency are reduced and stance times are increased, joint kinematics are not significantly different when sprinting with weighted vests, which lends support to the biomechanical specificity of this training mode (Cronin and Hansen 2006).

Specific speed development

Sprinting is a highly complex skilled movement involving high degrees of activation of multiple muscle groups (Ross et al. 2001). Speed is also categorised as a relatively closed skill, with predictable and planned motor patterns that can be reinforced via training (Young et al. 2001a). The relative sequencing of muscle activation and resulting movement mechanics are observed to change with sprint training (Ross et al. 2001). Dedicated neuromuscular training to develop the requisite inter-muscular co-ordination is therefore critical for improving the specific timing and execution of the motor patterns associated with high-velocity locomotion.

Acceleration phase speed development

From a kinetic and kinematic specificity viewpoint, training methods to develop acceleration should aim to replicate the characteristic stride mechanics of the acceleration phase, such as the greater hip and knee flexion at touchdown and greater knee extensor involvement in propulsion (Cronin and Hansen 2006). In addition, the following elements should be emphasised during acceleration technique drills, particularly during the initial strides:

*   Rearward arm drive (ipsilateral side to the knee driving forwards) past midline of the body;
*   Contralateral arm swing in a forwards direction – analogous to the arm swing employed during the propulsion phase of a vertical jump;
*   Body lean angle approaching an angle of 45 degrees from the vertical at 'toe off' for standing starts, or in the range 30–40 degrees for rolling starts (Kugler and Janshen 2010);
*   'Full' extension of hip, knee and ankle so that there is a straight line from rear foot to the top of the head at 'toe off'.

Falling starts are a good tool to familiarise the player with the desired degree of forwards body lean employed during acceleration movements. The three-point crouch start similarly offers a means to develop co-ordination of arm action and leg drive from a flexed starting position. Progressions for standing start drills will also include a variety of starting strategies employed by players to achieve the desired forwards body lean and foot placement. For example, one such strategy involves stepping back, also known as the 'false step', in order to create a forwards lean and position the supporting foot behind the athlete's centre of mass (Frost et al. 2008). These movement strategies can also incorporate a preload action, such as a drop step, which can serve to enhance power output and thereby propulsion – in a similar fashion to the 'split step' employed by racquet sports players to improve first step acceleration (Gamble 2011b).

Another important consideration is the conditions from which acceleration and first-step quickness are initiated during matches (Young et al. 2001a). Players may be static or in motion (in a variety of directions) when they accelerate to intercept the trajectory of a ball or become involved in play. Players must therefore be capable of executing acceleration and developing short-distance speed from a variety of starting conditions (Cronin and Hansen 2006). For similar reasons, in addition to conventional standing starts, acceleration techniques should be developed from different postures and positions, and also rolling starts to develop the ability to accelerate whilst in motion. Finally, execution of these different acceleration techniques under reactive conditions should be included in order to develop the coupling of perception and action during acceleration movements (Gamble 2011b).

Maximal speed development

A key aspect of improving sprint running velocity is maximising the propulsive ground reaction force at each foot contact and limiting touchdown time (Hunter et al. 2005). Propulsive impulse generated by the athlete during touchdown, relative to their body mass, is the single biggest predictor of sprinting velocity over short distances (≈16m) (Hunter et al. 2005). Co-ordinating torque generation at the hip and knee and the orientation of the foot prior to and during touchdown is a complex neuromuscular skill – it follows that this should require dedicated training in order to develop it. Accordingly, high-velocity training aimed at enhancing motor unit recruitment (intra-muscular co-ordination) and inter-muscular co-ordination has been shown to elicit improvements in speed performance (Delecluse et al. 1995). Indeed, conventional sprint training appears to be the superior method for producing short-term improvements in technique and speed (Kristensen et al. 2006).

Particular technical aspects of straight-line sprinting can also be coached and reinforced by appropriate technique drills (Cissik 2005). By their nature, such drills are self-paced and carried out at submaximal speed. Examples include walking drills such as 'A' drills (developing static balance), and 'B' drills (dynamic balance development from a static base of support) commonly employed in track athletics. A variety of progressions exist for these drills, which include bounding or skipping variations. It is critical to develop the ability to maintain a stable balanced position from which to generate and direct ground force reaction forces to produce propulsion. Similarly, these drills offer a means to develop the required postural control and co-ordination to maintain vertical stiffness throughout the lower limb kinetic chain and torso during the stance phase and avoid any collapse during each foot contact (Nummela et al. 2007). The other role served by these technique drills is to instruct and reinforce correct 'recovery' mechanics during the transition between the end of the stance phase (that is, 'toe off') and the early–middle part of the swing phase. Specifically, these drills emphasise flexing the leg as it travels under the body in order to reduce the moment of inertia (van Ingen Schenau et al. 1994).

While the technique drills described allow particular aspects of sprinting mechanics to be emphasised, such drills remain markedly different from the kinematics and movement velocities characteristic of high-speed running. Therefore, in order to allow carry-over to performance, these technique drills must ultimately be progressed to actual sprinting

(Cissik 2005). It is important that players are regularly exposed to sprinting at maximal velocity, as neuromuscular co-ordination patterns for individual muscles are observed to differ when running at different velocities (Higashihara *et al.* 2010). Sprint practice undertaken by players in different positions should also reflect the velocities and distances encountered during competitive matches. Furthermore, for sports that involve carrying or dribbling a ball, specific practice of high-speed locomotion accommodating the ball or implement of the sport should also be accounted for when designing speed-training sessions (Fujii *et al.* 2010; Sheppard and Young 2006).

Elements of agility development

A categorical definition of agility has recently been offered: 'rapid whole-body move-ment with change of velocity or direction in response to a stimulus' (Sheppard and Young 2006). In the context of team sports, agility therefore comprises not only change of direc-tion abilities but also perception and decision-making. In much the same way as speed expression, agility in the context of team sports is multifactorial (Gamble 2011c). There are also additional aspects to consider in the case of change of direction movements, such as the need to decelerate and accelerate in various directions. Fundamentally, team sports agility likewise comprises reaction to game-related cues, 'perception–action coupling' and decision-making elements (Sheppard and Young 2006).

There are two major schools of thought regarding 'sports agility' development (Bloomfield *et al.* 2007). One approach involves relatively closed skill practice of move-ment mechanics, often using specialised commercially available equipment such as ladders, mini-hurdles and resistance belts. Others advocate a more open skill approach in which agility movements are conducted in a training environment that is less structured and thereby closer to match conditions (Bloomfield *et al.* 2007).

Strength and speed-strength training modes

Lateral movements are a characteristic aspect of movement during team sports performance. In particular, evasive manoeuvres that occur in competitive play are frequently initiated with a lateral step (Twist and Benicky 1996). Similarly, the sidestep cutting action (rapid change of direction to evade a defensive opponent) involves hip abduction and generation of medial-lateral ground reaction forces to create lateral propulsion (McLean *et al.* 2004). Speed-strength development in these different planes of motion would therefore appear important to develop lateral acceleration in much the same way as sagittal plane speed-strength exercises are employed to improve straight-line acceleration (Hedrick 1999).

It is reported that standard bilateral strength and power measures (squat, loaded and unloaded vertical jump) typically are not strongly related with change of direction perfor-mance (Sheppard and Young 2006). Hang power clean scores of Australian rules football players were similarly unrelated to these players' scores on a change of direction measure (Hori *et al.* 2008). The bilateral and predominantly sagittal plane movement that character-ises exercises typically used for speed-strength development therefore appear inadequate for developing the requisite strength capabilities for change of direction movements. Strength (both concentric and eccentric), speed-strength and reactive strength qualities required for change of direction movements may be better developed via appropriate unilateral strength

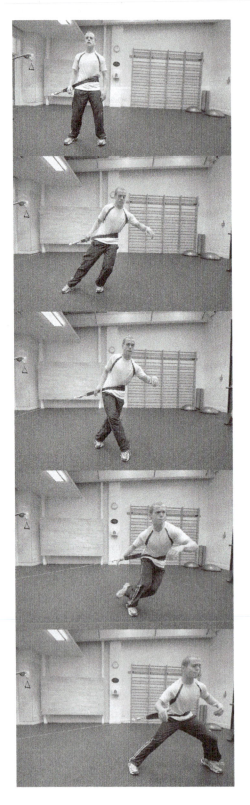

Figure 7.1
Cable resisted cross–over lateral lunge

and plyometric training exercises (Twist and Benicky 1996). Similarly such training should necessarily feature force-generation and propulsion movements in the relevant planes of motion. This is an area that warrants further research.

Depending on the duration of ground contact during these movements, slow SSC elements will also contribute to performance. Slow SSC elements (300–500ms) are likely to be more important than fast SSC (100–200ms) due to the relatively longer foot contacts involved in change of direction movements in comparison to sprinting. Reactive strength measures (for example, drop jump test scores) do appear to have stronger statistical relationship with change of direction performance than concentric strength measures, which typically show no significant relation to change of direction ability (Sheppard and Young 2006). For this reason, it is suggested that specific training to develop these muscular properties, such as bilateral and unilateral drop jump training, have the potential to improve change of direction abilities (Young and Farrow 2006). Such training to develop reactive strength should also feature single-leg plyometric drills that involve reversing direction and incorporate lateral movement in order to account for the relevant movements involved in change of direction.

Postural control and stability

Lumbopelvic stability and neuromuscular control aspects that include whole-body proprioception and balance all contribute to the ability to change direction efficiently. The player's awareness of, and ability to control, the position of their centre of mass is critical in allowing them to efficiently perform agility movements (Yaggie and Campbell 2006). The ability to retain lumbopelvic stability and strong trunk posture would seem to be crucial to maintain proper lower limb mechanics and efficient transfer of force from the ground

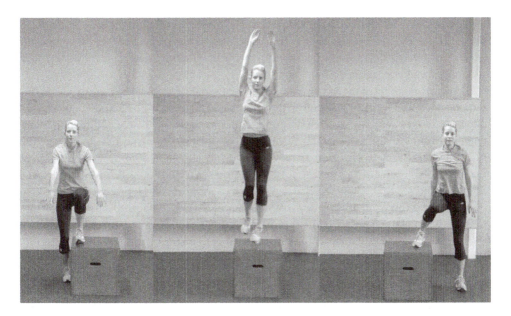

Figure 7.2 Alternate leg lateral box skips

upwards to generate change of direction movement (Kibler *et al.* 2006). Dynamic balance capacities are also important to allow the player to more effectively dissipate impact forces involved in deceleration and change of direction movements (Myer *et al.* 2006a).

Whatever starting posture movements are initiated from, acceleration, deceleration and changes in direction require appropriate postural adjustments (Young and Farrow 2006). A key aspect of postural control with respect to change of direction movement is controlling the position and orientation of the trunk with respect to the pelvis (Kibler *et al.* 2006). For example, during a lateral cutting manoeuvre the player typically leans into the new direction of movement as they cut with their outside foot, in order to maximise horizontal propulsion. Similarly, optimal execution of movement requires the player to maintain tension through a stable torso in order to transmit forces generated through the ground to effectively transfer these ground reaction forces into movement (Young and Farrow 2006). As such, stabilisation and strength through the lumbopelvic region would appear critical to optimal function of the kinetic chain (from base of support to extremities) involved during athletic movements in general, and change of direction movements in particular (Kibler *et al.* 2006).

Planned change of direction movements enable the athlete to anticipate, which allows the required postural adjustments to be made much more easily. In the case of unanticipated cutting movements that are executed in response to an external cue, these postural adjustments are harder to make, which in turn affects loading on lower limb joints (Besier *et al.* 2001). It follows that postural adjustments under reactive conditions should be incorporated into players' training (Besier *et al.* 2001; Craig 2004).

Change of direction movement skills development

Specific change of direction training has been shown to carry over to change of direction performance tests – particularly those involving similar cutting angles (Young *et al.* 2001a). Drills that integrate specific lateral and cutting movements allow technique to be developed and specific neuromuscular patterns to be reinforced (Craig 2004). This approach is analogous to the programmed conditioning methods for agility development described by Bloomfield and colleagues (2007).

By the nature of team sports, players are frequently required to decelerate sharply, as they respond to the movement of team-mates, opponents and the ball (Lakomy and Haydon 2004). A player's ability to decelerate is important in executing change of direction movements (Griffiths 2005), as they must first brake their forward momentum before propelling the body into the new direction of movement (McLean *et al.* 2004). Despite this, deceleration is not commonly addressed during training for team sports (Lakomy and Hayden 2004; Griffiths 2005). Targeted neuromuscular training to develop technical aspects of deceleration is therefore an area that may warrant investigation for team sports players.

Initially simple cones may be used to mark changes of direction. It has been identified that the specialised equipment commonly used in conjunction with programmed 'agility' conditioning methods are in fact not crucial to the success of these training modes (Gamble 2011c). Drills involving specialised equipment can be readily substituted for equivalent drills that develop similar movement skills without any significant impairment of performance improvements observed following training (Bloomfield *et al.* 2007). For example, in place of ladders the line markings on the pitch or court can be used to guide footwork drills. Indeed, this approach may be preferable as players will be less inclined to look at the floor when these drills are performed without ladder apparatus.

This can be progressed to using static poles or standing players to simulate a defender. A recent study found that the presence of even a static dummy 'defender' had a marked influence upon sidestep cutting mechanics (McLean *et al.* 2004). The simulated defender (a model skeleton) caused the players to perform more forceful cutting movements (greater ground reaction forces), accompanied by more hip flexion and abduction as well as greater (flexion and valgus) angles at the knee (McLean *et al.* 2004). These self-paced drills can be progressed by incorporating game-related skill movements (Twist and Benicky 1996).

A further progression is to initiate cutting movements in response to a particular external cue. Movement mechanics and joint kinematics during pre-planned and unan-ticipated cutting movements are significantly different (Besier *et al.* 2001). It follows that unanticipated cutting must be addressed in training, in order for neuromuscular control and co-ordination abilities to carry over to agility movements executed in match situa-tions. This need for perception–action coupling and decision-making elements is explored further in a later section.

Arm action is an often overlooked component of agility that can have a pronounced effect on the athlete's efficiency of movement when changing direction (Brown and Vescovi 2003). A key aspect during the sidestep cutting action (manoeuvre commonly used to evade an opponent) is driving the inside arm in the opposite direction to assist driving the inside leg towards the new direction of movement as the player executes the 'cut' with their outside foot. After this first stride in the new direction, similar backward arm drive by the opposite (outside) arm then assists in rotating the body and bringing the outside leg through to drive towards the new direction of movement. In both the initial cutting stride and second stride it is important that the arm drive is kept tight to the body, in order to reduce unwanted inertia and to direct the acceleration forces in the desired direction (Brown and Vescovi 2003). These elements must be addressed by specific movement prac-tice in much the same way as any other movement skill.

For sports that involve carrying a ball (American football, rugby football) or holding an implement (field hockey, lacrosse, ice hockey) there are indications that skill sports athletes exhibit enhanced agility when holding the implement of their sport (Kraemer and Gomez 2001). This is something that must be considered when designing agility training in these sports. With progression of training, it follows that drills can become more sport-specific by incorporating a ball or sports implement in the drill (Jeffreys 2006; Sheppard and Young 2006).

Transfer training for agility development

There is an important distinction between change of direction abilities during move-ments that are pre-planned (such as manoeuvring around fixed obstacles) and sport-specific agility executed in response to game-specific cues (movement of the ball, opponents or team-mates) (Sheppard and Young 2006; Young and Farrow 2006). During the initial stages of training to develop agility, change of direction movements that feature in agility performance can be developed by repetition of specific movement skill drills that are self-paced and negotiate fixed obstacles (cones, slalom poles, and so on). This change of direction training is essentially closed skill practice as movements are pre-planned and do not require any reaction or decision-making (Sheppard and Young 2006).

However, the defining characteristic of agility is that change of direction or velocity occurs in response to an external stimulus (Sheppard and Young 2006). As such in order to develop agility, planned change of direction movements executed in a static practice environment must be progressed to open skill conditions (i.e. requiring response to a stimulus) (Craig 2004). Requiring the athlete to initiate movements and changes of direction in response to external cues provides specific agility training as opposed to pre-planned change of direction movements (Young and Farrow 2006). Such training is important to improve reaction time and the ability to interpret cues from the environment in order to make postural adjustments and improve movement execution. These abilities also have implications in terms of injury prevention: loads sustained at the knee are reported to be significantly increased during unanticipated cutting movements (Besier *et al.* 2001). Appropriate dynamic neuromuscular training emphasising postural control and correct lower limb alignment during unanticipated cutting manoeuvres (such as against a 'live' opponent) therefore appears necessary in order to protect against non-contact knee injury (Besier *et al.* 2001).

How this transition to specific agility development can practically be achieved is by progressively removing the player's ability to anticipate movement responses (Besier *et al.* 2001). This progression can be viewed as a continuum of motor learning drills with closed movement skill practice at one extreme, and an entirely random open skill environment at the opposite end of the spectrum. In between these two extremes, strength and conditioning specialists can implement a continuum of drills that expose the player to a progressively increasing perceptual challenge. Examples of progressions include self-paced to maximal execution speed; progressing from fixed obstacles to initiating pre-planned movement on command; simple reaction (single response) to complex reaction (multiple movement responses); and finally incorporating decision-making and read-and-react drills against a 'live' opponent.

With advances in agility training, appropriate constraints associated with the particular sport should also be replicated in the training environment, such as opposing players and dimensions of the playing area (Handford *et al.* 1997). Similarly, making the cues in read-and-react drills game-related and incorporating decision-making that is specific to the sport may further help translate change of direction speed into sport-specific agility (Handford *et al.* 1997; Young *et al.* 2001a). In designing these open skill 'read-and-react' drills, sport-specific cues and movement responses must first be identified for the sport and playing position (Jeffreys 2006). These abilities to anticipate and process cues from the game environment in order to make decisions quickly are identified as a key factor in the faster movement times of more skilled players (Young and Farrow 2006). However, at the open skill end of the spectrum it may be argued that such advanced cognitive skill acquisition is better suited to the domain of technical and/or tactical practice and competitive play, under the instruction of the sports coach.

Summary

A number of individual qualities contribute to expression of speed qualities. Speed-strength development appears important in enabling players to overcome their own inertia when initiating high-velocity movements; however, modified versions of conventional speed-strength training modes may offer superior transfer to speed performance. Plyometric training can develop stretch-shortening cycle components that contribute to speed performance – specifically, slow SSC during acceleration and fast SSC for maximal speed; such training should have appropriate emphasis on unilateral and horizontal bounding exercises.

In addition to improving force-generating capacity via speed-strength training, acceleration abilities can also be developed by employing specific acceleration training modes. Whether developing acceleration or maximal speed, neuromuscular aspects – in particular inter-muscular co-ordination – can be developed via specific technical training, which will necessarily include actual sprinting over appropriate distances. In view of the multi-factorial nature of speed expression, an integrated approach to players' speed training that accounts for each of the aspects described would appear to be the best route to optimal development of overall speed performance.

In much the same way as straight-line speed development, multiple components contribute to agility performance in team sports. Again, dedicated training for each of the components described is required to fully exploit all of the identified factors that may contribute to improving agility performance. Postural control, neuromuscular skill, lateral acceleration, deceleration and reactive strength qualities are all implicated in successful execution of the change of direction movements involved in agility performance. Addressing the perceptual aspects, stimulus-response, and decision-making elements that characterise agility represents an additional challenge that must be accounted for in order to specifically develop agility. Essentially, developing all these elements will comprise both approaches typically taken to sports agility development (Bloomfield *et al.* 2007) – including aspects of closed skill practice and ultimately progression to an open skill practice environment.

8

LUMBOPELVIC 'CORE' STABILITY

Introduction

Core stability training has become an integral part of training for all athletes with the aim of improving performance (Carter *et al.* 2006; Liemohn *et al.* 2005), and core exercises are commonly prescribed for therapeutic training applications (Brown 2006). Specificity of training has a number of implications with regard to the transfer of core training modes to different training outcomes, for example performance versus injury prevention or rehabilitation.

Core stability is described in the sports medicine literature as 'the product of motor control and muscular capacity of the lumbo-pelvic-hip complex' (Leetun *et al.* 2004). In musculoskeletal terms this comprises the spine, pelvis and hip joints, and proximal lower limb – in addition to all associated musculature (Kibler *et al.* 2006). For example, there are 29 individual muscles that attach on the pelvis. Furthermore, the combination of muscles that provide lumbopelvic stability in a particular posture or movement is shown to vary depending on factors such as posture and the constraints of the task (Juker *et al.* 1998). The global term 'core' could therefore refer to any of a number of independent components that contribute to providing stability to the lumbopelvic region under various conditions (Mendiguchia *et al.* 2011).

Training the 'core' is therefore considerably more complex than the global term core training implies. Given the complexity of the structures and joints of the lumbar spine, pelvis and hip girdle, and the number of different muscles involved, it perhaps should not be surprising that developing lumbopelvic stability comprises a host of different factors. In reality, the term 'core training' has become an all-purpose label for any exercise that addresses some aspect of *lumbopelvic stability* (Gamble 2007a).

This ambiguity is likely behind the confusion regarding the effectiveness of 'core training' for different health and performance goals (Stanton *et al.* 2004; Tse *et al.* 2005). Training for lumbopelvic stability is typically undertaken with one of two objectives: improving performance and injury prevention (Kibler *et al.* 2006). The efficacy of 'core training' modes for injury prevention is documented; however, support for the role of training for lumbopelvic stability for performance enhancement has proven to be more elusive.

The various functions of the 'core'

When stripped of muscle and left to rely upon passive (bone and ligament) support, the human spine will collapse under 20lb (≈9kg) of load (Barr *et al.* 2005). This illustrates that the spine depends heavily upon the active stability provided by various muscles (Cholewicki and McGill 1996). The combination of systems and muscles that act to provide stability varies with posture, the direction of movement and magnitude of loading on the spine (Juker *et al.* 1998). Hence, a wide variety of muscles contribute to different degrees according to the demands of the situation.

In addition to providing spine stability under static conditions, lumbopelvic stability is identified as critical for whole-body dynamic balance (Anderson and Behm 2005). Most of the muscles that move and stabilise the limbs attach proximally to the lumbo-pelvic-hip complex. The muscles of the 'core' collectively function as synergists for athletic activity (McGill 2010). The 'core' region is therefore described as the 'anatomical base for motion' (Kibler *et al.* 2006). Movements in sports occur in multiple directions; there is accordingly a demand for lumbopelvic stability in all planes of motion (Leetun *et al.* 2004).

Furthermore, the lumbar spine is the site through which various compressive and shearing forces are transmitted during activity (Cholewicki and McGill 1996; Stephenson and Swank 2004). Co-contraction of various lumbopelvic muscles serves to stiffen the spine and trunk region (McGill 2010). This serves to allow efficient transfer of forces from the ground to produce movement and/or generate torque at the extremities (Behm *et al.* 2005; McGill 2006c).

It has been demonstrated that submaximal levels of muscle activation are usually adequate to provide effective spine stabilisation (Cholewicki and McGill 1996). Continuous submaximal muscle activation therefore appears to be crucial in maintaining spine stability for most daily tasks (McGill 2007b). Measures of trunk muscle endurance therefore show the greatest relationship with spine stability and incidence of pain or injury (McGill 2006b). Conversely, under higher-force conditions the larger muscles must brace the trunk whilst generating propulsion and resisting unwanted motion; this in turn demands various strength qualities.

Components of lumbopelvic stability

There are a number of different systems which can contribute to providing stability to the lumbo-pelvic-hip complex under a given set of conditions. Each of these components can be involved in various combinations, depending upon the constraints of the task and the loading conditions involved. Key factors that will determine the contribution from each system include the following:

* postural aspects – in particular whether the athlete is in a weight-bearing stance;
* the degree of any upper limb involvement;
* what motion is occurring at the trunk and extremities;
* the internal and external loading conditions imposed upon the athlete.

Deep postural muscles of the lumbar spine and pelvic girdle

The deep lumbar spine stabiliser muscles have attachments at segmental level (Anderson and Behm 2005; Barr *et al.* 2005). The most widely recognised of these muscles are transversus abdominis and multifidus; however, these muscles also include other muscles, such as rotatores (McGill 2007a). These muscles are small, which limits their torque-generating capacity, and are thus mainly concerned with providing local support. Hence these deep postural muscles have been collectively termed the 'local stabilising system' (Carter *et al.* 2006; Liemohn *et al.* 2005).

A reflection of the postural function of these muscles is that they are observed to fire at a low level ($\approx$10–30 per cent of maximum) in a tonic fashion for prolonged periods; that is, these muscles do not fatigue in the same way as the more superficial muscles (Barr *et al.* 2005). These muscles are also shown to contain a high density of receptors (McGill 2007a). This reflects their role in collectively providing proprioceptive sense of the position and orientation of the pelvis and lumbar spine.

Segmental control of the lumbar vertebrae and the orientation of the pelvis also strongly influences the loading imposed on the lumbar spine and the activity of these muscles is identified as critical for spine stability (Cholewicki and McGill 1996). The importance of these muscles can be inferred from the finding that these muscles are atrophied in individuals with chronic lower back pain (Barr *et al.* 2005; Danneels *et al.* 2001).

The capacity to control lumbar spine posture, and the positioning and orientation of the pelvis in particular, serves a critical role in determining the ability of other muscles that stabilise the lumbo-pelvic-hip complex to function (Workman *et al.* 2008). In particular, an anterior pelvic tilt is to be avoided given that this adversely affects the function of other muscles especially the muscles of the hip girdle. A posture characterised by an anterior tilt of the pelvis (and the lumbar spine lordosis that results) is also associated with low back pain and groin pain and/or injury (Waryasz 2010).

Maintaining 'neutral' lumbar spine posture, and controlling the position and orientation of the pelvis in all three planes/axes of motions, is therefore critical to any activity. Engaging the deep local stabiliser muscles must be viewed as fundamental to all activities undertaken in training and competition, regardless of what other subsystems are recruited on top.

The cues or techniques that are employed when teaching athletes to engage the deep postural muscles will however have a profound effect on spine and lumbopelvic stability. Specifically any technique that encourages abdominal hollowing or cues that involve 'drawing the belly button closer to the spine' should be avoided (McGill 2007c). The cues or techniques coached to athletes should therefore ensure that the shape or surface geometry of the abdomen is unchanged as they engage the deep postural muscles. In this way these muscles can be recruited in a way that does not compromise the function of the larger muscles that will be required to brace the trunk during higher-force athletic activities.

Muscles and connective tissue structures of the trunk

The muscular component of this subsystem includes the larger and more superficial muscles of the abdomen, including rectus abdominis and internal and external obliques, and the muscles of the back, which include the large extensor muscles longissimus and iliocostalis. These muscles, together with the thoracolumbar fascia (the abdominal fascia at the front, the lumbodorsal fascia at the back), collectively form a 'corset' structure (McGill 2007a).

Co-activation of these various muscles causes tension to be applied via the connective tissue structures, which serves to create a rigid corset surrounding the trunk (McGill 2007a). This natural corset of muscles and connective tissues acts in this way to brace the trunk and lumbar spine. During this bracing action the co-contraction of internal and external obliques, together with transverse abdominis, provides a cross-bracing effect that generates hoop stiffness and stability along various axes (McGill 2007c).

The larger abdominal muscles also assist with generating movement at the trunk; for example, the internal and external obliques are implicated in both twisting and lateral bending movement (McGill 2007a). That said, typically such movement predominantly originates from the supporting limb(s).

Muscles of the shoulder complex

Due to their attachment to the lumbodorsal fascia, the larger muscles of the shoulder girdle (for example, latissimus dorsi, trapezius) are able to contribute to providing tension and rigidity to the 'corset' structure described above (Pool-Goudzwaard *et al.* 1998). In this way the muscles of the shoulder girdle, particularly those associated with the articulation between scapula and thorax, contribute to bracing the trunk during high-force activities (McGill 2007a).

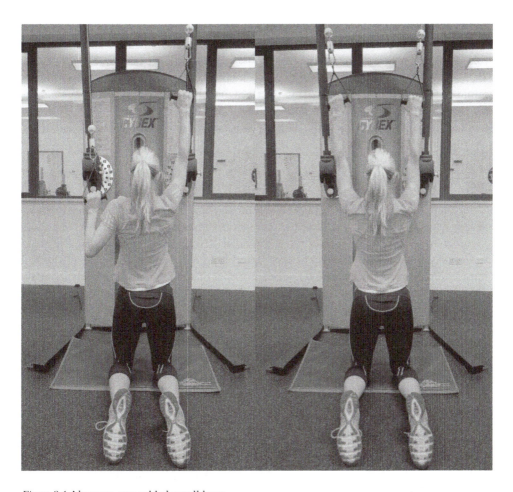

Figure 8.1 Alternate arm cable lat pulldown

In addition, when the athlete is load-bearing through the upper limb(s) the muscles of the scapula and rotator cuff are implicated in stabilising the shoulder girdle, and in turn the trunk region as a whole. During closed chain upper limb actions particularly, for example a push up exercise, these muscles will allow the athlete to anchor the shoulder girdle from the supporting upper limb, in much the same way as described below with regards to the muscles of the hip girdle.

Muscles of the hip girdle

The hips serve as the anatomical base of support for the pelvis and trunk. One of the primary functions of the muscles of the hip girdle is to stabilise the pelvis from the supporting lower limb (Kibler *et al.* 2006). Although the ligamentous structures of the hip provide a great deal more support than is the case with the shoulder (glenohumeral) joint, the muscles of the hip girdle nevertheless work in a way that is analogous to the rotator cuff muscles of the shoulder (Fabrocini and Mercaldo 2003). These hip muscles essentially allow the athlete to anchor the pelvis from the supporting lower limb, which in turn provides a stable platform for the lumbar spine and the trunk as a whole (McGill 2007a).

The other major function of the hip muscles is generating and transmitting forces to the trunk from the supporting limb(s) in order to generate movement. In addition to their role in normal walking and running gait, these muscles are crucial to generating torque and movement during pivoting and twisting actions. For example, gluteal activation was found to have a significant role during the throwing action in a study of baseball pitchers (Oliver and Keeley 2010). Activation of gluteal muscles (gluteus maximus and gluteus medius) was also found to directly relate to pelvis kinematics (rate of axial rotation) during the throwing action.

Summary

Lumbopelvic stability is clearly multidimensional; McGill (2006) has elucidated that the diverse muscle groups which combine to support the lumbar spine must be in balance in order to ensure optimal stability is provided. Given the complexity of the structures and joints of the lumbar spine, pelvis and hip girdle, and the number of different muscles involved, it perhaps should not be surprising that developing lumbopelvic stability comprises a host of different factors (Gamble 2007).

The function of the core relies upon the integration of a number of different components (Borghuis *et al.* 2008). Neuromuscular control aspects that govern the recruitment of these various systems and co-ordination of individual muscles are therefore critical. For example, maintenance of lumbopelvic stability during dynamic movements is underpinned by the firing of various core muscles in preparation for movement (Barr *et al.* 2005; Leetun *et al.* 2004). Hereby, the muscles providing the base of support are activated before the muscles involved in the particular movement (Anderson and Behm 2005).

These anticipatory postural adjustments help to prevent unwanted trunk motion and provide a stable base of support during movement. The neuromuscular system must govern function of stabilising muscles not only in anticipation of expected direction and magnitude of forces, but also in reaction to sudden movement or loading (Barr *et al.* 2005). A reflection of the importance of neuromuscular control is that individuals with chronic lower back pain exhibit impaired neuromuscular feedback and delayed muscle reaction, which is accompanied by reduced capacity to sense the orientation of their spine and pelvis (Barr *et al.* 2005; Rogers 2006).

Demands placed on the 'core' when engaging in team sports

In accordance with the variety of functions served by the respective subsystems that provide lumbopelvic stability, there is equally a demand for endurance, strength and power for the respective muscle groups involved (Willardson 2007). For example, the challenge of maintaining postural integrity whilst sustaining and/or generating external forces will require both strength and endurance of different lumbopelvic muscles (Barr *et al.* 2005).

Furthermore, depending on the sport, these various neuromuscular control and strength capabilities are required under both static and dynamic conditions. Co-contraction of muscles to stiffen or buttress the spine when performing activities under load will require strength under quasi-isometric conditions. Throwing and striking activities often require muscles of the trunk to assist with generating twisting torque, which demands concentric speed-strength. Conversely, deceleration and change of direction movements involve considerable eccentric loading of the muscles of the trunk and hip girdle as they work to resist movement generated by the athlete's own inertia. Finally, maintaining lumbopelvic posture and spine stability requires endurance and in particular the ability to maintain function under challenged breathing conditions.

Lumbopelvic stability and injury

The postural muscles that prevent excessive spine motion at segmental level, and help maintain desired pelvis and lumbar spine posture, act to reduce the stresses placed upon the lumbar spine and thereby protect against injury (Danneels *et al.* 2001; McGill 2006c). In addition, the larger more superficial muscles that brace the trunk and resist external forces under conditions of higher loading also serve to spare the spine (McGill 2006c).

Lumbopelvic instability can be both the cause (McGill 2006c) and result of injury (Hamill *et al.* 2008). Weakness or impairment at any point in this integrated system of support can lead to damage to structural tissues, resulting in injury and pain (Barr *et al.* 2005). As such, low or unbalanced scores on various tests of muscle function indicative of poor lumbopelvic stability are frequently identified as risk factors for injury (McGill 2006b). Impaired passive stability and disrupted motor patterns (compromising active stabilisation) are also commonly observed following injury (McGill 2006b; Montgomery and Haak 1999). For example, neuromuscular deficits in core stability and hip muscle function are often seen among subjects with low back pain (Hamill *et al.* 2008). Addressing these aspects via appropriate training can therefore serve a dual protective role in terms of both guarding against initial injury for healthy athletes and reducing the risk of re-injury in those with a history of low back pain.

A number of studies support the assertion that training different aspects of lumbopelvic stability has a role to play in reducing incidence of injury (Barr *et al.* 2005; Cusi *et al.* 2001; Hides *et al.* 2001; Tse *et al.* 2005). For example, scores of trunk muscle endurance are consistently shown to correlate with incidence of low back pain or injury (McGill 2006b). Lumbopelvic training that incorporated Swiss ball exercises was shown to successfully improve these measures of spine stability (extensor and side bridge endurance times) in sedentary individuals (Carter *et al.* 2006).

The need for targeted interventions to reduce incidence of back injury is underlined by the observation that the lower back is frequently reported as the third most common site of injury in sports, after the ankle and knee (Nadler *et al.* 2000). Low back pain and injury is reportedly commonplace among both recreational and competitive athletes and can severely impair the athlete's ability to train and compete (Montgomery and Haak 1999). Back injury is particularly prevalent in female athletes – injury data from NCAA collegiate athletes during the 1997/98 season indicated almost twice the number of lower back injuries in females compared to male athletes (Nadler *et al.* 2002).

In addition to injuries directly involving the spine, lumbopelvic stability has implications for injury risk and function of the joints of the lower extremity, via the *kinetic chain* of lower limb joints from the supporting foot to the lumbar spine (Leetun *et al.* 2004; Nadler *et al.* 2000). Consequently, deficits in lumbopelvic stability are identified as playing a role in the mechanism of knee ligament injury in particular (Hewett and Myer 2011). The role of lumbopelvic control and different aspects of core stability have therefore been highlighted as critical areas for investigation and interventions aimed at correcting neuromuscular control deficits that predispose athletes to lower limb injury.

Contribution of the 'core' to neuromuscular control of the lower limb

Muscles of the lumbo-pelvic-hip complex serve to provide 'proximal control' to the lower limb kinetic chain (Mendiguchia *et al.* 2011). Over recent years a number of studies in the sports medicine literature have identified factors relating to lumbopelvic stability in the mechanism for lower limb injury (Zazulak *et al.* 2007). The contribution of lumbopelvic stability and control of positioning and motion of the trunk in relation to the supporting lower limb has recently been implicated in the mechanism for knee injury for female athletes specifically (Hewett *et al.* 2009).

Differences in control of trunk posture in female athletes compared to males have been identified during different athletic tasks. For example, female athletes characteristically execute landing movements in an upright stance; there is some suggestion that it is likely that female athletes exhibit associated differences in trunk and hip muscle recruitment and activation, albeit these data are not yet available (Mendiguchia *et al.* 2011). These postural traits are identified as placing the knee ligaments, in particular the anterior cruciate ligament or ACL, at particular risk of injury (Leetun *et al.* 2004). Similarly, an impaired ability to control the positioning and motion of the trunk and thereby the athlete's centre of mass during change of direction movements is shown to adversely affect torques generated at the lower limb joints (Hewett and Myer 2011). Deficits in lateral stability of the trunk in particular have been implicated as a major risk factor for knee ligament injury with female team sports players during pivoting and cutting change of direction movements (Zazulak *et al.* 2007).

Based upon these findings it would appear that the trunk postures adopted by athletes in general, and females in particular, have the potential not only to modify the loading on lower limb joints during athletic activities but also to influence lower limb biomechanics. Training interventions to modify postural control strategies allow more favourable positioning of the trunk and head over the supporting limb(s) during relevant landing and change of direction activities might therefore also confer improvements in lower limb kinetics and kinematics (Mendiguchia *et al.* 2011). The hip musculature plays a key role in supporting and controlling motion at the trunk (Hewett and Myer 2011). Therefore, in addition to the lateral trunk muscles, developing strength and function of the muscles of the hip girdle, in particular the abductor muscles, should be a priority (Mendiguchia *et al.* 2011). Preliminary evidence from investigations supports the efficacy of training to develop hip and trunk neuromuscular control as a means to address knee injury risk factors (Myer *et al.* 2008).

Core function and performance

The lumbopelvic region represents a vital link in the kinetic chains, incorporating all joints and body segments from base of support to extremities, that are involved in athletic movements (Kibler *et al.* 2006). From this viewpoint, stabilisation of the lumbopelvic region would appear critical during athletic activities and sports skill tasks. Co-contraction of various muscles serves to stiffen the core region to facilitate efficient transmission of forces (McGill 2010). For example, a double spike in trunk muscle activation is observed during striking movements: the initial peak is observed as the athlete initiates the striking action; and the second peak serves to maximise force as the athlete connects with the target object (McGill *et al.* 2010).

As well as providing a stable base for motion at the distal segments (the limbs), the 'core' can also be the origin from which rotational torques are generated and transferred to the extremities (Kibler *et al.* 2006). For example, during an overarm throw the sequential rotation of the hips and trunk serves to generate angular momentum, which is transmitted to torque generation at the shoulder joint and ultimately the throwing arm (Aguinaldo *et al.* 2007). It follows that appropriate development of lumbopelvic stability and strength should be reflected in enhanced athletic and sports performance. Based upon such assertions coaches continue to routinely prescribe 'core' training with the specific aim of improving sports performance.

Despite this, a positive link between core training interventions and improvements in measures of athletic performance has yet to be established in the research literature (Stanton *et al.* 2004; Tse *et al.* 2005). In part this reflects that there a very few studies that have investigated this relationship (Hibbs *et al.* 2008). Another factor is the lack of consistency in terms of what constituted core training in the studies, and the nature of exercises employed (Gamble 2007a). Typically, investigators have failed to differentiate between core *endurance* and core *strength*. Assessments of core stability have similarly been conducted under conditions which represent a very limited load challenge for a trained athlete. Despite this, some of these tests have still reported significant, albeit weak to moderate, relationships with different measures of performance (Nesser *et al.* 2008; Okada *et al.* 2011).

The training interventions employed in the majority of the limited number of studies undertaken to date have likely been of insufficient intensity to elicit increases in strength (Nuzzo *et al.* 2008). This factor alone may explain the lack of any gains in performance reported by some studies (Stanton *et al.* 2004; Tse *et al.* 2005). It has been identified that more challenging training modes, equating to higher relative intensity and force demands, will be required to specifically develop the core *strength* required for athletic performance (McGill 2010). Preliminary support for this is provided by recent studies featuring more demanding core training interventions which have reported improvements in sports performance (throwing velocity) (Saeterbakken *et al.* 2011).

In order to maintain whole-body stability whilst sustaining and/or generating external forces, athletes require both strength and endurance for these muscles (Barr *et al.* 2005). These capabilities are required under a variety of static and dynamic conditions during competition. Furthermore, movements in athletic events and team sports occur in multiple directions; accordingly, players must possess lumbopelvic stability in all three planes of motion (Leetun *et al.* 2004).

An integrated approach to training the 'core'

As has been described, there are various different subsystems involved in providing lumbopelvic stability, and there are a variety of roles that these muscles are required to fulfil during athletic movement. It is therefore increasingly recognised that in addition to developing lumbopelvic stability and endurance, the optimal approach to training the 'core' should also comprise training to develop different strength qualities (Hibbs *et al.* 2008). Furthermore, these stability, endurance and strength qualities are expressed in a variety of postures and movements. It is logical that these diverse training goals will require a range of different training methods to be employed during the course of an athlete's physical preparation.

Postural stability neuromuscular training

Some authors have questioned the need for dedicated training for the postural muscles that provide local stability (Willardson 2007), based on the contention that these muscles will automatically be recruited simultaneously when athletes perform higher-intensity core exercises and more challenging exercises in the gym. It has, however, been emphasised that the deep postural muscles that provide local support and stability must not be neglected when training to develop athletes' 'core' strength and/or stability in order to avoid a scenario whereby the larger more superficial muscles attempt to compensate at the cost of restricted and impaired movement (Hibbs *et al.* 2008).

It is generally recognised that there is a need for dedicated training to develop the postural muscles and neuromuscular control capacities involved with precise control of lumbopelvic posture and maintaining whole-body equilibrium (Hibbs *et al.* 2008). This form of training comprises 'low threshold' postural movements that primarily demand endurance and motor control, which distinguishes this form of training from more intensive core training that essentially provides a strength challenge (McGill 2010).

As described in a previous section, the cues and techniques that are employed to help engage the relevant deep postural muscles when performing this form of training play a decisive role. Specifically, any cues that cause hollowing of the abdominal wall, which compromises the function of the more superficial muscles that brace the trunk, should be avoided (McGill 2006c).

'Low threshold' core exercises

These training modes comprise the more basic static floor exercises and exercises typically employed in corrective training and rehabilitation. Examples include the quadruped or 'bird-dog' exercise (McGill 2007b), supine bridge, and prone hip extension (Lewis *et al.* 2009). These exercises primarily focus on the deep lumbar stabilisers and low-intensity exercises for the hip musculature. Essentially, these exercises can be viewed as a tool to develop the athlete's motor control and recruitment of deep postural muscles and muscles of the hip girdle (Hibbs *et al.* 2008; McGill 2010). Another objective of these exercises is to develop proprioception and particularly the ability to sense lumbar spine positioning and orientation of the pelvis (Carter *et al.* 2006). The emphasis when performing these exercises is on maintaining a neutral spine posture and holding the pelvis stable.

The coaching cues employed when athletes perform these exercises appear to exert a strong influence on patterns of muscle activation and recruitment of accessory muscles. For example, the timing and degree of gluteal muscle activation when female subjects were given verbal cues to engage these muscles prior to performing a prone hip extension exercise were shown to be significantly different than when these subjects performed the same exercise without any cues (Lewis and Sahrmann 2009). The ranges of motion employed when performing these exercises also influence muscle activation and joint forces incurred (Lewis *et al.* 2009).

A critical element common to all training modes employed to develop these capabilities is the inclusion of a static hold during the exercise. This static hold element has been found to differentiate rehabilitation training modes that proved successful in developing the deep postural muscles, including multifidus (Danneels *et al.* 2001). With respect to repetition schemes, static hold durations of less than ten seconds are advocated for developing endurance in a way that avoids the adverse effects of oxygen starvation and acidosis (McGill 2010). The instruction to take a full breath during these static hold phases is designed to emphasise maintaining stabiliser muscle activation in a way that is independent of breathing patterns. The ability to maintain muscle activation during challenged breathing is a key indicator of effective versus ineffective stabiliser motor control patterns (McGill 2007a). In addition, this deep breath facilitates (partial) relaxation of the larger superficial abdominal muscles (particularly rectus abdominis), which encourages proper activation of the local lumbar stabilisers and deeper abdominal wall muscles.

One study investigated the acute effects of performing a variety of low-intensity lumbopelvic stability exercises (Crow *et al.* 2012). The exercises selected were designed to activate the gluteal muscles, and included the quadruped, supine bridge and prone single-leg hip extension. These exercises were completed prior to performing a maximal unloaded jump squat, and higher power outputs were observed in the elite team sports players studied, compared to performing either no warm-up or a warm-up on a vibration platform (Crow *et al.* 2012). It therefore appears that these exercises might serve a potentiating effect when employed as part of the warm-up prior to training and competition.

Postural control and proprioceptive training

The importance of sensorimotor control capacities in relation to core stability has been highlighted (Borghuis *et al.* 2008). Accordingly, proprioceptive training interventions employed in isolation can elicit improvements in standard measures of core stability and postural control (Romero-Franco *et al.* 2012). Proprioceptive training modes featuring domed balance training devices are similarly reported to positively influence lower limb biomechanics and the associated loading on lower limb joints (Myer *et al.* 2006a, 2006b).

This is particularly relevant to certain athlete populations, for example female athletes, who characteristically exhibit suboptimal postural traits during athletic activities (Mendiguchia *et al.* 2011).

Some of the exercises involved in developing these elements will have aspects in common with the training modes described in Chapter 3. In addition, specific balance and proprioceptive exercises can be employed which replicate the particular movements involved in the sport. For example, the implementation of a range of sprinting-specific proprioceptive exercises incorporating domed balance training devices and Swiss balls has been described for track sprinters (Romero-Franco *et al.* 2012). The training intervention employed was successful in eliciting improvements in measures of postural sway and control of centre of mass.

Lumbopelvic strength and higher load stability training modes

During the higher load training modes described in the following sections it is vital that the deep postural muscles are engaged. Conceptually the deep postural muscles represent the core of the 'core', with the larger muscles and connective tissues forming the outer layers on top. Much the same cues to those employed during postural training described above can be used to engage these muscles, and this will help to ensure pelvis and lumbar spine alignment is maintained so that the larger muscles of the hip girdle and trunk are able to function optimally. Co-contraction of these larger muscles acts to stiffen the torso to help maintain postural integrity under the loading conditions imposed by the particular exercise (McGill 2010).

The selection of higher load core strength and/or stability exercises should predominantly be executed with the spine in a neutral position, as opposed to exercises such as abdominal curls or crunches that involve repeated spine flexion. Training in a neutral spine/pelvis position better reflects the posture employed during the majority of speed and change of direction movements (McGill 2010). Furthermore, this approach also avoids a potential mechanism for low back pain and injury (McGill 2007b). The cumulative stresses from performing repetitive spine flexion and extension movements over time can exceed the failure limits of these tissues (McGill 2010). The significant hip flexor (for example, psoas) involvement that typically occurs with abdominal 'curl' or sit up exercises (Juker *et al.* 1998) also imposes considerable compressive loading on the lumbar spine (McGill 2007b). An investigation into spine loads and trunk muscle activation (that is, injury risk versus benefit) for a variety of exercises identified the sit up as having the highest compressive spine load relative to abdominal muscle activation of all the exercises studied (Axler and McGill 1997).

Static trunk stability exercises

As discussed in the previous section, exercise selection will effectively comprise progressions and variations of the front plank, bridge and side bridge exercises. There are numerous means to progress the stabilisation and strength stimulus with these exercises, with various permutations. For example, the stability challenge can be increased by incorporating contralateral limb movement to challenge equilibrium, and/or performing the exercises on a labile surface (for example, stability ball, domed training device). Performing a given exercise on a labile (that is, unstable) surface increases the stability challenge which in turn increases the level of trunk muscle activity – activation of external obliques in particular has been shown to be enhanced in the exercises studied (Vera-Garcia *et al.* 2000). Any combination of these progressions can be employed in the design of static core strength and/or stability exercises.

Variations of bridging exercises are widely advocated to develop the capacity to engage the muscles of the hip girdle whilst concurrently activating the stabilisers of the trunk (McGill 2006f). The efficacy and importance of the side bridge exercise has similarly been advocated previously (Gamble 2007a) based upon EMG data (Behm *et al.* 2005) and lower

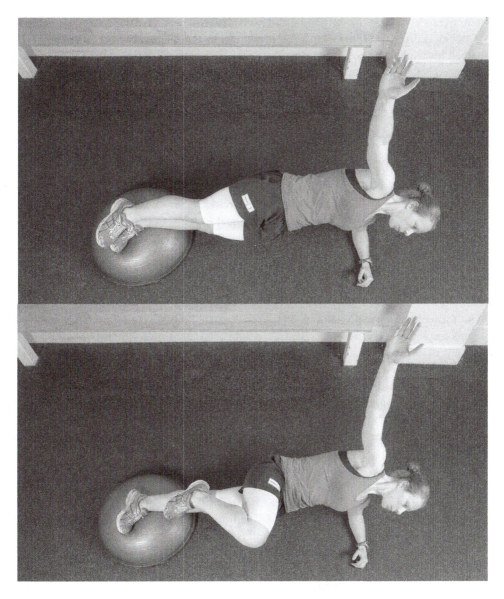

Figure 8.2 Side bridge on domed device

back compressive loads recorded during this exercise (Axler and McGill 1997). Where possible, exercise selection should favour exercises that report a high level of activation of a broad range of trunk muscles and relatively low compressive load penalty on the spine, although inevitably there will be some trade-off between these two factors.

Hip strengthening exercises

Exercise modes will include modified versions of standard exercises employed in clinical and rehabilitation settings, such as the supine bridge exercise. For example, a loaded version of the supine bridge, termed the barbell hip thrust, has become popular over recent years (Contreras *et al.* 2011). As well as the addition of external resistance, modifications associated with eccentric training approaches might also be considered. One example, using the barbell loaded bridge exercise, is that the eccentric movement might be performed on a single leg before returning to two legs for the concentric portion of the exercise.

Torsional stability training modes

As with the static trunk stability exercises described, exercise selection will predominantly feature advanced versions of standard exercises (that is, plank, bridge, side bridge). The front plank in particular is amenable to challenging torsional stability, which is reflected in its use in movement screens employed with athletes to assess this capacity (McGill 2006a). The torsional stability challenge with these exercises is mainly achieved by manipulating the points of contact – that is, moving from equal weight-bearing to a unilateral base of support. This can be done in combination with labile supporting surfaces, for example by employing domed devices or stability balls.

Unilateral resisted training modes

This form of lumbopelvic training comprises alternate limb or single-limb resisted movements employing cable resistance or free weights, executed in a weight-bearing posture. Hereby, the athlete is required to maintain postural integrity under conditions of external loading. These exercises specifically challenge the ability to brace the trunk and hip girdle in order to maintain a stationary and stable posture as the athlete performs the resisted movement with upper or lower limb(s). This form of stabilising challenge therefore features elements of both torsional stability and isometric trunk and hip muscle strength.

For example, a variety of upper limb resistance exercises performed in standing have been investigated as a trunk muscle strength training modality (Tarnanen *et al.* 2012). A previous study had noted significant levels of activation recorded from selected core muscles during alternate limb and unilateral resistance exercises (Behm *et al.* 2005). It has, therefore, been proposed that this approach might offer a superior means to elicit trunk muscle activation in the range required for gains in strength, in contrast to the relatively lower muscle-activation levels observed with common floor-based core stability exercises. In support of this contention, a range of unilateral cable-resisted upper limb exercises were reported to elicit activation levels greater than 60 per cent of maximum for selected trunk and back muscles, on both contralateral and ipsilateral side to the upper limb performing the resisted movement (Tarnanen *et al.* 2012).

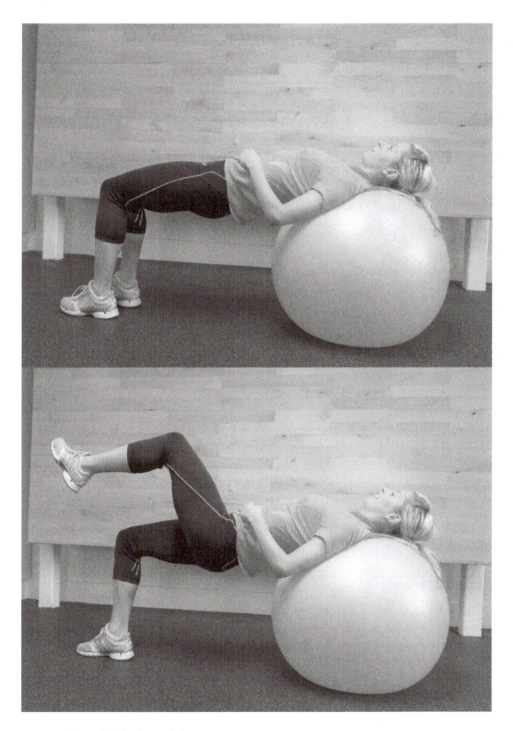

Figure 8.3 Swiss ball bridge with leg raise

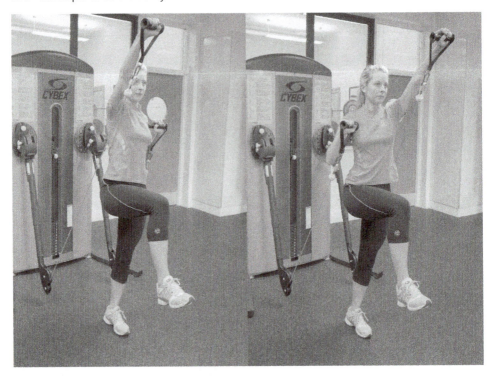

Figure 8.4 Single-leg alternate arm cable press

The importance of movement specificity has been emphasised for this form of training (Hibbs *et al.* 2008). Specifically, the recruitment and sequence of activation of trunk muscles should correspond to what occurs during movement in the sport. There is a degree of feed-forward control of trunk muscle activation, corresponding to the anticipated stabilisation challenge (Hibbs *et al.* 2008). Accordingly, in order to optimise carry-over of neural adaptations following training, the design of core strengthening exercises should aim to reflect the type of loading conditions the player is exposed to during movements encountered in their sport.

Rotational training

It has been identified that it is important to differentiate between twisting and twisting torque (McGill 2010). The combination of twisting movements performed under load can be particularly injurious for the spine. In general, the safest and best approach may be to separate twisting exercises from exercises involving rotational torques. Specifically, twisting movements should be performed under limited load, and performed chiefly by generating torque from the hips with a neutral and braced spine (McGill 2010).

While it is important to be strong and stable during movements where the hips and shoulders are aligned, it is equally critical that the athlete is able to retain lumbopelvic

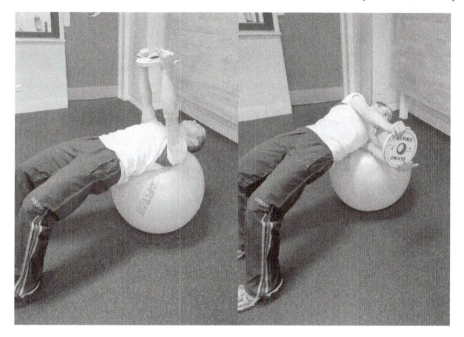

Figure 8.5 Swiss ball Russian twist

stability and posture when the pelvis and shoulders are moving independently of each other. This situation occurs not only during the flight phase when running, but also during the pivoting and twisting movements involved in change of direction activities. From this point of view, it would appear vital that exercise selection for stabilisation exercises progresses to movements where the motion of the shoulders is dissociated from the hips, and vice versa.

Conclusions

A systematic approach to athletic training for the 'core' requires that the strength and conditioning specialist accounts for all the different aspects described that underpin lumbopelvic stability. For example, low threshold core stability and postural control exercises should be performed on a daily basis, alongside a variety of higher load training modes designed to elicit greater levels of muscle activation and increase core strength. Whereas the latter core strength exercises can be integrated into the athlete's strength training workouts in the weights room, the low-intensity exercises for the local stabilisers require high degrees of concentration and focused mental attention. As such they are not amenable to the high levels of activity and psychological arousal that are characteristic of a weights room setting. Accordingly, it is recommended that these low-intensity exercises might be undertaken as a stand-alone session. Alternatively, exercises of this type have been successfully employed as part of the warm-up or prior to a workout or other training session.

As with all training, lumbopelvic stability training should incorporate progression and specificity (Cissik 2002; Stephenson and Swank 2004). In the case of dynamic lumbopelvic stability training particularly, intensity of loading and exercise selection should be implemented within the context of the athlete's periodised training plan (Stephenson and Swank 2004). Furthermore, the approach taken should reflect the needs of the individual athlete, based upon their training and injury history (Stephenson and Swank 2004). This will necessarily include relevant screening or fitness test data – such as the relationship between flexor, extensor and side bridge test endurance times (McGill 2004).

Practices on competition day, such as warm-up and athletes' activity while waiting to perform, should also not be overlooked as these appear to be key factors with respect to lumbopelvic function and lumbar spine health. A particular concern for non-starting players in team sports is the increase in lumbar spine stiffness observed from sitting on the bench waiting to enter into the game – reversing any positive effects of pre-match warm-up (Green *et al.* 2002). As such the musculature that provides lumbopelvic stability should not be overlooked during warm-up – particularly in the case of non-starting players.

9

TRAINING FOR INJURY PREVENTION

Identifying risk factors

Introduction

A major application of training for athletic preparation is to help guard against injury, and ultimately reduce the frequency and severity of injuries sustained by players in the sport. From this viewpoint one of the positive outcomes of strength training is increasing the strength and structural integrity of muscle and bone, and associated connective tissues. This effectively serves to increase the failure limits of these tissues.

Sport-specific physical conditioning can favourably influence injury risk when playing team sports. One general protective effect is that appropriately conditioned players are more resistant to the neuromuscular fatigue that renders athletes susceptible to injury (Hawkins *et al.* 2001; Murphy *et al.* 2003; Verral *et al.* 2005). The importance of this is illustrated in the common trend in many sports for higher injury rates in the latter stages of matches when players are fatigued (Best *et al.* 2005; Brooks *et al.* 2005a; Hawkins and Fuller 1999; Hawkins *et al.* 2001). Participating in metabolic conditioning appropriate to the sport serves to help guard against the negative effects of neuromuscular fatigue (Heidt *et al.* 2000; Verral *et al.* 2005).

In addition to these general protective effects of strength training and metabolic conditioning to raise players' resistance to the stresses and effects of fatigue incurred during games, another application of training is to specifically guard against the particular injuries associated with the sport (Kraemer and Fleck 2005). Specific neuromuscular and strength training interventions can be employed to target the particular risk factors and injury mechanisms associated with a certain type of injury in the sport. Therefore the logical first step when designing sport-specific injury prevention training is identifying the injuries that are characteristic of the particular sport and playing position, and the relevant risk factors associated with these injuries. Likewise, another relevant consideration is the intrinsic risk factors that might predispose each individual player to certain injuries.

Injury risk factors for team sports players

Injury risk can be stratified into intrinsic risk factors associated with the individual player and extrinsic risk factors that concern the environment in which the player trains and competes (Arnason *et al.* 2004; Quarrie *et al.* 2001). A logical first step in designing injury prevention programmes is to identify both the intrinsic risk factors specific to the individual player and the extrinsic factors associated with competing in the sport (Murphy *et al.*

2003). Once predisposing factors and typical mechanisms for injury are identified, specific preventative measures can then be taken in order to address these intrinsic and extrinsic risk factors (Arnason *et al.* 2004; Bahr and Krosshaug 2005).

Intrinsic injury risk factors

Profiling each individual player in the team offers a means to identify intrinsic risk factors. Relevant information will include age, ethnicity, gender, anthropometric characteristics, medical history (including previous and current injury status), training status and a musculoskeletal assessment that includes dynamic tests of mobility and stability. For example, age can be a predictor of general injury risk (Murphy *et al.* 2003) – older players were reported to suffer higher frequency of injuries in a cohort of senior soccer players in Iceland (Arnason *et al.* 2004). Players of black ethnic origin are identified as being more prone to certain muscle injuries – particularly hamstring muscle strains (Woods *et al.* 2004). Team sports players with high body mass index are shown to be at greater risk for certain injuries, such as non-contact ankle sprains (McHugh *et al.* 2006).

Gender is a major intrinsic risk factor for team sports injuries: female players sustain a significantly greater number of lower limb injuries (Murphy *et al.* 2003). This female gender risk factor is particularly evident for knee injury – females are two to ten times more likely to suffer ACL injury when participating in sport (Silvers and Mandelbaum 2007). Examination of NCAA injury data shows that the rate of ACL injury among female collegiate soccer and basketball players has remained constant (and consistently higher than males) over recent years, whereas rates of ACL injury in male collegiate soccer have declined over the same period 1990–2002 (Agel *et al.* 2005). This phenomenon of higher injury rates among female players endures despite considerable research attention and numerous injury prevention strategies designed to address the heightened risk of knee injury among female athletes.

Previous injury is identified as a key intrinsic risk factor that predisposes players to subsequent injury (Meeuwisse *et al.* 2003; Murphy *et al.* 2003; Quarrie *et al.* 2001). For example, senior soccer players who reported previous injuries were found to be four to seven times more likely to suffer injury – particularly repeat incidence of a prior injury (Arnason *et al.* 2004). Inadequate rehabilitation and premature return to play following injury are similarly identified as intrinsic risk factors (Murphy *et al.* 2003). The consequences of re-injury also tend to be more severe in terms of days lost post-injury in comparison to new injuries (Brooks *et al.* 2005a, 2005b).

Individual screening and functional assessment can identify intrinsic musculoskeletal risk factors (musculoskeletal and movement screening is covered in more detail in Chapter 2). Measures of joint laxity are associated with injury risk – higher levels of laxity indicative of mechanical instability are linked to increased injury incidence (Murphy *et al.* 2003). Muscle flexibility scores represent another intrinsic injury risk factor. The average pre-season hamstring and quadriceps flexibility scores of soccer players who went on to sustain hamstring and quadriceps injury during the season were lower than those who remained injury-free (Witvrouw *et al.* 2003). A similar association between decreased scores on hip range of motion and subsequent incidence of adductor muscle strains in soccer players is also reported (Arnason *et al.* 2004). Imbalances in measures of strength and flexibility are also suggested to be associated with injury risk (Knapik *et al.* 1991).

Extrinsic injury risk factors

Environment-related extrinsic risk factors concern the characteristic demands of the sport and associated training, level of competition, equipment, environmental conditions and the playing surface. The prevalence of certain types of injury tends to be characteristic of the particular sport. Players are also more likely to suffer injury during games than during practice (Murphy *et al.* 2003). Higher grades of competition within a particular sport are typically associated with greater incidence of injury in general, and also with more frequent occurrence of specific injuries – such as anterior cruciate ligament (ACL) injury (Orchard *et al.* 2001).

Errors in training design and implementation also represent major extrinsic injury risk factors. For example, poor lifting technique and incorrect movement mechanics that expose musculoskeletal structures to excessive strain can be caused by inappropriate instruction and poor coaching. Similar training errors include poor strength-training design that creates muscle imbalances or exacerbates pre-existing ones. Likewise, programming errors that impose excessive loading in terms of frequency or training volume can lead to non-functional overreaching which predisposes a player to overuse injury and injury due to residual neuromuscular fatigue.

Playing equipment may have a positive impact in terms of reducing contact injuries or a negative impact. Negative examples include football shoes that increase the traction between the shoe and playing surface in a way that resulted in a rise in ACL injuries (Lambson *et al.* 1996) and basketball shoes with air cells in the heel that were associated with four times greater incidence of ankle injuries, presumably by decreasing rearfoot stability (McKay *et al.* 2001). Positive examples include the introduction of mandatory full face masks in collegiate ice hockey that has served to dramatically reduce facial and dental injuries (Flik *et al.* 2005). Paradoxically, protective equipment may also lead to more aggressive play and risk-taking, which can in fact cause an increased number of injuries (Bahr and Krosshaug 2005). The interaction between environmental conditions and the playing surface is an important factor from an injury risk viewpoint – particularly with respect to the effect of weather conditions on resistance between the playing surface and the sports shoe (Orchard *et al.* 2001).

Epidemiological studies reporting injury data for representative groups participating in a particular team sport offer a means to help identify the extrinsic risk factors associated with the sport. Participation in a team sport involves inherent risk that may also vary for different playing positions; in turn this will tend to be reflected in the particular injuries reported. Injury surveillance data therefore provides a useful source of information about the relative incidence of different types and sites of injury in the sport. Such data may also offer further insight into specific risks associated with different playing positions, relative risk of injury during training versus competition, and the frequency and types of injury common to different phases of play (Shankar *et al.* 2007).

Representative injury data for selected team sports

Baseball

The majority of injuries associated with baseball concern the shoulder complex; the typical injury mechanism is linked to repetitively performing the throwing motion during practices and games. Common injuries reported involve the rotator cuff musculature, and onset is typically relatively insidious – hence most are classed as overuse injuries (Mullaney *et al.* 2005). An apparent critical factor with respect to incidence of shoulder impingement injury is that there is appropriate balance between those muscles that act to hold the head of the humerus in the shoulder socket and the muscles that accelerate the throwing arm.

Potential for damage would appear to be increased by deterioration of sound throwing technique due to the effects of fatigue. That said, pitchers were found to be quite resistant to fatigue-related changes in pitching kinematics and kinetics during a simulated game under controlled conditions (Escamilla *et al.* 2007). A study assessing muscular fatigue reported that the collegiate and minor league pitchers examined were similarly resilient on a variety of upper and lower limb strength-test measures with modest, albeit statistically significant, differences between pre-game and post-game force output scores (Mullaney *et al.* 2005). The lack of significant reduction in force output scores of the external rotator musculature found in this study may, however, have been a consequence of the fact that they contract in an eccentric fashion during the pitching action; force output tends to be much better maintained with repeated eccentric muscle contractions.

Similarly, issues associated with the relative timing of hip, trunk and shoulder rotation during the throwing action have also been identified as potential causative factors for shoulder and upper limb pain and injury in baseball (Aguinaldo *et al.* 2007). Specifically, the magnitude and sequential timing of rotation between hip, trunk and shoulder determines how angular momentum is transferred from these segments to the shoulder and distal upper limb joints. If the timing of this sequential motion is not optimal, there will be a loss of angular momentum for which the player must compensate by generating greater torques at the shoulder and upper limb in order to maintain throwing velocity (Aguinaldo *et al.* 2007). This scenario is suggested to influence the incidence of shoulder and elbow pain and injury, particularly among less skilled players, as greater torques generated at the upper limb joints will place increased strain upon these joints and connective tissue structures. One study identified that the relative timing of trunk rotation in the pitching action differentiated professional players from pitchers at college, high school and youth level (Aguinaldo *et al.* 2007). Professional players were found to initiate trunk rotation much later in the pitching cycle, and in turn these players reported lower internal rotation torques at the pitching shoulder in comparison to college and high school players.

Baseball pitchers often exhibit altered range of motion and strength ratios on their dominant (throwing arm) side compared to their non-dominant side. Specifically, a common finding is reduced range of motion in internal rotation accompanied with increased external rotation on the dominant versus non-dominant side (Mullaney *et al.* 2005). These changes in flexibility are mirrored by adaptations in muscular strength for these opposing movements. Pitchers commonly achieve higher force output in internal rotation but exhibit compromised external rotation force measured on their throwing arm in comparison to the contralateral side (Mullaney *et al.* 2005). Similarly, compromised strength scores are reported for specific tests of rotator cuff muscle strength – specifically supraspinatus – in these players.

A common complaint among young baseball players concerns damage to the epiphyseal cartilage at the head of the humerus (Sabick *et al.* 2005). A condition called 'Little League shoulder', or sometimes termed humeral epiphysiolysis, is prevalent among young pitchers – essentially arising from repeated trauma to the growth plate at the neck of the humerus.

Key factors in the incidence of this injury appear to be the combination of high rotational stresses and distraction forces during the throwing action, and weakness of the developing musculoskeletal system (Sabick *et al.* 2005). It has been suggested that it is the torsional forces during throwing in particular which are likely to be the major cause of damage to the epiphysis, given that growth plates are less resilient to this type of loading.

Soccer

Available data indicate that an elite male soccer player can expect to sustain one performance-limiting injury each season (Junge and Dvorak 2004). Senior players competing in the top two divisions in Iceland were reported to sustain 24.6 injuries per 1,000 player hours during matches and 2.1 injuries per 1,000 hours in training (Arnason *et al.* 2004). A study of four English professional soccer clubs reported injury incidence of 27.7 injuries per 1,000 player hours during matches and 3.4 injuries per 1,000 player hours for training (Hawkins and Fuller 1999). The incidence of injury during both matches and training among youth players at the same English professional clubs was markedly higher – 37.2 and 4.1 injuries/1,000 player hours for matches and training respectively (Hawkins and Fuller 1999).

Injuries commonly reported in soccer are lower limb – typically involving ankle and knee joints, and the thigh and calf musculature (Junge and Dvorak 2004). Lower limb injuries comprised 82 per cent of all injuries during a season of competition in the senior elite leagues in Iceland (Arnason *et al.* 2004) and 87 per cent of all injuries in English professional soccer (Hawkins *et al.* 2001). In an earlier study of English professional soccer the most common sites of lower limb injuries were the thigh (23 per cent of total), ankle (17 per cent), knee (14 per cent) and lower leg (13 per cent) (Hawkins and Fuller 1999). The majority of injuries observed were muscle strains (41 per cent of total injuries); sprains (20 per cent) and contusions (20 per cent) were the next most common types of injury.

A high incidence of muscle strains is reported in soccer: 8.4 injuries per 1,000 match hours and 0.8 injuries per 1,000 training hours were recorded during a season of competition at elite senior level in Iceland (Arnason *et al.* 2004). Due to the demands of the sport, soccer players are at particular risk for both hamstring (Verral *et al.* 2005) and adductor muscle injuries (Arnason *et al.* 2004; Nicholas and Tyler 2002). Joint and ligament sprains are likewise relatively common: reported at 5.5 injuries per 1,000 match hours and 0.4 injuries per 1,000 training hours in Icelandic senior elite soccer, most involving knee or ankle (Arnason *et al.* 2004). Over three-quarters of knee ligament injuries recorded in English professional soccer were to the medial collateral ligament (MCL) (Hawkins and Fuller 1999; Hawkins *et al.* 2001). However, severe knee ligament injuries in soccer most often involve the anterior cruciate ligament (ACL) (Arnason *et al.* 2004; Hawkins and Fuller 1999).

On average, injuries reported in English professional soccer resulted in 24.2 days lost to training and competition (Hawkins *et al.* 2001). Around a third of injuries reportedly result from bodily contact with another player (Junge and Dvorak 2004) – player contact was identified in 41 per cent of all injuries in English professional soccer (Hawkins and Fuller 1999). Both senior professionals and youth players are also reported to sustain more injuries to their dominant leg – reflecting players' greater use of their dominant leg when tackling and being tackled (Hawkins and Fuller 1999; Hawkins *et al.* 2001). Non-contact injuries are typically incurred when running or changing direction.

Studies of soccer players typically report a high incidence of re-injury; repeat injuries make up between a fifth and a quarter of all injuries sustained (Hawkins and Fuller 1999; Junge and Dvorak 2004). Such findings indicate that previous injury is a major risk factor for subsequent injury in soccer (Arnason *et al.* 2004). The severity of re-injuries with respect to time lost also tends to be greater than with the original injury (Hawkins *et al.* 2001). There is therefore a suggestion that rehabilitation undertaken in elite-level soccer – particularly following ankle sprains and posterior thigh strains – is insufficient or incomplete (Hawkins and Fuller 1999; Junge and Dvorak 2004).

Training injuries in English professional soccer appear to peak in July, coinciding with the end of pre-season training, whereas match injuries show a peak at the start of the playing season in August (Hawkins *et al.* 2001). This has led to suggestions that the content and effectiveness of pre-season physical preparation and adherence to off-season maintenance training may be inadequate. Conversely, the number of injuries among youth players also tends to rise towards the end of the playing season (Hawkins and Fuller 1999). In this case, cumulative fatigue associated with the burden of a large number of matches may play a role in the injury patterns observed with these young players.

Depending on the injury definition, overall injury rates for elite senior female soccer players appear to be similar to the corresponding data reported for males. Rates of 'traumatic' (as opposed to overuse) injury reported during matches in the German national league were 23.3 per 1,000 player hours during matches and 2.8 per 1,000 player hours during training (Faude *et al.* 2005). Reported match and training injury incidence among professional female soccer players in the United States were lower, possibly due to the different methods used in collecting injury data (Giza *et al.* 2005). The majority of injuries reported in elite senior women's soccer are lower limb – comprising between 60 per cent (Giza *et al.* 2005) and 80 per cent of total injuries (Faude *et al.* 2005). A study of female high school soccer players in the United States reported that all injuries sustained by 300 participating players (ages 14–18 years) during a season of play were to the lower limb (Heidt *et al.* 2000).

For the most part, injuries sustained by female soccer players appear evenly distributed between thigh, knee and ankle (Faude *et al.* 2005); however, a study of professional women's soccer in the United States has reported a relatively large number of head and/or facial injuries (Giza *et al.* 2005). Another study indicated that female soccer players may be prone to lower back injury (Nadler *et al.* 2002). This is supported by the surprisingly large number of back injuries reported by female players in the German national league (Faude *et al.* 2005). Women's soccer appears to involve a higher number of (lower limb) joint and/or ligament sprains but a lower proportion of muscle strains in comparison to men's soccer (Faude *et al.* 2005; Giza *et al.* 2005).

Another apparent difference is that injuries sustained by female soccer players are also more likely to be severe (Heidt *et al.* 2000). Of particular concern is the high incidence of ACL injury among female soccer players, especially during matches – reported to be in the region of 0.90 (Giza *et al.* 2005) to 2.2 ACL injuries per 1,000 player match hours (Faude *et al.* 2005) in elite senior women's soccer. A review of NCAA injury data also revealed that female collegiate soccer players sustained significantly more ACL injuries than male collegiate soccer players (Agel *et al.* 2005). Furthermore, a greater proportion of these ACL injuries sustained by female collegiate soccer players resulted from non-contact mechanisms compared to the corresponding data for male players.

Volleyball

The incidence of injury in volleyball is estimated at 4.1 injuries per 1,000 player hours during matches and 1.8 per 1,000 player hours during training (Verhagen *et al.* 2004). The majority of acute injuries reported in volleyball involve the lower limb and the most common type of injury is ligament strain. Ankle was the reported site of injury comprising 41 out of the 100 injuries reported in male and female volleyball players during the course of a season in Holland (Verhagen *et al.* 2004) – ankle inversion sprains in particular are very common (Stasinopoulos 2004). Nearly two-thirds of ankle sprains reportedly occur when players are at the net, sometimes due to contact with team-mates or opponents upon landing (Verhagen *et al.* 2004).

In contrast to the data for men's volleyball, female volleyball players appear to suffer a similar number of injuries during practice and competition. Injury rates during NCAA competition in the United States, although slightly greater (4.58 per 1,000 exposures), were not markedly higher than those during practice (4.1 injuries per 1,000 exposures) (Agel *et al.* 2007c). Ankle ligament sprains comprised 44.1 per cent of game injuries and 29.4 per cent of injuries during practice; the greater number of ankle injuries in games is partly due to the larger proportion of ankle injuries involving player contact during competition versus practice. Shoulder injuries are also quite commonly reported during games and practices in women's volleyball – particularly muscle and/or tendon strain injury (Agel *et al.* 2007c).

There appears to be a particular risk of re-injury following ankle sprains in volleyball (Verhagen *et al.* 2004) – a quarter of players reporting ankle injury had sustained an ankle injury during the preceding twelve months. Volleyball is also associated with particular overuse injuries most often involving the shoulder or lower back, with knee injuries being the third most common overuse injury reported by volleyball players (Verhagen *et al.* 2004).

Elite volleyball players appear to exhibit various musculoskeletal issues associated with the shoulder on their dominant side, which are identified as risk factors for overuse shoulder injury (Wang and Cochrane 2001). A study of elite volleyball players reported high incidence of a range of disorders, including: (dominant versus non-dominant side) muscular imbalance; restricted shoulder mobility; impaired eccentric strength; relative weakness in external rotation; and scapular asymmetry. Of these conditions, the imbalance between concentric internal rotator muscle strength and eccentric external rotator strength on the dominant side was shown to be significantly related with reported incidence of shoulder injury and pain in elite English volleyball players (Wang and Cochrane 2001).

Another reportedly common condition among volleyball players is patellar tendinosis – a knee joint extensor overuse injury more commonly known as 'jumper's knee' (Gisslen *et al.* 2005). The incidence of this overuse injury is likely to be underestimated by injury surveillance studies, as players will tend to continue to play matches despite experiencing pain (Verhagen *et al.* 2004). 'Jumper's knee' afflicts a large proportion of volleyball players over the course of their career and is even reported to be quite prevalent among elite junior players (Gisslen *et al.* 2005).

Basketball

A study of injury surveillance data from collegiate basketball in the United States reported the incidence of injuries during games to be 9.9 injuries per 1,000 athlete exposures during

NCAA competition (Dick *et al.* 2007b). This is markedly higher than a study of men's intercollegiate basketball in Canada, which reported an overall injury rate of 4.94 injuries per 1,000 athlete exposures (Meeuwisse *et al.* 2003). This latter study also noted that injury rates for minor injuries (causing less than seven sessions to be missed) were similar between games and practices in Canadian collegiate competition, but the incidence of more severe injuries was 3.7 times higher during games than during practice. The rates of injury reported during practices in NCAA competition is 4.3 per 1,000 athlete exposures (Dick *et al.* 2007b).

The majority of injuries reported in NCAA men's basketball involved the lower limb, with ankle ligament sprains comprising 26.2 per cent of game injuries and 26.8 per cent of practice injuries (Dick *et al.* 2007b). The ankle was also the most frequently reported site of injuries in Canadian collegiate basketball but injuries to the knee resulted in the most time out of participation (Meeuwisse *et al.* 2003). Knee injuries similarly made up a substantial number of injuries (approximately 10 per cent of all game and practice injuries) reported in NCAA basketball – most commonly 'internal knee derangement' (ligament and/or cartilage injury) or patellar injuries (Dick *et al.* 2007b). Although not generally classed as a contact sport, a third of the injuries reported in Canadian intercollegiate basketball resulted from contact with another player (Meeuwisse *et al.* 2003). That said, ACL injuries in men's intercollegiate basketball are more commonly non-contact (Agel *et al.* 2005, Dick *et al.* 2007b). Most injuries were reported to occur in the 'key' area of the court and of all the playing positions the most injuries were recorded by centres (Meeuwisse *et al.* 2003).

The reported rate of injury during matches in women's collegiate basketball in the United States was 7.68 injuries per 1,000 athlete exposures (Agel *et al.* 2007b). This value appears to be lower (3.66 injuries per 1,000 athlete exposures during games) among female players competing at high school level (Borowski *et al.* 2008). The majority of injuries in women's basketball involve the lower limb, representing over 60 per cent of all injuries sustained in women's collegiate basketball in the United States (Agel *et al.* 2007b). A study of high school basketball reported that 35.9 per cent of injuries sustained by female players involved the ankle and/or foot region, and the knee (18.2 per cent of all injuries) was the second most common site of injury (Borowski *et al.* 2008). An earlier study reported that the lower back is the third most prevalent site of injury in women's basketball (Nadler *et al.* 2002). More recent injury reporting studies from women's collegiate and high school basketball in the United States reported the head and/or face to be the third most prevalent site of injury (Agel *et al.* 2007b, Borowski *et al.* 2008).

The most reported single injury in women's basketball at high school level is knee ligament sprain (Borowski *et al.* 2008). At collegiate level, knee 'internal derangement' injury is the second most reported injury in both games and practices (ankle ligament injury is the most common) (Agel *et al.* 2007b). In women's basketball knee injuries were reported to comprise up to 91 per cent of season-ending injuries (Ford *et al.* 2003). NCAA injury data spanning 1990–2002 report that the rate of ACL injury was significantly higher for female collegiate basketball players than males (Agel *et al.* 2005). The majority (ranging from 64.3 per cent–89.7 per cent of total depending on the year) of ACL injuries sustained by female collegiate players were the result of non-contact mechanisms. The pattern of ankle injuries monitored during a playing season in female professional basketball peaked during the initial two months (particularly the first month) following the start of the season

(Kofotolis and Kellis 2007). This would appear to indicate inadequate or inappropriate physical preparation of players during pre-season.

A high proportion of injuries in female basketball involve player-to-player contact, representing 46 per cent of all injuries sustained during games of female collegiate basketball in the United States (Agel *et al.* 2007b). Similarly, a study of Greek female professional basketball in Europe identified that the majority of ankle sprains during matches occurred within the 'key' area of the court (that is, the scoring zone in front of the posts) (Kofotolis and Kellis 2007). This was attributed to the greater number of ankle sprain injuries involving player-to-player contact within these areas. In accordance with this, the playing positions which most frequently engage in contesting possession within the 'key' area of the court were also reported to suffer the highest incidence of ankle injury in female professional basketball in Europe (Kofotolis and Kellis 2007).

Netball

There is a paucity of published studies documenting injury incidence in netball, particularly at elite level (Gamble 2011). Based upon the available studies, the majority of injuries in netball involve the lower limb (McManus *et al.* 2006) and the predominant type of injury is ligament sprain or disruption (Hume and Steele 2000; Stevenson *et al.* 2000). The majority of injuries are sustained during competitive matches rather than practices (Saunders and Otago 2009). The ankle is the most frequent reported site of injury for both recreational and elite players, followed by the knee (McManus *et al.* 2006; Saunders and Otago 2009). In particular, lateral ankle sprain has previously been identified as the single injury most commonly reported in netball (Hopper *et al.* 1999). This injury in netball is typically associated with landing in a plantar-flexed foot position, combined with forced inversion upon landing.

Ankle injuries sustained in netball are reported to be frequently associated with landing and also player-to-player contact (Hume and Steele 2000; Saunders and Otago 2009). The prevalence of ankle injuries in netball (Hopper *et al.* 1999) combined with the high rate of recurrence with this injury (Swenson *et al.* 2009) may predispose netball players to the syndrome known as 'chronic ankle instability' (Holmes and Delahunt 2009). A study of netball indicated almost half of injuries sustained by players during state championships were recurrences of previous injuries (Hume and Steele 2000).

American football

A recent and comprehensive injury surveillance study for American football reported an injury rate in high school and college football in the United States that is almost twice that of basketball (the second most popular sport among males in these age groups) (Shankar *et al.* 2007). This was supported by injury surveillance data from NCAA competition in the United States which reported 36 injuries per 1,000 athlete exposures for games – three and a half times the rate reported for NCAA men's basketball (Dick *et al.* 2007a). There was a greater relative injury incidence overall for collegiate versus high school football (Shankar *et al.* 2007). Unsurprisingly a high incidence of contact injuries is reported – the majority being sustained when tackling or being tackled (Shankar *et al.* 2007).

The sites and types of injury appear to be broadly similar between high school and collegiate football. One study reported injuries to the knee (16.4 per cent of all injuries) were most common in collegiate football, followed by the shoulder (13.2 per cent of total) and then ankle (12.7 per cent) (Shankar *et al.* 2007). NCAA data indicated a similar pattern; however, the ankle ranked as the second most common site of game injuries (Dick *et al.* 2007a). In high school football, knee (15.2 per cent of all injuries) and ankle (also 15.2 per cent of total) were the most frequent sites of injury, followed by the shoulder (12.4 per cent of total injuries). Concussions made up a significant number of game injuries in NCAA men's football (Dick *et al.* 2007a). There is similarly a high reported incidence of concussions in high school football (Shankar *et al.* 2007).

Competitive play accounts for a considerably higher rate of injury than practice sessions at both high school (*c.* four times greater injury rate) and collegiate level (nearly eight times higher) (Shankar *et al.* 2007). The injury rate during practices for NCAA players was reported to be approximately 4 injuries per 1,000 athlete exposures for practice in the fall (autumn), whereas during spring practice the rate was appreciably higher – approximately 10 injuries per 1,000 athlete exposures (Dick *et al.* 2007a). During games there are a lower proportion of muscle and/or tendon strains (high school: 10 per cent during games versus 24 per cent during practices; college: 14 per cent games versus 25 per cent practices) (Shankar *et al.* 2007). Conversely, a higher proportion of ligament sprains is reported during competitive play (high school: 33 per cent during games versus 29 per cent practices; college: 39 per cent games versus 25 per cent practices) (Shankar *et al.* 2007).

Most injuries during practices are ligament sprains and muscle and/or tendon strains, which jointly comprised 53 per cent of reported practice injuries in high school football and 50 per cent of total collegiate football practice injuries (Shankar *et al.* 2007). Injuries during practices in high school football are less severe, with a faster return to play than those sustained during competition. It has been identified that practices during the spring season have a two- or three-fold higher injury rate in collegiate football (Dick *et al.* 2007a), with a particular increase in the number in severe injuries (Albright *et al.* 2004). This appears to be a consequence of players striving to compete for selection for the upcoming fall (autumn) season. The same study noted that of all strings of players (in terms of ranking order for selection) the 'non-players' (those rated as unlikely to be selected) sustained by far the greatest number of injuries during practices (Albright *et al.* 2004). This is likely a reflection of their typical role as 'cannon fodder' during practices.

For both high school and collegiate football, running plays are reported to account for the greatest number of injuries during games (Shankar *et al.* 2007). Running plays are also reported to result in more severe injuries, with the greatest number of season-ending injuries occurring during running plays. In keeping with this, the most frequently injured playing positions reported in high school football are offensive linemen and running backs, and linebackers are the most injured defensive positions (Shankar *et al.* 2007). At collegiate level, although these playing positions continue to be among the most injured positions, wide receivers also have a similarly high incidence of injury (12.3 per cent of total injuries) to running backs (12.1 per cent of total). Regardless of playing level, running backs reported the highest incidence of ankle injury of any playing position (Shankar *et al.* 2007). The data for match injuries indicate that passing plays most commonly result in injuries to wide receivers (offence) and cornerbacks (defence) – unsurprising given the high involvement of these playing positions in such plays (Shankar *et al.* 2007).

Rugby union football

Due to the contact nature of the sport, rugby union football has a high reported incidence of injury. Risk of injury also appears to increase as players progress towards higher levels of competition (Quarrie *et al.* 2001). The most extensive epidemiological study to date in professional rugby union was undertaken in the United Kingdom, with full participation of all English Premiership clubs over two seasons (Brooks *et al.* 2005a). Overall incidence of injury during domestic matches was reported to be 91 injuries per 1,000 player-hours – considerably higher than is reported for other professional team sports. Incidence of injury reported at international level is higher still – 97.9 per 1,000 player-hours during the 2003 World Cup competition (Best *et al.* 2005).

Perhaps unsurprisingly, contact injuries comprise the majority of injuries recorded during match-play (72 per cent) in professional rugby union (Brooks *et al.* 2005a). This is similar to findings reported in elite junior rugby union in Australia (McManus and Cross 2004). Forward positions (responsible for contesting possession) have a higher incidence of contact injuries due to their involvement in set-piece phases (scrum, line-out and kick-off). Similarly, forwards sustain a higher number of contact injuries when contesting possession at rucks or mauls, whereas contact injuries sustained by the back positions are more typically 'tackle injuries' – that is, occurring when tackling or being tackled (Brooks *et al.* 2005a). As a group, backs are reported to sustain a greater number of non-contact injuries during domestic senior professional matches – this was also reported to be the case in elite junior rugby union in Australia (McManus and Cross 2004).

The lower limb is the most frequent site of injury in rugby union football and the most frequent reported lower limb injury in professional domestic rugby is thigh haematoma (Brooks *et al.* 2005a), albeit the severity of such injuries was typically minor in terms of time lost. Hamstring injuries were the second most common injury during matches, reflecting their high incidence among players in the back positions. Knee injuries represent the most costly injuries in professional rugby union: the moderately high incidence of knee injuries combined with their high average severity accounts for the fact that these injuries result in the greatest number of days' absence from training and competition of any injury type (Brooks *et al.* 2005a; Dallalana *et al.* 2007). A high proportion of knee injuries reported in matches (72 per cent) are sustained during contact (Dallalana *et al.* 2007). Tackle situations – particularly being tackled – account for a large number of the ACL (72 per cent) and MCL (46 per cent) injuries that occur during matches. Shoulder injuries have the second highest average severity in terms of days absence per injury (Brooks *et al.* 2005a) – reflecting that this is the typical site of impact when tackling opposing players (Gamble 2004b).

The different playing positions in rugby union have designated and quite special-ised roles during play, and as such there is a greater distinction between positions – for example in comparison to rugby league (Gamble 2004b). This is reflected in marked differences between individual playing positions in terms of type, incidence and severity of injury sustained during matches (Brooks *et al.* 2005a). For example, fly half (back) and hooker (forward) positions reported the highest frequency of injury during domestic professional matches, whereas the most severe injuries tended to involve right locks and open-side flankers (forwards). Overall, the playing positions at most risk (in terms of both frequency and severity of injury reported) appear to be hooker (forward) and outside centre (back) in these domestic professional games. Data from international (2003 World Cup) competition indicated injury rates were highest for Number 8, open-side flanker (forwards) and outside centre (back) positions (Best *et al.* 2005). Similarly, the Number 8 and flanker positions were found to be the playing positions most at risk of injury in an elite junior rugby union squad competing in the Australian National Championships (McManus and Cross 2004).

Unsurprisingly, there is a much lower relative incidence of injury reported in professional rugby union during training – regardless of the type of training (Brooks *et al.* 2005b). Conversely, the severity of training injuries in terms of days lost is greater than that for injuries sustained during matches. The majority of training injuries reported are lower limb and mainly comprise either muscle and/or tendon strains or ligament sprains. Contact skills practices involve the highest injury rate; however, running conditioning also accounts for a large proportion of training injuries and non-contact injuries comprise a higher percentage (57 per cent) of the total training injuries reported (Brooks *et al.* 2005b). Strength training shows the lowest injury rates of all training modes, albeit the greater number of lumbar disc and/or nerve root injuries reported by forwards (as compared to backs) are attributed to strength training (Brooks *et al.* 2005b).

Rugby league football

As is the case with rugby union, the majority of injuries sustained during matches in rugby league football are tackle injuries (Gabbett 2004). The act of being tackled in particular is a leading cause of injury in senior professional rugby league, as it is in rugby union. At amateur level, tackling (as opposed to being tackled) appears to account for a greater proportion of the total injuries during matches – possibly due to lower levels of defensive skills (Gabbett 2004).

Another finding in common with rugby union is that injury rates in rugby league increase at higher levels of competition (Gabbett 2004). The head and neck are the most common sites of injury reported during matches among rugby league players (Gabbett 2004). Muscular injuries are the most common types of injuries during rugby league matches at all levels of competition.

Rugby league football has a lesser emphasis on set-piece phases of play and possession is not contested after each tackle is made; consequently playing positions in rugby league are more homogeneous in comparison to rugby union. Even so, as a group the forward positions tend to make and receive more tackles during a match and this is reflected in higher overall incidence of injury among forwards compared to backs at all levels of competition (Gabbett 2004).

Rugby league football studies also report that injury rates during training are much lower than in matches (Gabbett 2004). The majority of reported training injuries sustained by rugby league players are lower limb, with most being muscle strains. This mirrors the findings reported in professional rugby union football. A study of rugby league players showed that the use of skill-based conditioning games may reduce the incidence of training injuries during conditioning activities – in comparison to traditional running-based conditioning without any game skills element (Gabbett 2002).

Australian rules football

A study of the Australian Football League over three seasons (1997–2000) reported that the incidence of new injuries during matches was 25.7 injuries per 1,000 player hours (Orchard and Seward 2002). There was also a high reported frequency of recurrence of previous injuries. The thigh was the most frequently reported site of injury in the Australian Football League; the most common injury type being muscle strains (Orchard and Seward 2002). Hamstring muscle injuries are a particular concern for the sport (Verral et al. 2005), especially given the very high (34 per cent) recurrence rate reported for this injury as compared to the 17 per cent overall recurrence rate for all injuries in this study.

Following hamstring muscle strains, ACL ligament sprains are the next most prevalent injury reported in the Australian Football League – the majority of which are attributed to a non-contact mechanism (Orchard and Seward 2002). The relative incidence of complete ACL tears during matches in the Australian Football League was reported to be 0.82 ACL injuries per 1,000 player-match exposures and 0.62 injuries per 1,000 player-match exposures for non-contact ACL tears specifically (Orchard et al. 2001). A history of ACL reconstruction was identified as a significant intrinsic risk factor for these injuries in Australian rules football players. Extrinsic risk factors identified as affecting ACL injury incidence in Australian Football League matches included weather conditions over the period preceding a game. Specifically, 28-day evaporation values and rainfall over the year prior to the game were identified as influencing frequency of ACL tears – likely due to the associated impact upon shoe-playing surface traction when there were particularly dry pitch conditions (Orchard et al. 2001).

Ice hockey

A study of Division One collegiate men's ice hockey in the United States reported injury rates during matches as 13.8 per 1,000 player exposures and 2.2 per 1,000 player exposures during practice (Flik et al. 2005). The majority of injuries reported were attributed to contact – occurring during collisions with opponents (32.8 per cent of all injuries) or the perimeter boards surrounding the playing area (18.6 per cent of total injuries). The most common sites of injuries reported with these players were knee and/or leg (22 per cent of total), head (19 per cent of total), and shoulder (15 per cent) (Flik et al. 2005).

Concussion was the single most frequently reported injury in American collegiate men's ice hockey – representing 18.6 per cent of all reported injuries – the majority of which occurred during competitive matches (Flik et al. 2005). Illegal activity – specifically elbowing – was identified as being the cause of many concussions during games. Forwards sustained the most concussions – suffering twice the number of concussion injuries reported by defensemen (Flik et al. 2005). MCL strains were the second most frequently reported injury in the study – all of them occurring during games. Another frequently reported injury that is particularly severe in terms of time lost is syndesmotic or 'high ankle' sprain – an injury that appears to be much more common in ice hockey than other sports. This reported incidence of ankle syndesmotic sprain injury appears fairly evenly distributed between games and practices (Flik et al. 2005).

It has been reported that overall injury incidence did not appear to differ significantly between collegiate men's and women's ice hockey in Canada (Schick and Meeuwisse 2003).

However, the women's collegiate ice hockey players featured in the study had played far fewer games. When match data were compared, injury rates were significantly higher: 22.4 injuries per 1,000 match exposures for men versus 10.43 injuries per 1,000 match exposures for female collegiate ice hockey players (Schick and Meeuwisse 2003). Injury surveillance data over four seasons following the start of NCAA women's ice hockey competition in the United States in 2001 reported 12.6 injuries per 1,000 athlete exposures in games, compared to 2.5 injuries per 1,000 athlete exposures during practices (Agel *et al.* 2007b). These data are broadly similar to the injury data previously reported for women's collegiate competition in Canada (Schick and Meeuwisse 2003).

Female ice hockey has key differences in the playing rules: games are shorter in length and the rules prohibit intentional body checking. Despite this, the vast majority of injuries that were reported in female ice hockey (96 per cent of the total) were categorised as contact injuries (Schick and Meeuwisse 2003). NCAA data mirrored this finding with approximately half of all injuries sustained during women's collegiate ice hockey involving player contact (Agel *et al.* 2007a). Even so, data from Canadian collegiate competition indicated the severity of injuries suffered in collegiate women's ice hockey was less in terms of time lost subsequent to injury – the male collegiate players in the study reportedly sustained a much higher number of injuries which were categorised as severe (resulted in more than fourteen missed sessions following injury) (Schick and Meeuwisse 2003).

As is the case with male players, the most common injury in women's collegiate ice hockey in Canada was reported to be concussion; the next most common injuries were ankle sprains and adductor muscle strains (Schick and Meeuwisse 2003). NCAA data were broadly similar – concussions being the most common injury (21.6 per cent of total injuries), with knee internal derangement (12.9 per cent of total) and shoulder – specifically acromioclavicular joint injury – (6.8 per cent of total) being next common (Agel *et al.* 2007b). Canadian male collegiate players also suffered a number of facial injuries, which were not reported at all during collegiate women's ice hockey participation in Canada (Schick and Meeuwisse 2003).

Analysis of risk factors for injury prevention training interventions

In addition to players' routine strength training, particular strength and neuromuscular training exercises may also be prescribed to specifically guard against common injuries reported in the sport. This specific injury prevention role for strength training has not received the research attention it would appear to merit. Too often, specific strength exercises are only prescribed for team sports players once an injury has already occurred (Wagner 2003). Although there are a growing number of studies detailing injury data for different sports, there are very few that assess injury prevention strategies for sports. For example, despite soccer's status as the most popular sport in the world, a review of the literature pertaining to injury prevention for soccer players found only four relevant studies that met inclusion criteria (Olsen *et al.* 2004).

The process of specific training prescription should begin with a needs analysis of the particular sport, including research into the injuries commonly sustained during competition. After examining injury data for the sport, the injury history of each player and any ongoing injury concerns will then help to highlight the specific needs of each individual.

Such analysis of the sport combined with an assessment of the individual will identify what areas of the body are prone to what type of injury.

Once identified, the design of the injury prevention intervention programme should aim to systematically address risk factors for each specific injury identified for the sport and the athlete (Nicholas and Tyler 2002). Such preventative measures can only be taken by first gaining an understanding of the causative factors and injury mechanisms that are characteristic of the particular injury (Bahr and Krosshaug 2005). Such data for injuries that are representative of different team sports are increasingly available (Junge and Dvorak 2004) – and these are summarised in the next section.

Risk factors and injury mechanisms for identified injuries

Ankle complex

The lower leg is the most frequent site of injury in the majority of sports (Thacker *et al.* 2003). Ankle sprains comprise up to a third of all injuries sustained during participation in sports (Osborne and Rizzo 2003). Once injured, the risk of subsequent re-injury to the ankle is greatly increased (Osborne and Rizzo 2003). Elite and recreational basketball players with a history of ankle injury were reported to have a five times greater likelihood of sustaining an ankle injury (McKay *et al.* 2001). Collegiate American football players who had suffered previous ankle injury are similarly reported to suffer six times higher ankle injury incidence (Tyler *et al.* 2006).

Ankle inversion sprain injury

Ligament laxity is commonly observed following ankle sprain injuries, which results in decreased mechanical stability provided to the ankle joint (Wikstrom *et al.* 2007). In addition to this reduced mechanical stability post-injury, neuromuscular and proprioceptive function is frequently also impaired; the function of afferent sensors originating in the joint are often disrupted following ankle ligament injury (Lephart *et al.* 1998). A consequence of this interference in somatosensory feedback is that the player is less able to sense joint position and motion at the ankle joint (Hertel 2008). This disruption of proprioception and neural control post-injury is termed 'functional ankle instability', and is associated with deficits in postural balance and 'dynamic stabilisation' (see Chapter 3) (Wikstrom *et al.* 2007).

In severe cases, recurrent ankle injury can lead to chronic ankle instability (CAI), which describes a pattern of recurrent ankle sprain injury with persisting symptoms of instability, such as episodes of the ankle giving way during normal activities. Various sensorimotor and mechanical deficits have been identified in those suffering with chronic ankle instability (Holmes and Delahunt 2009). This typically includes a combination of both mechanical instability, resulting from physical changes to joint and connective tissue structures from the initial injury or injuries, and functional instability due to reduced proprioception and kinaesthetic sense and a diminished ability to sense and regulate force output (Hertel 2008).

Mechanical and functional instability of the ankle following injury is demonstrated by the observation that corrective taping or external bracing to provide added stability are effective in reducing subsequent injury incidence (McKeon and Mattacola 2008). External support in the form of strapping or ankle braces is, however, only effective in reducing injury in athletes who have previously sustained ankle sprains (Osborne and Rizzo 2003; Stasinopoulos 2004). Furthermore, the protective effect of external support offered by bracing appears to diminish with recurrent exposure to ankle sprain injury. Volleyball players with four or more previous ankle sprains appear to experience no benefit from external ankle bracing (Stasinopoulos 2004).

The first-time incidence of ankle injuries (for players without any history of lower limb joint injury) appears to be influenced by gender, with a trend for more ankle inversion sprains suffered by female high school and collegiate players (Beynnon et al. 2005). The female basketball players studied were reported to suffer a significantly greater number of first-time ankle inversion injuries than male basketball players. Among female players, the type of field team sport they participate in also appears to influence first-time incidence of ankle sprain injury: female basketball players report more first-time ankle sprains than female lacrosse players (Beynnon et al. 2005). This does not appear to be the case for male high school and collegiate players.

A large proportion of ankle inversion sprains in team sports occur when landing with a plantar-flexed ankle position in combination with forced inversion upon touchdown. Often the mechanism for ankle injuries sustained during landing involves contact with another player (Kofotolis and Kellis 2007). For example, in volleyball ankle injuries often occur as a result of landing on the foot of a team-mate or opponent in the area proximal to the net (Verhagen et al. 2004). In the same way, landing – often onto the foot of another player – was reported to account for almost half the ankle injuries sustained by elite and recreational basketball players (McKay et al. 2001).

A common injury mechanism for non-contact ankle injuries is twisting or turning the ankle when changing direction (McKay et al. 2001). As a consequence of the associated impairment of mechanical and functional stability players with previous ankle injury are more vulnerable to these injuries. The combination of high body mass index and a history of previous ankle injury appears to render players at further heightened risk of non-contact ankle injury. Collegiate American football players with both high body mass index and history of ankle injury are reported to be at nineteen times greater risk compared to players with normal body mass index and no previous ankle injury (Tyler et al. 2006). The greater inertia of heavier players challenges their ability to control their own momentum during change of direction movements to a greater extent and increases forces exerted on the supporting foot and ankle. The interaction of these greater forces with the lingering mechanical and functional instability of the previously injured ankle can then place the player's capacity to dynamically stabilise the ankle closer to its failure limits (Tyler et al. 2006).

Syndesmotic high ankle sprain injury

Although less common than lateral ankle sprain, syndesmotic or high ankle sprains comprise a considerable number of ankle injuries sustained in contact sports (Williams et al. 2007) – notably high incidence is reported in ice hockey (Flik et al. 2005). This injury involves the ligaments associated with the distal tibia and fibula. The classic injury mechanism for syndesmotic ankle sprain involves application of an external rotation force while the ankle is dorsiflexed and the foot is pronated – the key factor being that the talus is forcefully rotated with respect to the lower leg (Williams *et al.* 2007). Syndesmotic ankle sprains typically result in more time lost subsequent to injury in comparison to lateral inversion sprains. Particularly severe disruption of the ligaments (categorised as grade III syndesmotic injury) can require surgical intervention. Lack of awareness has been identified as a factor in syndesmotic ankle sprain injuries being underdiagnosed until recently. Similarly, there is currently a lack of data regarding these injuries – particularly with respect to rehabilitation and prevention of syndesmotic ankle sprain injuries (Williams *et al.* 2007).

Knee

Knee ligament injury

Knee injuries are among the most debilitating injuries to which team sports players are exposed (Thacker *et al.* 2003). Of all injuries, knee injury – particularly to the ACL and MCL – is associated with the longest enforced absences from practice and competition (Thacker *et al.* 2003). In two-thirds of cases complete ACL rupture is accompanied by damage to knee cartilage, causing further impairment of function and mechanical instability (Silvers and Mandelbaum 2007). At their most severe, injuries to the knee can even be career ending – particularly in the case of ACL injury. Following reconstructive surgery to repair complete ACL rupture long-term pathology is also often seen, including premature onset of osteoarthritis in later life (Silvers and Mandelbaum 2007). Unlike ankle injuries for which external bracing has been shown to help reduce risk of repeat injury, prophylactic bracing for the knee has not been demonstrated to have any positive impact upon injury rates (Hewett et al. 2006b; Silvers and Mandelbaum 2007). This underlines the importance of training interventions to address knee ligament injury risk (Hewett *et al.* 2005).

A history of previous knee ligament injury is a major risk factor for suffering subsequent injuries. Following injury, the knee often exhibits mechanical instability due to physical changes, such as increases in joint laxity, as well as functional instability due to disrupted somatosensory and proprioceptive function (Ingersoll *et al.* 2008). These factors lead to a significantly increased risk of re-injury (Murphy *et al.* 2003). Those who are ACL-deficient or have a reconstructed ACL following surgical intervention exhibit impairments in somatosensory function, some of which persist for an indefinite period (Ingersoll *et al.* 2008). The disruption of proprioceptive function also appears to endure longer at smaller angles (15 degrees) of knee flexion (Lephart *et al.* 1998). Neural inhibition affecting the quadriceps and hamstring muscles in particular is also observed post-ACL injury, which affects both strength and function (Ingersoll *et al.* 2008). The twelve-month period following surgical ACL reconstruction has been identified as a critical phase during which players are susceptible to repeat injuries to the same knee (Orchard *et al.* 2001). Beyond this period, players continue to be more prone to suffering another ACL injury; and this risk concerns both the uninjured and previously reconstructed knee equally.

Team sports players are particularly liable to suffer injuries to the knee; these can occur with or without direct contact. In particular, ACL rupture commonly results from a non-contact injury mechanism (Chappell *et al.* 2002) – more than two-thirds of ACL injuries occur in the absence of direct physical contact from other players (Hewett *et al.* 1999,

2006a). Non-contact knee injuries commonly occur when deceleration is combined with change of direction with the foot planted (Silvers and Mandelbaum 2007). This risk is greater when landing or changing direction with the lower limb in a relatively extended position (Ford *et al.* 2003; Hewett *et al.* 2006b, Quatman *et al.* 2006). The elements of jumping, landing and changing direction that feature in team sports therefore expose players to knee injury risk.

Collision sports such as football and rugby football have the added risk of contact knee injury. Players in these sports must perform multidirectional movements under resistance from opponents and also sustain direct impact during tackles, and this is reflected in greater incidence of contact ACL injuries and MCL injuries in particular (Thacker *et al.* 2003). This is illustrated by NCAA injury data reporting greater incidence of ACL injury in male collegiate lacrosse in comparison to soccer and basketball, which was attributed to the differing levels of direct physical contact permitted in these sports (Mihata *et al.* 2006).

Sidestep cutting movements are identified as increasing knee valgus and internal tibia moments of force and anterior loading on the knee (Kaila 2007), all of which place the ACL under strain. During sidestep cutting movements specifically, it is this valgus loading rather than anterior shear forces in a sagittal plane that is the more likely cause of ACL rupture, in view of the relative magnitude of strain involved (Silvers and Mandelbaum 2007). These torsional forces and potential risk of ACL rupture are greater if the sidestep cutting manoeuvre is executed with the tibia internally rotated and/or the planted foot is in a pronated position (Silvers and Mandelbaum 2007).

Joint kinematics and associated loads are shown to differ considerably between unanticipated versus pre-planned sidestep cutting movements. Specifically, although knee flexion and/or extension moments do not appear to be markedly different, valgus and internal rotation moments of force at the knee joint were significantly greater during sidestep cutting movements initiated in reaction to an external cue (versus pre-planned) (Besier *et al.* 2001). The fact that players are unable to pre-plan postural adjustments under unanticipated conditions therefore results in altered lower limb kinematics and joint loads, which in turn pose greater potential risk of injury to both ACL and MCL (Besier *et al.* 2001). Team sports players are thus exposed to particular knee injury risk – for example, when performing evasive sidestep cutting manoeuvres to avoid opposing players (McLean *et al.* 2004).

It is widely documented that female players suffer significantly higher ACL injury incidence – between two and ten times greater reported incidence depending on the sport (Silvers and Mandelbaum 2007). Various anatomical and biomechanical factors have been suggested to contribute to the higher knee injury rates demonstrated by adolescent and adult female team sports players (Ford *et al.* 2003; Noyes *et al.* 2005). A cadaveric study of mechanical properties of the human knee report that at low knee flexion angles the female knee possesses significantly less passive joint stiffness (25 per cent) under torsional loads and also greater joint laxity in rotation (28 per cent) compared to those of males (Hsu *et al.* 2006). This apparently inherent reduced mechanical stability of the knee joint in female players is often also compounded by adverse lower limb biomechanics.

Part of the disparity between genders may in part originate in growth and maturation effects, on the basis that such differences in ACL injury rates are not apparent prior to puberty (Hewett *et al.* 2006b). Increases in lever length of the lower limbs during puberty are compounded by increases in body mass, which are not accompanied by any natural gains in strength in female athletes. As a result, the female player faces greater challenges controlling motion of the trunk and exerting proximal control of the lower limb following puberty. Female athletes therefore often exhibit 'ligament dominance' – that is, in the absence of active muscular stabilisation they are over-reliant on ligaments to support the lower limb joints (Ford *et al.* 2003). As a consequence of these changes, female athletes also exhibit characteristic postural control traits and lower limb biomechanics during standard athletic tasks, which place them at greater risk of knee ligament injury (Barber-Westin *et al.* 2006; Quatman *et al.* 2006).

For example, female players are reported to have a marked tendency compared with males to execute athletic movements in an upright posture with the lower limb relatively extended and the upper leg in an inwardly rotated position (Leetun *et al.* 2004). This places the knee joint in a less mechanically stable position; this is reported to occur frequently in female athletes, particularly when landing or changing direction (Thacker *et al.* 2003). When studied during pre-planned sidestep cutting movements it was similarly noted that female subjects showed markedly different hip, knee and ankle and/or foot joint angles and more variable knee rotation motion, compared with males (McLean *et al.* 2004).

These postural traits during landing and sidestep cutting mean more force must be absorbed through the knee and ankle joints, and it is evident that female athletes also typically fail to fully recruit the hip musculature to assist and help control lower limb motion (Hewett *et al.* 2006b; Landry *et al.* 2007). The role of lumbopelvic control and hip muscle function in providing proximal neuromuscular control to the lower limb has been highlighted (Mendiguchia *et al.* 2011); this has been directly implicated in the mechanisms for ACL injury (Hewett and Myer 2011).

The role of the lumbo-pelvic-hip complex with respect to ACL injury also includes the capacity to control the position and motion of the trunk during athletic movements (Myer *et al.* 2008). A prospective study identified that a measure of lateral trunk strength was a significant predictor of female but not male athletes who suffered knee ligament injury and ACL injury in the study period (Zazulak *et al.* 2007). The capacity to control lateral lean of the trunk was strongly associated with ACL injury incidence in the female athletes studied (Zazulak *et al.* 2007). This is supported by a recent investigation of video captures of ACL injuries: analysis of video footage identified that lateral trunk lean in combination with increased abduction angle at the knee joint was present in the female athletes as they sustained ACL injury (Hewett *et al.* 2009). This pattern was not found in equivalent video captures of male athletes suffering ACL injury.

Neuromuscular recruitment patterns also appear to differ in females (Hewett *et al.* 2006b). For example, female players have a greater tendency for preferential recruitment of quadriceps over hamstrings; this phenomenon is known as 'quadriceps dominance' (Ford *et al.* 2003). The action of the quadriceps can increase anterior shear at the knee joint, and in turn increase the strain on the ACL (Silvers and Mandelbaum 2007). In contrast, the hamstrings compress the knee joint and oppose anterior shear forces during weight-bearing closed-chain movements; as a result of these functions the hamstrings muscle group is described as an 'ACL-agonist' (Hewett *et al.* 1999). This quadriceps-dominant muscle recruitment strategy is therefore potentially injurious to the ACL in female players.

Similarly, differences in gastrocnemius recruitment during unanticipated sidestep cutting have also been reported between female and male adolescent soccer players (Landry *et al.* 2007). Activation of the gastrocnemius, particularly in combination with quadriceps activation, has the potential to increase strain on the ACL. Female players displayed both higher overall activation of the gastrocnemius and an apparent imbalance in recruitment between medial and lateral gastrocnemius, with relatively greater activation of lateral gastrocnemius (Landry *et al.* 2007).

Patellar tendinopathy

Aside from injuries to the knee ligaments and joint cartilage, chronic overuse injuries associated with the patellar tendon are also common in jumping sports particularly. Incidence of patellar tendinitis or 'jumper's knee' is notably high among volleyball players (Gisslen *et al.* 2005). Although debilitating, players will often continue to train and compete while suffering symptoms of this overuse injury (Verhagen *et al.* 2004). Particularly serious cases can be career threatening, and surgical intervention may be required (Kettunen *et al.* 2002).

Understanding of the underlying pathology of patellar tendinopathy is incomplete – from relevant studies it appears to not be an inflammatory condition. Patellar tendinopathy appears to be multifactorial – a range of musculoskeletal factors may be present, and the specific combination appears to vary between individual cases. The consensus is that suboptimal tracking of the patella and associated stresses on connective tissues play a role in the mechanism for this injury (Cowan *et al.* 2009). Accordingly, patellar tendinopathy is commonly associated with sports that involve high knee extensor torques and repeated jumping movements (Visnes and Barr 2007).

Risk factors for patellar tendonitis include reduced flexibility of the hamstring and quadriceps muscles, which is postulated to increase strain on the tendons (Witvrouw *et al.* 2001). Muscular imbalances or reduced eccentric strength are also identified as potential risk factors. Imbalances in function of muscles and/or connective tissue structures medial and lateral to the knee joint have the potential to disrupt the tracking of the patella. Symptomatic subjects are often identified as having altered activation and possibly atrophy of the VMO versus vastus lateralis muscle; however, this is not always the case (Cowan *et al.* 2009). The function of hip muscles that contribute to lumbopelvic stability and proximal control of the lower limb are also identified as possible factors in the development of patellar tendinopathy (Cowan *et al.* 2009). For example, isokinetic concentric and eccentric torques in hip external rotation and eccentric hip abduction torques have been reported to be impaired in subjects with patellofemoral pain (Boling *et al.* 2009). Deficits in lateral trunk flexion isometric strength have likewise been reported in those suffering patellofemoral pain (Cowan *et al.* 2009).

Neuromuscular control issues relating to lower limb biomechanics are similarly implicated with this injury (Cowan *et al.* 2009). In the presence of some or all of these risk factors, players who perform high volumes of games and practices involving repetitive execution of a particular movement (classically jumping activities) tend to experience an insidious and progressive onset of symptoms of patellar tendinitis.

Hamstrings

Hamstring injuries are commonly reported to be the most prevalent form of noncontact injury in team sports such as soccer, rugby football, American football and Australian rules football (Opar *et al.* 2012). An injury surveillance study of the English professional soccer leagues identified hamstring injury to be the single most frequent injury diagnosis (12 per cent of total injuries), with particularly high incidence in the Premier League (28 per cent of total) mostly occurring during running activities (Woods *et al.* 2004). Data from professional rugby union in England support this observation: the majority of hamstring injuries were sustained when running, although those sustained while kicking are often the most severe (Brooks *et al.* 2006). Incidence of hamstring injury within the sport is often higher among playing positions that most frequently engage in high-speed running and change of direction activities. For example, in rugby union a higher incidence of hamstring injuries in matches (but not training) is reported for backs in comparison to the forward positions (Brooks *et al.* 2006).

The majority of hamstring injuries (53 per cent) reported in English professional soccer concerned the biceps femoris muscle (Woods *et al.* 2004), which is a finding common to most sports (Opar *et al.* 2012). The typical site of hamstring strain injury is close to the muscle–tendon junction (Peterson and Holmich 2005). These injuries may be insidious in onset, resulting from cumulative muscle damage, or the mechanism for injury may be a single triggering event (Opar *et al.* 2012). Hamstring injuries are commonly sustained when engaged in running activity (Woods *et al.* 2004; Brooks *et al.* 2006). The end of the swing phase and beginning of the stance phase are identified as the points in the gait cycle where players are most prone to hamstring injury when running (Opar *et al.* 2012). These phases feature high eccentric loads while the hamstring muscle is stretched to its full length; and it is also here that the transition between eccentric action to decelerate the leg and concentric action to generate propulsion occurs (Woods *et al.* 2004). It has also been suggested that the hamstring muscle is most vulnerable to strain injury during this switch between eccentric and concentric action (Peterson and Holmich 2005).

A number of modifiable risk factors have been identified with respect to first-time hamstring injury. These include deficits in flexibility, lumbopelvic posture, conditions of fatigue and imbalances in muscle strength and function (Opar *et al.* 2012). Conditions involving high eccentric forces in combination with strain loads, such as during kicking tasks, are also associated with increased risk of hamstring strain injury (Opar *et al.* 2012). A greater incidence of hamstring injuries has been reported for players entering the game as substitutes versus starting players in English professional rugby union (Brooks *et al.* 2006). Similarly, the occurrence of severe hamstring injuries immediately was also reported to be greater following the half-time break. These findings indicate that insufficient warm-up is an additional risk factor for hamstring injury.

Pre-season hamstring flexibility scores of Belgian soccer players who went on to sustain hamstring muscle injury during the season were found to be significantly lower than those who did not suffer hamstring injury (Witvrouw *et al.* 2003). This is not a consistent finding, however; the data regarding the association between hamstring flexibility and risk of first-time hamstring injury from other studies have been more equivocal (Opar *et al.* 2012). Reduced hamstring flexibility has been identified in players following hamstring injury (Croisier 2004) and this does appear to contribute to the greater risk of recurrent hamstring injury (Opar *et al.* 2012). In addition, reduced hip flexor flexibility was identified as a risk factor that was related to the increased rate of hamstring injury reported for Australian rules football players who were over the age of 25 (Gabbe *et al.* 2006).

Lumbopelvic posture, and specifically the presence of anterior pelvic tilt, is also identified as placing the hamstrings under additional strain and thereby at risk (Opar *et al.* 2012).

In the absence of effective lumbopelvic stabilisation from postural lumbopelvic and hip muscles, the hamstring muscles are required to work to help stabilise the pelvis whilst simultaneously fulfilling their locomotor function. Not only is this inefficient use of loco-motor muscles but it also accelerates the onset of fatigue: both of these factors can make the hamstrings more susceptible to injury. Video analysis of hamstring injuries in Australian rules football has also identified that a common injury mechanism is running with the trunk in a forward flexed position (Verral *et al.* 2005). This often occurs in the act of accel-erating or reaching to pick up or catch a ball. A lumbopelvic posture with the pelvis in an anteriorly tilted position can also place the hamstrings in an elongated position, potentially imposing greater strain on the hamstring muscles (Croisier *et al.* 2004).

The rising incidence of hamstring injuries towards the end of the playing period is a scenario common to team sports including rugby football and soccer (Brooks *et al.* 2006; Woods *et al.* 2004), which strongly suggests a fatigue effect. The impact of residual fatigue is also evident in the observation that the incidence of hamstring injury during a match is reportedly greater when a higher volume of training was undertaken in the week preceding the match (Brooks *et al.* 2006). A fatigued muscle can sustain less loading whilst being stretched (Croisier *et al.* 2004). This effect of fatigue on the ability of the muscle to absorb energy is complicated by the fact that the biceps femoris hamstring muscle receives dual innervation – from this arises the theoretical possibility of differential effects of fatigue within the same muscle (Croisier *et al.* 2004). Parts of the muscle innervated from one source might be at a more advanced state of fatigue, hence operating with different contractile properties to other parts of the muscle. The high incidence of hamstring injury in team sports is believed to be in part due to the require-ment to perform repeated bouts of high-intensity work during the course of extended playing periods (Verral *et al.* 2005).

The association between imbalances in strength and function with hamstring strain injury has been investigated in soccer players at elite level. Bilateral asymmetry (that is, difference between dominant and non-dominant lower limb) between concentric and eccentric strength of both hamstrings and quadriceps, the ratio between quadriceps versus hamstrings concentric strength scores and a 'mixed ratio' of concentric quadriceps versus eccentric hamstrings strength have all been used to evaluate strength imbalances. A study of professional soccer players identified that imbalances in two or more of the isokinetic test measures listed above when measured during pre-season was related to incidence of hamstring strain injury during the subsequent playing season (Croisier *et al.* 2008).

History of previous injury is a major risk factor for hamstring injury (Verral *et al.* 2005). A large proportion of the hamstring strains reported in team sports such as soccer are recurrent injuries (Arnason *et al.* 2008). There is accordingly a high rate of re-injury reported with hamstring strain injuries in team sports. Re-injury rates reported in the literature range from 14 to 63 per cent, depending on the sport, the severity of the initial hamstring injury, and the length of the follow-up period (up to two years) (Peterson and Holmich 2005; de Visser *et al.* 2012). Furthermore, repeat injuries sustained are often more severe than the initial injury (Brooks *et al.* 2006). The first month following return to play appears a critical period: it was during this time interval that over half (59 per cent) of the total re-injuries were reported to occur in data from English professional rugby union (Brooks *et al.* 2006). The failure of standard rehabilitation programmes employed in sport to reduce the rates of re-injury over the past three decades, despite extensive research attention during this period, has recently been highlighted in the literature (Mendiguchia *et al.* 2012).

Following injury, a variety of structural and functional changes may be observed (Opar *et al.* 2012). For example, scar tissue formation may be observed in scans of the hamstrings muscle up to one year following return to competition post-injury (Mendiguchia *et al.* 2012). Alterations in muscle activation are also evident following hamstring strain injury (Sole *et al.* 2012). Such changes are often accompanied by changes in the length–tension relationship of the previously injured muscle. The increased risk of re-injury, even after extensive rehabilitation has been followed and full function appears to have returned, are attributed to these persisting effects on the hamstrings muscle length–tension relationship (Opar *et al.* 2012).

There is some suggestion that a proportion of posterior thigh injuries presenting clinically as hamstring strains are in fact of lumbar spine origin – as indicated by a negative MRI scan for hamstring muscle strain injury (Orchard *et al.* 2004). It is believed this is a consequence of the L5–S1 nerve supply of the hamstring muscles (for the same reason, athletes may also present with calf muscle pain). Impingement or entrapment of the nerve root in the lumbar spine region may cause symptoms characteristic of muscle injury (Orchard *et al.* 2004).

The groin triangle

Adductor or 'groin strain' injury is commonly reported in many team sports – in particular ice hockey, soccer and Australian Rules football (Maffey and Emery 2007; Nicholas and Tyler 2002). A further complication with players presenting with groin pain is that medical staff, trainers and coaches must also be vigilant for more serious conditions such as osteitis pubis and sports hernia (Lynch and Renstrom 1999). Likewise, potentially serious medical conditions that can produce similar symptoms must also first be ruled out.

Injuries to the groin that are typically reported in team sports can be divided into acute injuries with a sudden onset and overuse injuries. Acute injuries are usually associated with greater time loss, in terms of forcing players to miss practices and matches, whereas in the case of overuse injury players often elect to continue to train and play despite persisting symptoms of groin pain (Engebretsen *et al.* 2010). A common injury mechanism for acute adductor muscle injury identified with field sports players is sudden forceful external rotation of the hip whilst the upper leg is in an abducted position with the foot planted (O'Connor 2004). The high incidence of adductor muscle injury is attributed to the elements of multidirectional acceleration and change of direction at high speed that are common to many team sports. The adductor muscles' role in stabilising and decelerating the lower limb also involves a high degree of eccentric loading, and this has similarly been implicated in the high incidence of strain injury (Tyler *et al.* 2001).

Previous injury is consistently reported as a risk factor for groin injury (Engebretsen *et al.* 2010). For example, a study of professional ice hockey players reported that a history of previous injury within the preceding year was a significant risk factor for suffering further adductor muscle strain injury (Emery and Meeuwisse 2001). Groin injury is also associated with a high rate of recurrence (Arnason *et al.* 2004; Maffey and Emery 2007; Nicholas and Tyler 2002), and traditional passive rehabilitation methods appear relatively ineffectual for treating groin pain. It has therefore been identified that in order to be effective, interventions should feature active strengthening exercises to restore strength and function of the adductor muscles (Tyler *et al.* 2002).

Adductor muscle weakness measured by clinical isometric strength assessment during pre-season was identified as a risk factor that was associated with the incidence of new groin injuries suffered by male soccer players during the subsequent playing season (Engebretsen *et al.* 2010). Imbalance between adductor and abductor muscle strength measures is also identified as a major risk factor for adductor muscle strain injury (Nicholas and Tyler 2002). A study of a professional ice hockey team reported that if a player's pre-season adductor strength test scores were less than 80 per cent of their strength scores for abduction they had a significantly higher incidence of adductor muscle strain during the subsequent season (Tyler *et al.* 2001).

Similarly, players who start the season in a deconditioned state appear more prone to suffering adductor strain injury (Maffey and Emery 2007). Players who had failed to complete a certain number of off-season training sessions suffered a higher incidence of adductor muscle injuries when they reported to pre-season training camp (Emery and Meeuwisse 2001). This strongly suggests that fatigue is a risk factor for adductor strain injury, in much the same way as it is for hamstring strains.

Similar to the findings concerning hamstring injury risk, a relationship has been identified between impaired adductor muscle flexibility and risk of adductor muscle strain. Baseline scores of passive hip range of motion in abduction were found to be associated with subsequent incidence of adductor muscle injury in soccer players (Arnason *et al.* 2004). This association was not found in a study of professional ice hockey players, suggesting the influence of adductor muscle flexibility on injury risk may depend upon the sport (Tyler *et al.* 2001).

Deficits in lumbopelvic stability have also been identified as a risk factor for adductor strain injury (Maffey and Emery 2007). Impaired function of deep lumbar stabiliser muscles has been implicated in players with a long-term history of groin pain. Deficiencies in the way in which force is transmitted from the locomotor muscles to the torso, as a result of suboptimal function of muscles that stabilise the pelvis and lower limb, may expose the adductor muscles to injury risk (Maffey and Emery 2007). In the presence of instability at the pelvis or lower limb malalignment, the adductor muscles may try to compensate, thus placing them under additional strain (Lynch and Renstrom 1999). It has therefore been suggested that treatment for groin pain should include active strengthening for the hip and abdominal muscles that help provide lumbopelvic stability.

Lumbar spine

After the ankle and knee, the lower back is commonly reported to be the third most common site of injury in sports (Nadler *et al.* 2000). This is particularly the case in sports involving striking or throwing movements which require rotation of the hips, pelvis and spine (Harris-Hayes *et al.* 2009). Female athletes in particular also appear prone to low back pain and injury. A study of injury incidence among NCAA collegiate athletes for the 1997/98 season indicated almost twice the number of lower back injuries in females (Nadler *et al.* 2002).

The mechanism for low back pain and injury is often cumulative; there may or may not be a single triggering event (McGill 2007b). Similarly, a distinction must be made between acute back pain or injury and chronic conditions. Acute episodes of low back pain respond well to rest and treatment or even resolve spontaneously (Rogers 2006). Conversely, chronic lower back problems (lasting longer than three months) do not respond to rest or passive therapies; in these cases the consensus is that active approaches involving appropriate training interventions are most effective (Danneels *et al.* 2001).

The observation that when stripped of supporting musculature a cadaver human spine will buckle under 20lb (≈9kg) of load illustrates the contribution made by the various supporting muscles in providing active spine stability (Barr *et al.* 2005). Low back pain is often accompanied by disrupted motor patterns of various stabilising muscles (Rogers 2006). A common finding is that deep lumbar spine stabiliser muscles are atrophied in individuals with chronic lower back pain (Barr *et al.* 2005). Importantly this atrophy does appear to be reversible with appropriate training intervention, with associated improvements in low back pain symptoms (Hides *et al.* 2001). Individuals with chronic lower back pain also exhibit impaired neuromuscular feedback and delayed muscle reaction, which is accompanied by reduced capacity to sense the orientation of their spine and pelvis (Barr *et al.* 2005). There is some debate whether these functional deficits are primarily a cause or consequence of chronic low back pain (McGill 2007b).

Team sports require both strength and endurance for the muscles that stabilise the spine in all three planes of motion (Barr *et al.* 2005; Leetun *et al.* 2004). Weakness or impairment at any point in this integrated system of support can lead to damage to structural tissues (ligament and articular structures), causing injury and pain (Barr *et al.* 2005). Imbalances in strength and endurance of flexors and extensors of the trunk have also been implicated as a risk factor for low back pain (Rogers 2006). Endurance rather than absolute strength of trunk muscles has been identified as being the most decisive factor with regard to low back pain incidence (McGill 2007b).

The hip musculature serves a major role in stabilising the pelvis during all dynamic activities performed in an upright stance or weight-bearing through the lower limbs (Nadler *et al.* 2000). Impaired function of the hip extensors and hip abductors are observed with athletes who are suffering lower back pain (Nadler *et al.* 2002). Strength imbalances in these muscles are also implicated in lower back pain incidence, particularly in female athletes (Nadler *et al.* 2000). Isometric hip external rotation strength was identified as the single best predictor of lower back and lower extremity injury incidence in collegiate athletes (Leetun *et al.* 2004). Inflexible or weak hip rotators can also predispose the athlete to poor pelvic alignment; excessive lumbar spine motion can also occur in an attempt to compensate for impaired hip rotator function (Regan 2000). Both of these factors can lead to pain and the incidence of lumbar spine injury.

Shoulder complex

As a consequence of the high degree of mobility of the shoulder joint, it is heavily reliant on dynamic (that is, muscular) stability (Wagner 2003). Active stabilisation is provided by the co-ordinated function of a number of muscles, in particular those that control the articulation between the scapula and thorax, and the 'rotator cuff' of muscles at the glenohumeral joint (Myers and Oyama 2008). The co-ordination and synergistic function of the various stabilising muscles is controlled via an integrated sensorimotor system that relies upon afferent input from mechanoreceptors within the muscles and connective tissues structures.

Any disruption to these structures or alteration in function of the individual muscles that contribute to providing dynamic stabilisation will therefore have major consequences for the structural integrity of the shoulder complex and the corresponding risk of injury.

Acute shoulder injury

In collision sports, such as rugby football, American football and ice hockey, injuries to the shoulder represent a leading cause of lost participation in training and matches. In a study of professional rugby union in England the number of days lost to shoulder injuries was reportedly second only to knee injuries (Headey et al. 2007). Similarly high incidence of shoulder injury is reported in American football: half of all elite collegiate players participating in the 2004 NFL Combine reported history of shoulder injury; and of these players a third had previously undergone shoulder surgery (Kaplan et al. 2005). A study of ice hockey injuries in Finland likewise identified a high number of shoulder injuries among players of various ages, particularly those in the 20–24 and 25–29 age groups. The majority of the reported injuries (79 per cent) were the result of body checking or other collisions with players or the boards surrounding the ice rink (Molsa et al. 2003).

Contact shoulder injuries in collision sports most often occur during tackles. Accordingly, playing positions with the greatest exposure to tackle situations generally, and high-speed collisions in particular, typically report the highest incidence of shoulder injuries (Headey et al. 2007). Acromioclavicular (A-C) joint separations are the most commonly reported type of injury among elite collegiate American football players (Kaplan et al. 2005). Anterior instability is another common condition that was reported – predominantly affecting defensive positions among this sample of elite collegiate players (Kaplan et al. 2005). A study of English professional rugby also reported that the most common contact injuries sustained by players were A-C joint injuries (Headey et al. 2007). The most severe tackle injury involving the shoulder in English professional rugby union, in terms of time lost subsequent to injury, was shoulder dislocation (Headey et al. 2007). Rotator cuff tears and impingement injuries are also frequently reported among both English professional rugby players (Headey et al. 2007) and elite collegiate American football players (Kaplan et al. 2005). Rotator cuff tears appear to be most commonly sustained from direct impact on the shoulder as a result of a fall or collision with another player.

The incidence of shoulder injury in English professional rugby union football is reported to be highest in the final quarter of matches and during the latter stages of training sessions (Headey et al. 2007). This finding implies a fatigue element in the incidence of contact shoulder injuries in collision sports. It has also been proposed that repeated exposure to impact forces during collisions may lead to cumulative microtrauma, which in turn could potentially lead to impaired active and passive stability of the shoulder complex. Biochemical markers of muscle damage following a competitive rugby match showed that the degree of muscle damage was directly linked to the number of tackles each player had performed and sustained during the course of the match (Takarada 2003). Such muscle damage results in short-term reductions in function, which are fully restored after a period (several days) of recovery. The training status of the player also has a major effect on the degree of muscle damage following strenuous physical exertion (Takarada 2003).

There is a high rate of re-injury reported with shoulder injuries – 27 per cent of all shoulder injuries reported in a study of professional rugby union in England were recurrences of previous injuries (Headey *et al.* 2007). Following acute injury trauma and disruption to connective tissues and joint structures may be observed, which may result in reduced mechanical stability. Even in the absence of changes in mechanical stability there are typically changes in functional stability following injury due to persisting effects on sensorimotor function from the initial trauma (Myers and Oyama 2008). Sensorimotor deficits and alterations in function of the muscles that provide stability to the glenohumeral joint and control the articulation between scapula and thorax have major consequences for the integrity and dynamic stabilisation of the shoulder complex.

Recurrent injuries are also often more severe than new injuries in terms of time lost subsequent to the injury (Headey *et al.* 2007). This is likely a consequence of the persisting instability following injury leading to a reduced ability to maintain joint integrity, and resist external forces during collisions, once players have returned to training and competition. This high rate of re-injury appears particularly evident with dislocation and/or instability injuries; these injuries were reported to have a 62 per cent recurrence rate among English professional rugby union players (Headey *et al.* 2007). These findings also reflect difficulties in achieving effective injury rehabilitation in order to restore full function.

Overuse injuries of the shoulder complex

Overuse injuries of the shoulder complex can also be prevalent in team sports, particularly those that involve throwing and striking, such as baseball and volleyball. For example, imbalances and specific deficits in strength and function of particular rotator cuff muscles are characteristically found in overhead throwing and striking sports, which result in associated symptoms of pain and impingement (Wilk *et al.* 2002). Repeatedly performing ballistic throwing or striking movements during practice and competition can cause progressive weakness of the muscles that work eccentrically to decelerate the humerus and stabilise the glenohumeral joint, due to the cumulative stresses and microtrauma involved (Behnke 2001). For example, specific atrophy of the infraspinatus muscle accompanied by reduced external rotation strength scores is evident in beach volleyball players (Lajtai *et al.* 2009).

Strength ratios of internal and external rotator muscles of the shoulder are frequently employed to identify athletes at risk of overuse shoulder injury (Niederbracht *et al.* 2008). In particular, reduced eccentric strength of external rotator muscles relative to the concentric strength of internal rotators shows a significant association with shoulder pain and injury in overhead sports players (Wang and Cochrane 2001).

Aside from the development of imbalances or relative weaknesses, repetitious sports activity and eccentric overload can also lead to impaired sense of scapular position and control of scapula stabilisers (Wang and Cochrane 2001). Such disruption in scapulo-humeral rhythm (scapular movement and positioning in response to movement of the upper arm) can lead to glenohumeral joint instability (Brummitt and Meira 2006). This is suggested to be a common mechanism leading to pain and injury particularly in overhead athletes (for example, volleyball players) (Wang and Cochrane 2001).

Summary

Intrinsic risk factors have been described that can predispose a player to sustaining injury. As discussed, playing a given sport exposes players to conditions – 'extrinsic risk factors'

– that may expose them to certain injuries. Epidemiological data have been summarised that detail the incidence and severity of injuries that are characteristic of participation in different team sports. When a player who exhibits intrinsic risk factors is then exposed to extrinsic risk factors by competing in a particular sport, all that remains is for a triggering event to take place for an injury to result (Bahr and Krosshaug 2005). This triggering event pertains to the injury mechanism – typical injury mechanisms have been summarised for the injuries commonly identified in team sports.

Based upon this analysis, the next step is to design training interventions to address those of the above risk factors that are reversible and attempt to specifically guard against identified injury mechanisms. Such interventions have the dual aim of reducing overall injury incidence and reducing the severity of injuries sustained by players. Depending on the inciting event, some injuries – such as those resulting from contact with an opponent – are not avoidable; however, the severity of the damage that is sustained may be limited by prior preventative training (Bahr and Krosshaug 2005).

10

TRAINING FOR INJURY PREVENTION

Specific training interventions

Introduction

Sport-specific physical conditioning can favourably influence a player's injury risk profile when training and competing in the sport. One general protective effect is that appropriately conditioned players are more resistant to the neuromuscular fatigue that renders athletes susceptible to injury (Hawkins *et al.* 2001; Murphy *et al.* 2003; Verral *et al.* 2005). The importance of this is illustrated in the common trend in many sports for higher injury rates in the latter stages of matches when players are fatigued (Best *et al.* 2005; Brooks *et al.* 2005a; Hawkins and Fuller 1999; Hawkins *et al.* 2001). Participating in a pre-season conditioning programme was shown to reduce by more than half the injuries sustained by female high school soccer players during the subsequent season (Heidt *et al.* 2000). More sport-specific metabolic conditioning appears more effective in guarding against these negative effects of neuromuscular fatigue (Verral *et al.* 2005). In this way, the general protective effect of metabolic conditioning regarding injury risk exhibits specificity effects.

Strength training similarly serves a general protective effect in making the musculo-skeletal system stronger and thereby more resistant to the stresses incurred during games (Kraemer and Fleck 2005). The addition of strength training to the physical preparation of male collegiate soccer players was followed by an almost 50 per cent reduction in injury rates during subsequent playing seasons (Lehnhard *et al.* 1996). One aspect of this is that trained muscle is more resistant to the microtrauma caused by strenuous physical exertion and also recovers faster (Takarada 2003). The protective function of strength training also exhibits specificity, as it is restricted to the bones and connective tissues associated with the limbs and muscles employed during the training movement.

However, conventional training alone is not sufficient to address critical risk factors and neuromuscular control deficits identified for particular injuries. For example, a strength-training intervention in isolation had no significant impact upon the aberrant lower limb biomechanics that predispose female players to knee injury, despite significantly increasing strength levels (Herman *et al.* 2008). Targeted interventions have the potential to address such risk factors in order to specifically guard against certain injuries to which team sports players may be exposed.

Training for injury prevention comprises both safeguarding against first-time injury and also reducing the risk of recurrence of previous injuries. The previous chapter explored the risk factors relevant to the particular sport and playing position, and the intrinsic risk factors that affect each individual player. In this chapter we examine the specific neuromuscular and strength-training interventions that can be employed to address the risk factors and injury mechanisms identified for the particular injuries that are commonly seen in different team sports.

Approaching training for injury prevention

Often the injury prevention interventions that are employed both in studies and in the field are essentially the same as those which have reported success in a rehabilitation setting. This concerns not only the training mode and but also other training parameters – such as frequency, intensity and volume prescribed. For example, it is customary for many rehabilitation training interventions to be performed with a daily frequency – eccentric training regimens commonly prescribe training bouts to be performed twice daily (Rees et al. 2009). Unfortunately, due to the relative shortage of studies investigating injury prevention training interventions, a dose–response relationship has yet to be established (Engebretsen et al. 2008). However, this daily (or twice daily) frequency of training would seem contrary to what is known about the time course for adaptation of muscle and connective tissues, as well as what is known about the optimal range of training frequency to elicit neuromuscular adaptations from the strength training literature. It has been identified in the sports medicine literature that exercise prescription in a rehabilitation and injury prevention setting typically does not account for fundamental aspects of training design, such as variation, progression and periodisation (Rees et al. 2009).

In terms of exercise selection, it is also yet to be resolved what the optimal training modes might be for preventing specific injuries. While the training interventions that have shown to be effective for the rehabilitation of specific injuries would appear to be a sensible starting point, equally it should be acknowledged that an uninjured athlete has very different requirements and capabilities from an athlete who has recently sustained a particular injury. In support of this contention is the observation that the 'prophylactic' application of standard rehabilitation protocols for particular injuries do not appear to be particularly effective in reducing injury incidence for previously healthy athletes (Engebretsen et al. 2008; Kraemer and Knobloch 2009).

The study by Fredberg and colleagues (2008), for example, employed low-intensity body-weight resistance exercises derived from rehabilitation eccentric training protocols for Achilles and patellar tendinopathy. The training intervention failed to reduce subsequent injury incidence in the soccer players studied. In fact the injury rate of players who were asymptomatic at the start of the study but showed abnormalities in their Achilles and/ or patellar tendon in their ultrasound scans prior to the intervention was higher than the norm for the group in the subsequent season. These results indicate the training intervention not only failed to serve any preventative function but was also ineffective as an early treatment or rehabilitation modality (Fredberg et al. 2008).

Based upon these observations, it appears that when approaching injury prevention it is important to make a distinction between athletes who have a history of injury versus those with no previous incidence. Those who are at increased risk based on their injury history and/or ongoing deficits in function can be easily identified via questionnaires or interviews and grading players' responses using clinical assessment tools available in the sports medicine literature (Engebretsen et al. 2010). As described in Chapter 2, there are numerous clinical tests that can be employed for musculoskeletal assessment. There are also a number of assessments of neuromuscular control and function indicative of lower limb injury risk, detailed in Chapter 3. In the case of athletes who report prior incidence of a particular injury it is important to consider the specific risk factors identified for re-injury. From this viewpoint, it is similarly important to consider the neuromuscular and sensorimotor deficits that can result from particular injuries.

In this instance, the intervention employed to guard against (repeat) incidence of injury might be broadly similar to the approach employed during the latter stages of rehabilitation for that specific injury. However, it should be noted that standard preventative interventions that feature rehabilitation exercises are not shown to be effective in some studies, even among those identified as being at high risk based on previous injury or reduced function reported at baseline (Engebretsen *et al.* 2008). This suggests that the standard 'rehabilitation' approach to injury prevention training prescription may not be sufficient even for previously injured athletes.

In any case, injury prevention for previously healthy athletes (with respect to a particular injury) would appear to necessitate a less conservative and more progressive approach, rather than merely employing the same training prescription that is applied for rehabilitation. The threshold intensity or neuromuscular challenge required to elicit the desired adaptation is likely to be greater in a healthy versus an injured athlete. There will also be differences in motivation between injured and uninjured athletes. Healthy athletes will not have the same intrinsic motivation – undertaking the training intervention in order to relieve pain and other symptoms – that an injured athlete will. Likewise, in order to assist compliance in the longer term, as well as facilitating continued adaptation, it is likely that there will be need for reduced frequency and greater variation in terms of exercise prescription when employing this form of training with healthy athletes to reduce training monotony and boredom.

Integration of injury prevention training

Issues of adherence are frequently cited by investigations of injury prevention interventions in the sports medicine literature (Emery and Meeuwisse 2010). Poor compliance has been reported even among those identified as being at particular risk of injury, in some cases resulting in a failure to complete even the recommended minimum training frequency and volume required for a prophylactic effect (Engebretsen *et al.* 2008). In general, adherence is much better when injury prevention interventions are performed in a group setting, compared to when exercises are prescribed to be performed in the athlete's own time. Similarly, one approach that shows a great deal of promise in terms of resolving issues of compliance is to integrate the injury prevention intervention into the players' warm-up prior to training (Gilchrist *et al.* 2008).

It follows that injury prevention interventions should be performed in a group setting, with appropriate supervision where possible. Furthermore, compliance concerns not only adherence but also the quality of execution (Engebretsen *et al.* 2008), which will also be determined by the player's attention and directed mental effort when performing the exercises set. From this viewpoint, the greater the degree to which such interventions are incorporated into players' routine training, the better the level of compliance is likely to be. For example, rather than performing interventions to develop strength, muscle recruitment, and so on, as a stand-alone session, they should be integrated into the player's (supervised) strength training programme. Likewise, corrective neuromuscular training prescribed might be incorporated into speed and agility sessions, and dynamic balance and stabilisation exercises performed as part of the players' standard warm-up prior to training.

Intensity and progression of training variables

As discussed in the previous section, it is likely that the intensity of preventative or prophylactic training will need to exceed a threshold in order to elicit adaptation in healthy tissues. Furthermore, in accordance with the size principle, higher-intensity preventative training should aim to recruit the higher threshold motor units that will come into play when the player is operating at high velocity or against a high degree of external resistance, for example during bodily contact with opponents.

Similarly, healthy athletes will tend to adapt more quickly and therefore in order to avoid plateaus in the training response there will be a need for progression. Equally the required rate of progression of different training parameters will necessarily differ from what is typically seen in a rehabilitation setting. By definition, an injured athlete has limitations that are not present in an uninjured healthy athlete. It follows that the rate of progression for athletes with a prior history of a particular injury will initially be determined by set criteria, such as the return to baseline of specific neuromuscular and sensorimotor capacities.

Injury prevention training interventions

Ankle

Developing proprioceptive function and the active stability provided by muscles of the lower leg are key aspects of guarding against ankle injury for athletes with or without previous history of ankle sprains. Afferent input from mechanoreceptors within the muscles associated with the ankle joint serve the dominant role in providing the athlete with a sense of joint position and kinaesthetic awareness (Holmes and Delahunt 2009). Appropriate strength training and neuromuscular training offer a means to develop the proprioception provided by muscle mechanoreceptors. A variety of strength training and neuromuscular training interventions have been shown to improve measures of proprioception and ankle joint position sense specifically (Holmes and Delahunt 2009).

Much of the increased risk of re-injury with ankle sprains is attributed to a loss in proprioceptive function associated with the injured ankle. Taping the lower limb and ankle joint is often employed particularly for players with previous ankle sprain injury, in part as a means to augment proprioception due to the cutaneous stimulation provided (Hopper *et al.* 1999). Those with a history of ankle injury characteristically show deficits in sensorimotor control leading to 'functional instability' (Hertel 2008), and this may be combined with mechanical instability resulting from disruption to the ligaments and joint capsule from the initial injury. The syndrome termed chronic ankle instability (CAI) is a particularly severe example of this (Holmes and Delahunt 2009).

Clearly, addressing and correcting these deficits must be a starting point for interventions aimed at preventing re-injury. Those suffering with chronic ankle instability exhibit reduced proprioception, and in particular an impaired sense of ankle joint position in the frontal plane (Holmes and Delahunt 2009). Similarly, kinaesthetic sense during movement may be impaired in those with chronic ankle instability. Consequently, postural control and static balance are often both reported to be reduced in those with chronic ankle instability, and dynamic stabilisation is another aspect of neuromuscular control that is found to be affected (Holmes and Delahunt 2009).

Training to develop proprioception in the previously injured ankle is demonstrated to be effective in reducing the risk of re-injury (Osborne and Rizzo 2003; Stasinopoulos 2004). A targeted single-leg balance training intervention for high school football players deemed to be at high risk for non-contact ankle injury was successful in reducing injury rates to the extent that the injury risk factors of previous ankle injury history and high body mass index were entirely offset in these players (McHugh et al. 2007). A study of male soccer players with a history of previous ankle inversion injury reported that of three preventive interventions studied (strength training for evertor muscles, external bracing and proprioception training), only proprioceptive ankle disc training successfully reduced the rate of re-injury (Mohammadi et al. 2007). Training with a mini trampoline was reported to be equally effective as balance disc training for reducing postural sway indicative of functional ankle instability in recreational athletes with previous ankle sprain injury (Kidgell et al. 2007). Importantly, the protective effect of proprioceptive training appears to be maintained even with athletes with a previous history of numerous (more than three) ankle sprains, which does not appear to be the case with external bracing (Stasinopoulos 2004).

The training intervention most consistently found to be effective in the literature for preventing first-time ankle sprains as well as recurrent injuries is balance or proprioceptive training (McKeon and Mattacola 2008). For example, a balance training intervention that was effective in reducing the incidence of ankle sprain injuries in male and female high school soccer and basketball players with a history of ankle sprains also reported a strong positive trend ($p=0.059$) among players without prior ankle injury (McGuine and Keene 2006). The instances in the literature where equivocal results have been reported for athletes without any history of ankle injury may simply reflect that the proprioceptive training interventions employed in these studies was insufficiently challenging.

Players who have not suffered prior ankle injury will not exhibit the sensorimotor deficits associated with previous ankle injury, and given that the baseline level of function is higher, it follows that more basic balance training activities are unlikely to elicit significant improvements. For these players, more challenging training modes to develop dynamic postural control and dynamic stabilisation are likely to be more effective (Figure 10.2). The reader is referred to Chapter 3 for definitions and descriptions of these training modes.

The capacities required for maintaining equilibrium during normal gait and landing activities comprise both feed-forward motor control and afferent feedback from receptors in the joint, muscle and skin (Hertel 2008). Both of these components are implicated in the sensorimotor deficits observed with those suffering chronic ankle instability, and these abilities are therefore affected in these players. Previously injured players should therefore also progress to dynamic balance and dynamic stabilisation training modes, once baseline levels of sensorimotor function have been restored. Indeed, this may be a requirement for those with chronic ankle instability, in view of the limited effectiveness often reported with standard static balance training interventions in this subject population (McKeon and Hertel 2008). In support of this contention, a progressive balance training programme, featuring a variety of dynamic balance and dynamic stabilisation tasks under both pre-planned and reactive conditions, was reported to elicit significant improvements in function and measures of static and dynamic postural control in subjects suffering with chronic ankle instability (McKeon *et al.* 2008). Higher training frequency appears to be beneficial with proprioceptive or balance training interventions (McKeon and Mattacola 2008). It also appears that additional benefits are conferred when the proprioceptive training intervention is continued for a longer duration (McKeon and Hertel 2008b).

Deficits in strength of muscles that contribute to providing stability to the ankle following injury have been identified as a factor in functional instability. It is likely that transient reductions in strength are due in a large part to neural inhibition, as strength deficits typically resolve during the period following the initial injury (Hertel 2008). However, for players suffering with chronic ankle instability, strength deficits may persist. In contrast to clinical approaches that typically focus on the peroneal musculature, based upon the literature it is the invertor muscles which actually appear to be those most affected (Holmes and Delahunt 2009). Appropriate strength training to restore function and develop strength for these muscles is therefore recommended to help prevent re-injury. Closed chain single-limb support exercises performed under external resistance in a variety of planes are recommended for this purpose (Bellew and Dunn 2002). In general, these exercises should be performed without shoes (to remove the external support provided) and variations performed on labile surfaces such as foam mats might also be considered.

In view of the fact that the majority of ankle injuries occur when landing or changing direction, appropriate movement skills instruction and training is also identified as a possible means of reducing ankle injuries (McKay *et al.* 2001). This may be particularly beneficial for players who have a history of ankle sprains, in view of the fact that athletes have a tendency to exhibit altered motor control strategies following injury (Wikstrom *et al.* 2007). Retraining 'correct' movement mechanics would appear especially important for players showing these signs of functional ankle instability. In support of this, an intervention that consisted solely of instruction and practice of jumping and landing technique was equally effective at reducing injuries among female volleyball players as proprioceptive training and bracing (Stasinopoulos 2004). Corrective neuromuscular training to develop postural control and movement skills is discussed in detail in Chapter 3.

From the limited investigations into syndesmotic ankle injury that have been published there are guidelines with respect to stages of treatment and rehabilitation. There are currently no such guidelines for prevention strategies for this specific injury. In the absence of this information, a good starting point might be to follow the guidelines suggested for the final stage of rehabilitation, which includes strength and neuromuscular training similar to that employed to guard against lateral inversion sprain injuries.

Knee ligament injury

Interventions to reduce risk of knee ligament injury, and ACL injury prevention for female players in particular, typically focus on addressing documented biomechanical and neuromuscular risk factors via corrective training (McLean *et al.* 2004). Studies with male athletes are currently somewhat lacking but various neuromuscular training interventions have been shown to reduce incidence of ACL injury with female team sports players (Hewett *et al.* 1999; Mandelbaum *et al.* 2005). Effective interventions that are documented to reduce rates of ACL injury generally comprise multiple components, aimed at addressing a combination of neuromuscular training outcomes. A range of training modes are employed, including strength training, plyometrics, a variety of proprioceptive and balance training modes, and movement skills training (Hewett *et al.* 2006a). One such example is the Sportsmetrics protocol developed at the Cincinnati Sports Medicine Research and Education Foundation (Hewett *et al.* 1999). Recently, lumbopelvic training has also received increasing attention due to the reported association between neuromuscular deficits in the capacity to control trunk position and the mechanism of ACL injury with female athletes (Zazulak *et al.* 2007)

Strength training, in combination with other forms of neuromuscular training, is a common feature of most (but not all) successful knee injury prevention protocols. Exercise selection should generally focus on developing strength and recruitment of the proximal hip musculature (Myer *et al.* 2008) and specific development of the hamstring muscle group would also seem to be important. Reflex activation of the hamstrings originating from mechanoreceptors at the knee joint is identified as crucial to dynamic stabilisation of the knee joint (Lephart *et al.* 1998), reflecting the role of the hamstrings as an 'ACL agonist' during weight-bearing closed-chain movements (Hewett *et al.* 1999). The functional capacity of the hamstring muscles is therefore an important factor contributing to dynamic stabilisation of the knee. Hence, in addition to proprioceptive training, specific strengthening of the hamstrings would also appear to be important for developing the capacity to stabilise the knee during movement. This is particularly relevant to female players for whom hamstring strength typically plateaus early in their development: it is reported that hamstring strength measures of older age groups (13–17 years) do not differ significantly from those of 11-year-old females (Barber-Westin *et al.* 2006).

Effective training interventions for reducing risk and incidence of knee injury generally feature some form of corrective movement skills training (Silvers and Mandelbaum 2007). An apparently important feature of this training is the inclusion of specific coaching with feedback regarding 'safe' versus 'unsafe' biomechanics (such as posture and lower limb alignment) for athletic movements (Hewett *et al.* 2006a). Adjustments in movement mechanics have the potential to reduce torques imposed upon the knee ligaments (particularly ACL) when landing and during cutting movements (Myer *et al.* 2005). Postural control factors, such as degree of knee and hip flexion upon landing, affect the ability of soft tissues to absorb joint loading and capacity of relevant muscles (such as hamstrings) to generate protective forces upon lower limb joints (Lephart *et al.* 2005). Specific approaches to movement skills neuromuscular training are discussed in detail in Chapter 3.

The inclusion of high-intensity plyometric training also often differentiates successful interventions from other studies that did not report significant reductions in ACL injury incidence (Hewett *et al.* 2006a). This is likely due to a combination of factors which are protective for the knee joint. The first of these is the development of key components of sensorimotor control during landing and bounding movements, which includes both feedforward control and proprioceptive input (Hertel 2008). The second is the development of eccentric strength and also muscle activation both prior to touchdown and during the eccentric phase of landing and bounding movements (McBride *et al.* 2008). These training effects are likely to facilitate improvements in the ability to dissipate forces at the knee joint during landing tasks.

The mechanistic connection between trunk, hip and lower limb with specific reference to knee joint injury has been identified in the literature (Hewett and Myer 2011). The lumbo-pelvic-hip complex not only provides proximal control to the lower limb (Mendiguchia *et al.* 2011) but the position and motion of the trunk during athletic tasks

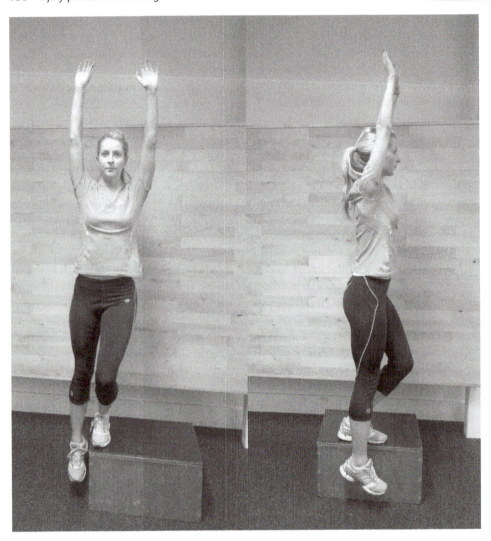

Figure 10.1 Low box single-leg knee and ankle flexion

also influences the stresses placed upon the knee joint. The latter factor has been specifically implicated in the mechanism for ACL injury for female athletes (Hewett *et al.* 2009). Specific neuromuscular training interventions to develop trunk and hip control have therefore been proposed as a preventative measure for reducing knee joint injury (Myer *et al.* 2008). Various forms of postural balance and single-leg stabilisation training have previously been shown to have beneficial impact on knee injury risk factors (Myer *et al.* 2006b). It has also been identified that interventions should focus on developing core strength and lateral stability provided to the trunk in particular (Zazulak *et al.* 2007). The reader is referred to Chapter 8 for a summary of training methods to develop different aspects of core strength and stability.

It is critical to address any deficits and functional instability for those who have suffered a previous knee ligament injury, particularly involving the ACL, in order to protect the player against recurrence of injury to both the previously injured and 'healthy' knee (Orchard *et al.* 2001). The disruption of somatosensory function and associated increased risk of re-injury appears to persist for a long duration for those with a surgically reconstructed ACL and also those who are ACL-deficient (Ingersoll *et al.* 2008). It follows that attention must be given to both recently injured players and also to those players who have been healthy for an extended period and report full function. Inhibition of muscle activation is also found in the injured limb of ACL-deficient and ACL-reconstructed subjects (Ingersoll *et al.* 2008). Interventions to help restore sensorimotor function and guard against re-injury should therefore include a combination of training modalities, including strength training and training modes to develop static postural balance, dynamic balance and dynamic stabilisation. It is important that exercises are performed with both limbs, as some of the changes following injury are also observed in the healthy contralateral limb (Ingersoll *et al.* 2008).

Patellar tendinopathy

Eccentric strength training is often employed for specific development of medial quadriceps (VMO) and patella tendon as part of the rehabilitation for patellar tendinopathy (Zwerver *et al.* 2007). A range of training modes have been employed, including controlled eccentric knee flexion movements as well as rapid drop squats or drop jump landings (Visnes and Barr 2007). Unilateral single-leg squat protocols have proven efficacy as rehabilitation tool. These exercises are typically performed on a decline surface, maintaining an upright posture with minimal forward torso lean and neutral lower limb alignment so that the supporting knee remains in line with the toes (Visnes and Barr 2007).

A biomechanical analysis identified that employing a decline surface with a minimum angle of 15 degrees serves to specifically load the patella tendon, which appears to explain the superior effectiveness of decline squats in comparison to eccentric squats performed on a flat surface (Zwerver *et al.* 2007). There does appear to be an optimal range of motion for the exercise – descending to a knee flexion angle of 60 degrees. Beyond this range, forces placed upon the patellofemoral joint increase to a greater extent than patellar tendon forces (Zwerver *et al.* 2007). In symptomatic athletes, the depth will initially be governed by pain experienced during the movement – it is typically recommended to work just into the range where the movement becomes painful (Visnes and Barr 2007). Within the specific range of motion, progression can be achieved by adding external load, for example using dumbbells held at the sides or supported upon the shoulders. Adding a 10kg load via a backpack was shown to increase knee moment of force by 23 per cent (Zwerver *et al.* 2007). It is important, however, that an upright torso posture is maintained when external loading is added, in order that appropriate moments of force through the lower limb joints are maintained during the movement.

Despite the effectiveness generally reported with eccentric training modalities as a rehabilitation tool for those suffering symptoms of patellar tendinopathy, data from one study suggest that standard rehabilitation eccentric training interventions may be less effective for players who are asymptomatic but exhibit abnormalities on ultrasonograph tendon scans indicative of increased risk for developing tendinopathy (Fredberg *et al.* 2008).

Furthermore, the data from studies to date do not indicate that standard eccentric training modes reduce the initial incidence of signs and symptoms of patellar tendinopathy. There is therefore no sound evidence to support the use of the majority of conventional eccentric training modes that are used for rehabilitation as a means to prevent first-time patellar tendinopathy injury.

It could, however, be speculated that a less conservative approach featuring higher eccentric loading and more progressive selection of exercise modes would elicit a greater level of adaptation and might therefore serve a greater protective effect. An investigation of tendon loading during eccentric training exercises identified a fluctuating pattern of loading and unloading on the tendon, which differed from the constant pattern observed during concentric training (Rees *et al.* 2009). It has been speculated that these fluctuations in tendon load, which differentiate eccentric training from conventional training modes, might be the specific stimulus that elicits remodelling of tendon structures. In addition, the fluctuations in tendon loading were attributed to greater difficulty in controlling muscle tension during the eccentric action (Rees *et al.* 2009). Specific changes in muscle activation during the eccentric phase of loaded jumping movements have previously been documented following training (Cormie *et al.* 2010a). It could therefore be speculated that exposure to eccentric loading under appropriate conditions might serve a protective effect by enhancing the player's capacity to control muscle activation and tension during the eccentric phase, thereby sparing the tendon. It follows that the eccentric training stimulus provided should aim to replicate the loading conditions and movements encountered during athletic activities.

The hip muscles' role in providing lumbopelvic stability and controlling lower limb alignment in single-leg stance and athletic movements, and the influence on knee joint loads have been identified as critical factors in the mechanisms of patellar tendinopathy (Boling *et al.* 2009; Cowan *et al.* 2009). In support of this contention, postural balance and dynamic stabilisation training modes have been shown to reduce the incidence of patellar tendinopathy among elite female soccer players (Kraemer and Knobloch 2009). Training to develop strength of lateral trunk and hip abductor muscles should similarly be a particular area of emphasis, in view of the reported relationship between reduced lateral trunk strength and patellar tendinopathy (Cowan *et al.* 2009). Developing flexibility of muscles of the hip and knee joint likewise would appear to be an important aspect for the prevention of patellar tendonitis, given the association found between reduced quadriceps and hamstrings flexibility scores and incidence of this injury (Witvrouw *et al.* 2001).

Hamstrings

The increased incidence of hamstring strain injury reported following breaks of play indicates the importance of a comprehensive warm-up appropriate for preparing players to perform the activities required in the training session or match to follow (Brooks *et al.* 2006). A warm muscle has distinctly different mechanical properties, particularly with regard to its viscoelasticity. Likewise, the type of warm-up undertaken can also impact upon neuromuscular function (Bradley *et al.* 2007; Little and Williams 2006a). It is important that this not be neglected for players who enter the play as substitutes, given the higher rate of injury reported in this scenario (Brooks *et al.* 2006).

Lumbopelvic posture and stability are also factors that can increase the strain on the hamstring muscles. A focus of training interventions should be correcting the anterior pelvic tilt, given the association with hamstring strain injury (Croisier 2004), particularly the adverse effects this posture appears to have on activation of the gluteal muscles (Mendiguchia *et al.* 2012). Preliminary evidence suggests that interventions to improve lumbopelvic stability serve a protective role in decreasing the strain on the hamstrings and thereby reducing the risk of injury (Mendiguchia *et al.* 2012). It is similarly suggested that exercises to develop strength and recruitment of the gluteal muscles should be a focus for preventative interventions as well as rehabilitation (Mendiguchia *et al.* 2012). In addition to their role in stabilising the pelvis from the supporting limb, the extensors of the hip – and the gluteal muscles in particular – work synergistically with the hamstrings to generate hip extension and thereby propulsion when running. Decreased activation and strength of the gluteal muscles following hamstring strain injury has likewise been implicated in the mechanism for re-injury (Mendiguchia *et al.* 2012). There is also a suggestion that 'stabilisation training' may serve a role in reducing rates of re-injury in those with prior hamstring strain injury and should therefore be included in rehabilitation and preventative interventions (de Visser *et al.* 2012).

Strength imbalances are implicated in the incidence of hamstring strain injury. An investigation that evaluated strength imbalances using isokinetic strength test measures in soccer players, in particular the 'mixed ratio' of concentric quadriceps versus eccentric hamstring strength, assessed the effects of corrective strength training on the subsequent rate of hamstring injury (Croisier *et al.* 2008). A sub-group of the players identified as having a strength imbalance when tested at pre-season performed corrective strength training to normalise the relevant strength ratios. The rate of hamstring strain injury for these players in the subsequent competition season was reduced to a level that was in line with players who exhibited no strength imbalance at baseline (Croisier *et al.* 2008). This finding supports the efficacy of corrective training to normalise strength imbalances in reducing hamstring injury risk.

Developing muscular strength offers a means to extend the functional limits of the hamstrings, in order that there is extra force-generating capacity in reserve when the muscles' function is impaired by fatigue. Alongside strength training, appropriate metabolic conditioning similarly has an important role in the prevention of fatigue-related hamstring injury by developing fatigue-resistance (Verral *et al.* 2005). This is supported by a study demonstrating significant reductions in hamstring injury following a programme of pre-season training incorporating sport-specific anaerobic interval training drills (Verral *et al.* 2005). The success of the training intervention in reducing hamstring injuries, and number of games missed due to hamstring injury, was attributed to the adoption of high-intensity sport-specific interval training in place of the submaximal aerobic training emphasis of previous seasons (Verral *et al.* 2005).

Although the data are somewhat equivocal, lack of flexibility has been identified as a risk predisposing soccer players to hamstring muscle strains (Witvrouw *et al.* 2003). Reduced flexibility following injury has also been identified as contributing to the risk of re-injury (Opar *et al.* 2012). The best application of flexibility training might therefore be in a corrective function for those who exhibit reduced hamstring flexibility scores or imbalances between dominant and non-dominant limbs. Stretches for the hip flexors should also be considered, in view of the association reported between reduced flexibility of the

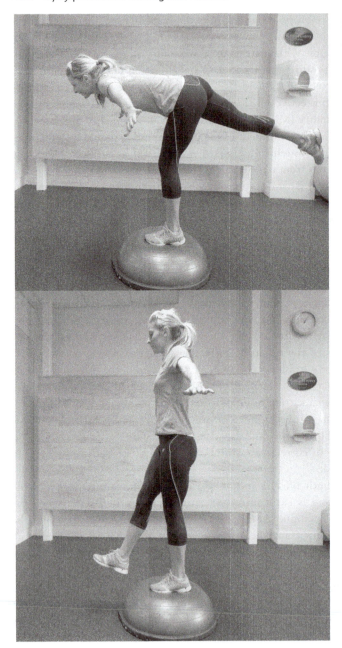

Figure 10.2
Single-leg hip flexion and
extension on domed device

hip flexor muscles and increased hamstring strain incidence in older players (Gabbe *et al.* 2006). Tightness of the hip flexors may also contribute to an anterior pelvic tilt, which is likewise associated with hamstring injury risk (Opar *et al.* 2012). Static stretching and partner-assisted flexibility training may be best performed during a cool-down after games and training or as a stand-alone flexibility training session, in order to avoid any potential adverse effects on performance (Gamble 2011e).

It has been identified that there is a tendency for athletes with a history of recurrent hamstring injury to show marked strength deficits. These athletes often show reduced scores with their previously injured limb on a range of isokinetic measures (particularly eccentric scores and mixed concentric:eccentric ratio measures) compared to the healthy contralateral limb (Croisier *et al.* 2002). It has been demonstrated that these deficits can be offset via corrective training, and doing so appeared to protect against sustaining further injury during a 12-month follow-up period (Croisier *et al.* 2002). Other authors have identified that the optimal angle – that is, knee joint angle at which the highest isokinetic concentric knee flexor torque was recorded – is significantly different for the previously injured leg versus the healthy contralateral limb in athletes with a history of recurrent hamstring injury (Brockett *et al.* 2004).

A number of authors suggest that eccentric strengthening exercises in particular may be important for hamstring strain injury prevention, especially for those with prior history of hamstring injury (Arnason *et al.* 2008; Brockett *et al.* 2004; Brooks *et al.* 2006). A potentially critical adaptation associated with eccentric training, which is not observed with conventional strength training modes, is eliciting a shift in the length–tension relationship (Brockett *et al.* 2001). Eccentric training therefore offers a means to correct changes in the optimal angle observed following injury so that muscle length associated with peak torque generation is moved closer towards pre-injury values, thereby helping to restore full function at longer muscle lengths to guard against re-injury (Brockett *et al.* 2004). Adaptations associated with eccentric training also serve a persisting protective effect that ameliorates eccentric muscle damage incurred during other activities undertaken during the period following the training intervention (Brockett *et al.* 2001); this phenomenon is termed the 'repeated bout effect'.

Injury prevention studies investigating the effects of eccentric training have typically employed the same corrective strength training modes as used in a rehabilitation setting. The 'Nordic hamstrings' exercise has been employed in the majority of studies; this exercise is performed in a kneeling position with the subject's feet secured by a partner; the subject resists their own momentum as they fall forwards. There is some evidence that eccentric training in this form may have a protective effect in reducing hamstring injuries in team sports players (Arnason *et al.* 2008; Brooks *et al.* 2006). However, the data from other studies are more equivocal and compliance with this form of training is often reported to be low (Opar *et al.* 2012).

It should, however, be recognised that conventional rehabilitation interventions employed following hamstring strain injury have proven to be ineffective in reducing the reported rates of re-injury over an extended period (Mendiguchia *et al.* 2012). In terms of exercise selection, it would equally appear to be critical that training modes are reflective of relevant movements in the sport, and that eccentric strength is developed at the required ranges of motion and muscle lengths. For example, specific development of eccentric strength at extended hamstring muscle lengths has been recommended (Croisier *et al.* 2002). Relevant postures and ranges of motion will include the critical terminal swing and early stance phases identified within the running gait cycle (Opar *et al.* 2012), as well as the locomotion and sports skill movements that are encountered in the sport. Based on these criteria, the Nordic hamstring exercise represents a highly nonspecific training mode. Employing this exercise alone is therefore unlikely to provide the comprehensive development of strength capabilities that is required, and more specific training modes should also be considered (Mendiguchia *et al.* 2012). For example, variations of the straight-legged deadlift (Figure 10.3) have been suggested to favour eccentric strength gains at relevant muscle lengths (Opar *et al.* 2012).

Adductor muscles

Strength training is recommended to protect against groin injury, in view of the association reported between adductor muscle weakness and injury (Engebretsen *et al.* 2010). In support of this, a pre-season strength training programme for the adductor muscles was reported to significantly reduce the incidence of adductor muscle strains in the following

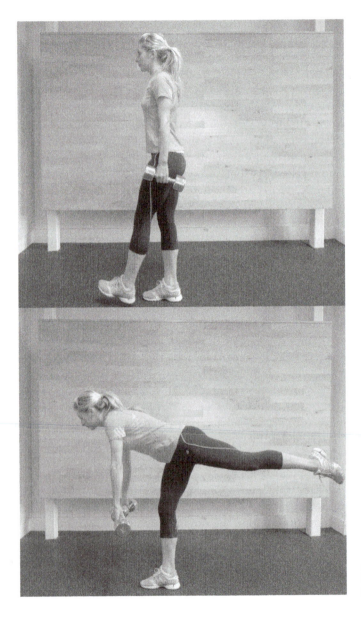

Figure 10.3
Single-leg dumbbell
straight-legged deadlift

season, in comparison to the rate of injury reported in the previous season (Tyler *et al.* 2002). Corrective strength training is recommended particularly for players with a relative weakness in their adduction versus abduction strength scores (Tyler *et al.* 2001). Targeted adductor muscle strengthening to correct identified strength imbalances has accordingly been shown to be effective in decreasing adductor strain injury incidence (Nicholas and Tyler 2002). Similarly, strength training for the adductor muscles has been identified as a critical component of interventions for those with a history of groin pain and injury (Tyler *et al.* 2002). In terms of exercise selection, given that the adductor muscles are primarily employed in closed kinetic chain activities, it follows that strength training for the adductors should similarly feature closed chain exercises.

Appropriate conditioning is also recommended as a means to protect against groin injury, based upon the findings that players with lower fitness scores suffer a greater incidence of groin strain injury (Maffey and Emery 2007). This protective effect of sport-specific conditioning in reducing injury also appears to show a dose–response relationship – that is, the more training that players had performed the lower the probability of injury (Emery and Meeuwisse 2001). Training interventions to specifically develop strength-endurance and increase fatigue-resistance of the adductor muscles might therefore also be recommended.

Although not a consistent finding, an association has been reported between impaired adductor muscle flexibility and risk of adductor muscle strain. Baseline scores of passive hip range of motion in abduction were found to be associated with subsequent incidence of adductor muscle injury in soccer players (Arnason *et al.* 2004). This association was not found in a study of professional ice hockey players, suggesting the influence of adductor muscle flexibility on injury risk may depend upon the sport (Tyler *et al.* 2001). Flexibility training is therefore recommended for 'at risk' sports such as soccer, and it may also be prudent to include these exercises for players in other sports.

As deficits in lumbopelvic stability are identified as a risk factor for groin strain injury, it is also recommended that training to develop lumbopelvic stability should be included in preventative training interventions. Corrective training to develop recruitment and function of the deep lumbar postural muscles and muscles of the hip complex is recommended,

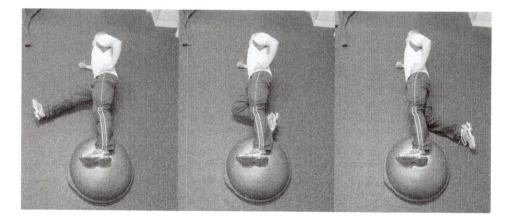

Figure 10.4 Side bridge 'wipers' on domed device

particularly for those with a history of groin pain and adductor strain injury (Maffey and Emery 2007). The reader is referred to Chapter 8 for information about specific training interventions.

Lumbar spine

Team sports players in particular have a need for both strength and endurance for the muscles that stabilise the spine in all three planes of motion (Barr *et al.* 2005; Leetun *et al.* 2004). Endurance rather than absolute strength of trunk muscles has been identified as being the most decisive factor with regard to low back pain incidence (McGill 2007b). Fundamentally, the postural muscles are designed to operate isometrically to provide stability to the lumbar spine. Accordingly, it has been identified that training modes that incorporate a static hold are found to be most effective in eliciting gains in cross-sectional area of deep lumbar stabilisers (multifidus) in patients with chronic low back pain (Danneels *et al.* 2001).

The muscles of the hip complex serve a major role in all dynamic activities performed in an upright stance (Nadler *et al.* 2000). The hip muscles are involved particularly in stabilising the pelvis during single-leg stance and the generation and transmission of forces from lower limb(s) to the spine. Correcting hip abductor strength imbalances via a core strengthening programme shows the potential to reduce subsequent lower back pain incidence (Nadler *et al.* 2002). Isometric hip external rotation strength was identified as the single best predictor of lower back and lower extremity injury incidence in collegiate athletes (Leetun *et al.* 2004). The importance of hip muscle function and the co-ordination between motion at the hips, pelvis and lumbar spine during throwing and striking sports skill movements has also been highlighted with respect to low back pain and injury (Harris-Hayes *et al.* 2009).

A critical aspect of injury prevention is neuromuscular and movement skills training to reinforce safe and 'spine-sparing' postures and movement patterns. A 'neutral' spine alignment is the most advantageous from the point of view of stability – when in a flexed position the lumbar spine is less able to resist both compressive and shear forces (McGill 2007b). Maintaining a neutral spine posture when performing athletic tasks is therefore beneficial for lumbar spine stability and helping to maintain the joint structures and connective tissues concerned within their failure limits. Accordingly, a key aspect of spine-sparing movement strategies is that motion occurs predominantly from the hips, rather than moving at the lumbar spine. Adopting these 'safe' postures and movement strategies not only spares the spine but also often facilitates superior athletic performance (McGill 2007b).

Corrective neuromuscular training to develop strength and recruitment of the deep postural muscles is also likely to be necessary for players with a history of lumbar spine pain and injury, based upon the finding that low back pain is often accompanied by disrupted motor patterns of various stabilising muscles (Rogers 2006). Similarly, a common finding is that deep lumbar spine stabiliser muscles are atrophied in individuals with chronic lower back pain (Barr *et al.* 2005). Importantly, this atrophy does appear to be reversible with appropriate training intervention, with associated improvements in low back pain symptoms (Hides *et al.* 2001). Individuals with chronic lower back pain also exhibit impaired neuromuscular feedback and delayed muscle reaction, which is accompanied by reduced capacity to sense the orientation of their spine and pelvis (Barr *et al.* 2005). The importance of 'proprioceptive' training to develop sensorimotor control has therefore been highlighted with respect to maintaining lumbar spine stability and reducing risk of pain and injury (Borghuis *et al.* 2008).

Specific training aimed at addressing the various functional deficits associated with low back pain and injury are likely to serve a protective function in guarding against both first-time incidence of injury, and recurrence injury in those with a history of low back pain. This should include developing strength and particularly endurance of muscles that provide lumbopelvic stability, addressing hip muscle weakness and imbalances, and developing proprioceptive awareness of lumbar posture and positioning of the pelvis (Rogers 2006). The various systems and muscles that provide stability to the lumbo-pelvic-hip complex work in different combinations depending on the posture and movement; a variety of exercises are therefore required (Axler and McGill 1997). Progressions should include exercises performed in standing postures and involving weight-bearing closed chain movements, in order to integrate the hip musculature and help develop balance and proprioception. The reader is referred to Chapter 8 for a full description of training approaches to develop lumbopelvic stability.

Neuromuscular and movement skills training that reinforces safe lumbar spine posture and emphasises moving the torso from the hips should be included in players' preparation (Barr *et al.* 2005; McGill 2007b). Maintaining the functional range of motion of muscles that cross the hip is also key to allowing these movement strategies and postures to be adopted. It follows that flexibility training for the hip and lower limb is another important aspect of training to help prevent low back pain and injury.

Shoulder complex

Acute shoulder injury

There is a suggestion of a fatigue element in the incidence of contact shoulder injuries in collision sports, based on the observation that injuries are commonly sustained during the latter stages of matches and training sessions (Headey *et al.* 2007). Similarly, transient reductions in function associated with microtrauma resulting from repeated collisions may also contribute to this finding in the case of matches and contact training sessions (Takarada 2003). One implication of this finding is that coaches in collision sports must allow for this by scheduling adequate recovery time following competitive matches and contact skills practices to guard against cumulative damage that may decrease function and predispose the player to more serious shoulder injury. Training interventions can also increase fatigue resistance and reduce the degree of muscle damage following strenuous physical exertion. Appropriate physical preparation, including strength training and contact skills conditioning, therefore has an important role in protecting against muscle damage, improving recovery of function and offsetting the effects of fatigue (Takarada 2003).

Targeted strength training interventions to develop strength and integrated function of the muscles that stabilise the joints of the shoulder girdle offers a means to enhance the structural integrity and failure limits of the shoulder. As a consequence of the high degree of mobility at the shoulder complex, it is heavily reliant upon the active stability provided by the integrated function of various muscles. As the majority of the range of motion during movement originates at the glenohumeral joint and from the articulation of the scapula and thorax (Myers and Oyama 2008), it follows that these areas should be the focus for training interventions. Both strength and strength-endurance should be addressed, in view of the observed influence of fatigue on shoulder injury incidence (Headey et al. 2007).

The optimal approach to preventive strength training for the shoulder complex will be in part dependent on the profile of the player. For example, if a particular imbalance has been identified, isolated exercises to strengthen particular muscles will be warranted (Beneka et al. 2006). If no imbalance has been identified, or pre-existing imbalances have been resolved, the use of more complex exercises has been advocated (Malliou et al. 2004). Such exercises allow muscles of the shoulder and upper limb to be recruited in a more integrated fashion (enabling sport-specific movements to be incorporated) and also facilitate greater gains in functional strength (Giannakopoulos et al. 2004). However, ongoing targeted strengthening for rotator cuff and scapula stabilisers should not be neglected for players in sports that are known to be particularly prone to shoulder injury (Gamble 2004b).

Resistance in the form of either free weights (such as dumbbells) or cable machines is generally preferable for these exercises as they avoid the adverse length–tension relationship associated with resistance bands or tubing, as well as providing greater ease of progressing load. Exercises for the scapula stabilisers should include rowing and pulling exercises that focus on retracting and adducting the scapula – for example, cable and dumbbell rows, cable lat pulldown exercise, and both standard and supine variations of the pull up – as well as exercises that focus on controlled scapular protraction, such as the 'push up plus' and dumbbell pull over exercises (Escamilla et al. 2009). Each of the four rotator cuff muscles is activated to varying degrees depending on the position of the upper limb and the constraints of the movement being performed (Decker et al. 2003; Takeda et al. 2002). It follows that exercise selection should reflect the movements and the loading conditions encountered during matches.

Given the high rate of re-injury and the severity of recurrent shoulder injuries it is critical that any residual deficits in function and sensorimotor control are addressed for players who have suffered previous shoulder injury (Headey et al. 2007). The reduced mechanical stability provided to the shoulder following traumatic injury, for example due to joint capsule and ligamentous laxity, increases the importance of active stabilisation but also poses challenges for proprioceptive function (Myers and Oyama 2008). It is therefore vital that sensorimotor training interventions are employed to help restore proprioceptive function in order to address the deficits in neuromuscular control and functional stability observed with players with previous shoulder injury. Prescription of specific exercises is discussed in the following section.

Overuse injuries of the shoulder complex

Chronic shoulder pain and injury are strongly associated with muscle imbalances or deficits in function of the rotator cuff of muscles that stabilise the glenohumeral joint and the muscles that control the articulation between the scapula and the thorax. For example, a relative weakness of external rotators is associated with overuse shoulder injury and is particularly prevalent among players in overhead sports (Wang and Cochrane 2001). Targeted strength training for the muscles that act on the glenohumeral joint and stabilise the scapula is therefore required, particularly for players in throwing and striking sports, to help avoid developing shoulder pain and overuse injury (Wagner 2003). This should include interventions to help correct or prevent the development of deficits in strength and strength-endurance that are characteristically observed in these sports.

Assessing the strength ratio between internal and external rotators is therefore a recommended starting point when addressing balance between muscles of the gleno-humeral joint (Beneka et al. 2006). This assessment can be undertaken using an isokinetic device if available (Giannakopoulos et al. 2004) or dumbbells if not (Beneka et al. 2006); in either case, both internal and external rotators are assessed in a position with the upper arm abducted at 90 degrees. Given that the external rotators act predominantly in an eccentric fashion when stabilising the glenohumeral joint during throwing and striking movements, it follows that eccentric strength or torque measurements are most relevant for these muscles (Niederbracht et al. 2008). The strength ratio expressed between internal rotators' concentric strength versus eccentric strength of external rotators is therefore suggested to be more valid. As alluded to previously, improving eccentric strength scores of the external rotators in relation to concentric strength of the internal rotators would appear to be the more critical issue (Niederbracht et al. 2008). Concentric strength improvements of external rotators are not always shown in following injury prevention training interventions. However, regardless of any lack of changes in concentric torque, eccentric strength measures are shown to improve in response to specific strength training for the external rotator muscles (Niederbracht et al. 2008).

Once identified, training modes can be selected to address rotator cuff muscle imbalances. A number of different exercises have been identified that elicit significant activation of each of the four rotator cuff muscles either alone or in combination (Escamilla et al. 2009). Isolated exercises with dumbbells, isokinetic training and multi-joint upper-body strength training exercises all have application to improving external versus internal peak torque ratios (Malliou et al. 2004). Once isolated exercises for specific development of rotator cuff muscles have been introduced, more complex exercises can be included in players' training which allow greater force development (Giannakopoulos et al. 2004). The muscles that control the articulation between the scapula and the thorax serve a crucial role in helping to achieve an optimal position and orientation of the socket in which the head of the humerus sits (Behnke 2001). A continuing focus on these muscles in players' physical development is therefore critical in order to maintain joint integrity and avoid impingement at the glenohumeral joint.

Functional problems with the shoulder complex are not always a result of activity: poor posture can also place the scapulae in a protracted position, creating a 'rounded' shoulder posture. Errors in physical preparation can have a similar effect on scapula position: unbalanced development of anterior (particularly chest) muscles can result in a protracted resting posture. Strength training for the middle and lower back muscles (rhomboids, middle and lower trapezius) that retract the scapulae can also serve an important role in correcting suboptimal postural traits. Appropriate exercises can strengthen these middle back muscles while actively stretching the shortened anterior muscles, helping to bring the resting position of the scapula back towards the desired position.

An impaired sense of scapula position and reduced ability to control the motion of the scapula about the wall of the thorax is a common finding among players who experience shoulder pain and injury in sports that involve repetitive throwing or striking (Wang and Cochrane 2001). This may be accompanied by reduced function affecting not only the rotator cuff muscles but also the prime movers of the gleno-humeral joint. The changes in sensorimotor control observed with overuse shoulder injuries are attributed to inhibition effects that result from the pain and the impinge-ment that is often associated with these conditions (Myers and Oyama 2008). Strength training offers a means to improve sensorimotor control and help to restore pain-free function. A range of exercises have been recommended for scapula stabilisation, including dumbbell and cable exercises (Brummitt and Meira 2006), which can be employed to develop strength and improve the capacity to control scapula positioning during movement. There will also be a need for corrective proprioceptive training for those athletes who exhibit suboptimal scapulo-humeral rhythm or shoulder reposi-tioning test scores during screening.

For overhead striking (as in volleyball) and throwing sports (baseball, softball, team handball) in particular, flexibility training to offset characteristic changes in internal versus external rotation range of motion appears warranted (Lintner et al. 2007). The common profile of baseball pitchers is for them to exhibit reduced internal rotation at the shoulder alongside increased range in external rotation (Mullaney et al. 2005). This is believed to be a consequence of repeatedly performing the throwing action during practices and games, often spanning a period of many years. Whereas the increased external rotation appears to be a structural (that is, bony) adaptation in the orientation of the humeral head and as such a relatively permanent adaptation, the reduction in internal rotation does appear to be modifiable. Professional baseball pitchers who had undertaken a programme of flexibility training targeted at addressing posterior capsule tightness over a prolonged period scored significantly higher on internal rotation range of motion measured on their dominant (throwing) arm (Lintner et al. 2007).

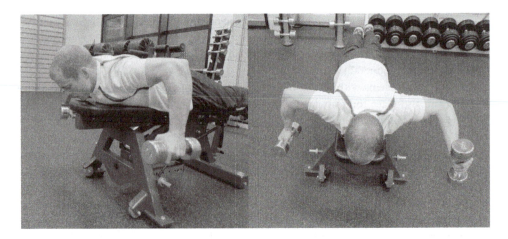

Figure 10.5 Prone dumbbell external rotation

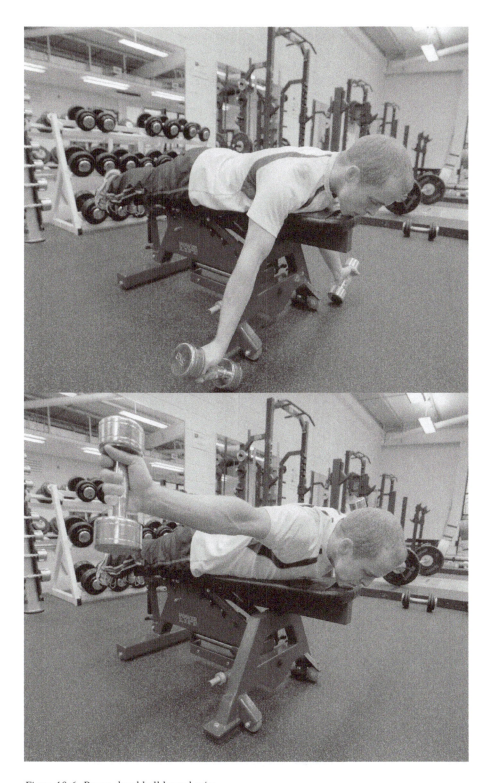

Figure 10.6 Prone dumbbell lateral raise

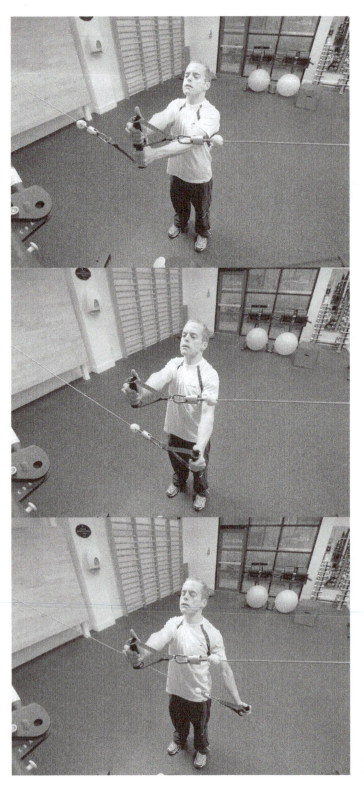

Figure 10.7
Alternate arm cable
reverse fly

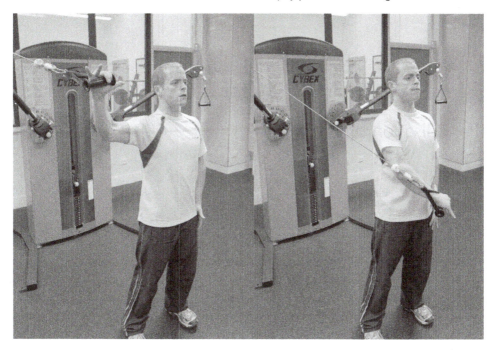

Figure 10.8 Cable diagonal pulley

Summary

The paucity of well-controlled injury studies make definitive recommendations with regard to evidence-based injury prevention training difficult, particularly in the case of muscle injuries such as hamstring strains (Peterson and Holmich 2005). In the absence of such studies, it is necessary to rely upon what is known about specific injury mechanisms and relevant modifiable risk factors for the particular injury.

Common themes include:

- Addressing functional stability by improving proprioception and neuromuscular control;
- Incorporating all parts of the lower limb kinetic chain – recognising the role of the hip musculature in providing proximal control to the lower limb and absorbing landing forces (Hewett *et al.* 2006a);
- Increasing muscle strength and correcting strength imbalances in order to increase in mechanical stability provided to a joint;
- Addressing muscle tightness and imbalances in mobility and flexibility via targeted flexibility training where deficits are identified.

In order to be most effective, the design of an injury prevention training intervention should not only be specific to the injury but also to the sport (Bahr and Krosshaug 2005). Practically, this means that exercise prescription should progress to exercises that reflect the specific conditions of the sport.

11

PLANNING AND SCHEDULING

Periodisation of training

Introduction

Training variation is fundamental to successful training prescription (Fleck 1999; Stone *et al.* 2000b; Willoughby 1993). Periodisation offers a framework for planned and systematic variation of training parameters (Brown and Greenwood 2005; Plisk and Stone 2003; Rhea *et al.* 2002; Stone *et al.* 2000b). Accordingly, it has been established that periodised training is able to elicit improved training responses in comparison to training groups with no variation in training load (Fleck 1999; Stone *et al.* 2000b; Willoughby 1993).

The consensus is therefore that periodised training offers superior development of strength, power, body composition and other performance variables (Fleck 1999; Stone *et al.* 1999a, 1999b, 2000b; Wathen *et al.* 2000; Willoughby 1993). Despite this there are very limited research data upon which to base decisions regarding the best approach to periodisation, particularly in the case of athlete populations (Fleck 1999; Cissik *et al.* 2008). The choice of periodisation schemes is therefore likely to be largely dictated by what is most appropriate for the competition calendar involved in the particular sport and what other training and technical practices the athlete is concurrently performing (Wathen *et al.* 2000).

In view of this, unique challenges are faced when attempting to apply periodisation to training design in team sports. Team sports players are required to perform high volumes of technical and/or tactical training, team practices and competitive matches. As a result, successful application of periodised training design for team sports requires considerable planning and skill (Gamble 2004b). Indeed there are numerous complications that represent an obstacle to effective application of periodised training in most team sports.

Despite these considerations, training variation provided by periodisation remains vitally important for team sports athletes. It follows that the approach to periodisation should be specific to the demands of the particular team sport, including the length of the competitive season and the number and frequency of fixtures involved. Selection of periodisation methods for different training mesocycles throughout the year should also reflect the needs of the respective phase of training (Plisk and Stone 2003).

Training variation

Training variation is acknowledged as serving a critical function in successful training prescription (Fleck 1999; Stone *et al.* 2000b; Willoughby 1993). According to either general adaptation syndrome (Selye 1956) or the more recent fitness–fatigue theory (Chiu and Barnes 2003), sustained exposure to the same training stimulus over time will fail to elicit further adaptation, and in time may lead to diminished performance (Wathen *et al.* 2000). One aspect of training variation is therefore avoiding plateaus in training adaptation or 'maladaptation' (negative impact on performance resulting from unplanned over-reaching or overtraining).

Another issue when planning athletes' training is that only two or three training goals can be emphasised at any one time (Zatsiorsky and Kraemer 2006). This is the case particularly with conflicting training goals that involve opposite hormonal responses (such as catabolic versus anabolic) and neuromuscular fatigue that interfere with training adaptation. Those sports that require a variety of training goals require that training is varied in a systematic way in order that different training goals are accounted for during different phases in the athlete's training year.

The degree of training variation required is also likely to be specific to the training experience of the individual (Plisk and Stone 2003). More basic periodisation schemes that involve less variety in training parameters are sufficient for younger athletes or those who do not have a long training history (Bompa 2000; Kraemer and Fleck 2005; Plisk and Stone 2003). This is not the case for more advanced athletes.

Periodisation of training

Periodisation was developed with the aim of manipulating the process of training adaptation, primarily in an effort to avoid the maladaptation phase and combat the risk of non-functional over-reaching or the more chronic state of overtraining or 'unexplained underperformance syndrome' (Wathen *et al.* 2000; Brown and Greenwood 2005). Periodisation offers a framework for planned and systematic variation of training prescribed to vary the training stimulus at regular intervals in order to prevent plateaus in training responses (Brown and Greenwood 2005; Plisk and Stone 2003; Rhea *et al.* 2002; Stone *et al.* 2000b).

Accordingly, it has been established that periodised training is able to elicit improved training responses in comparison to training groups with no variation in training load (Fleck 1999; Stone *et al.* 2000b; Willoughby 1993). However, very few studies of sufficient length assessing the effects of different approaches to periodised planning have been published (Fleck 1999). As such there are insufficient data upon which to base decisions when selecting the best approach to periodisation in order to plan athletes' training (Cissik *et al.* 2008).

One of the primary considerations when selecting the most appropriate periodisation scheme upon which to plan the training year is the competition calendar for the particular sport (Wathen *et al.* 2000). Another complication when scheduling athletes' training is the interaction of concurrent training and technical and/or tactical practices performed in the sport. In addition to scheduling concerns, the number and variety of training goals demanded in the sport are another key consideration.

Scheduling and transfer of training effects

In addition to avoiding potential negative effects of training monotony, use of periodisation schemes allows planning of training prescription to prioritise selected training goals at particular times in the training year. Periodisation and appropriate scheduling also offer the strength and conditioning specialist the facility to take advantage of the residual effects of preceding training cycles (Zatsiorsky and Kraemer 2006). Essentially, preceding phases of training can be used to 'potentiate' or enhance the athlete's response to the particular training prescribed in subsequent cycles. This 'superimposition' of training effects may be achieved via a coherent progression of training prescription during successive training cycles, and in particular the selection of training modes employed for different aspects of physical preparation. This is illustrated in Figure 11.1.

Periodising intensity, volume and content of training prescribed

In the traditional periodisation models, the training year or macrocycle is divided into an initial general preparation phase 'GPP', followed by special preparation phase(s) 'SPP' and culminating in the competition phase. The GPP is typically preceded by a period of active rest following the previous competition season and each phase within the training cycle may be separated and subdivided with 'transition' cycles (Wathen *et al.* 2000). The training goals for each cycle classically follow a particular sequence (Zatsiorsky and Kraemer 2006).

The goals during the general preparation phase are classically hypertrophy and/or strength-endurance and base metabolic conditioning to provide a foundation for the subsequent training phases in the year. Training goals then sequentially progress during the special preparation phase from general strength to strength/power and there is a shift to more intensive metabolic conditioning. The training goals that predominate during the competition phase will depend upon the sport; however, strength training is typically oriented towards power and power-endurance and metabolic conditioning becoming highly specific to the bioenergetics of the sport.

In accordance with the training goals for the respective phases of training, the early cycles in the training year or 'macrocycle' during the general preparation phase are characterised by higher training volumes and lower intensities (Wathen *et al.* 2000). Classically, as the training year progresses through the special preparation phase and into the competition phase, training intensity is increased with corresponding decreases in training volume. Whatever the periodisation scheme employed, intensity and volume will broadly show this diverging pattern (intensity progressively increasing and volume progressively decreasing) over the course of the training macrocycle. Another factor that comes into play during competition cycles is tapering of training frequency and volume for critical phases in the competition calendar to allow residual fatigue effects to subside in order that training effects can be fully expressed in the athlete's competition performance (Zatsiorsky and Kraemer 2006).

Periodic changes in exercise selection and conditioning modes are important in order to systematically change the training stimulus and thereby facilitate continued training adaptation (Zatsiorsky and Kraemer 2006). The classical model for periodised planning is for training modes to feature a progressive shift from 'general' training modes during general preparation cycles to increasingly 'specific' training modes, particularly as the athlete approaches key phases in the competition period. Accordingly, the general preparation phase is classically characterised by general strength training exercises and relatively non-specific metabolic conditioning modes including cross training. The special preparation phase in turn features a gradual progression towards the sport-specific strength training exercise selection and metabolic conditioning modes that characterise the competition

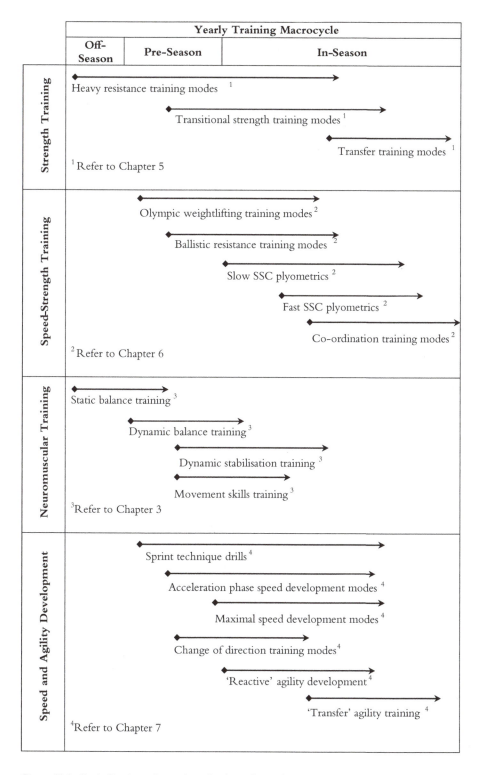

	Yearly Training Macrocycle		
	Off-Season	Pre-Season	In-Season

Strength Training

Heavy resistance training modes [1]

Transitional strength training modes [1]

Transfer training modes [1]

[1] Refer to Chapter 5

Speed-Strength Training

Olympic weightlifting training modes [2]

Ballistic resistance training modes [2]

Slow SSC plyometrics [2]

Fast SSC plyometrics [2]

Co-ordination training modes [2]

[2] Refer to Chapter 6

Neuromuscular Training

Static balance training [3]

Dynamic balance training [3]

Dynamic stabilisation training [3]

Movement skills training [3]

[3] Refer to Chapter 3

Speed and Agility Development

Sprint technique drills [4]

Acceleration phase speed development modes [4]

Maximal speed development modes [4]

Change of direction training modes [4]

'Reactive' agility development [4]

'Transfer' agility training [4]

[4] Refer to Chapter 7

Figure 11.1 Periodisation of exercise selection schematic

phase. This sequential shift towards the most specific strength training movements and conditioning modes is designed to translate the general or 'non-specific' strength qualities and conditioning base developed during earlier training cycles into sport-specific strength and fitness as the athlete enters the competition phase (Zatsiorsky and Kraemer 2006).

Approaching periodisation

When planning athletes' training it is customary to divide the 'macrocycle' (training year or biennial or quadrennial cycle in the case of Olympic sports) into smaller blocks called 'mesocycles' (Zatsiorsky and Kraemer 2006). Within each *mesocycle* are smaller blocks of time known as *microcycles*, which typically comprise a week or two-week block. Periodisation of training should consider planned variation and scheduling at levels from macrocycle, to mesocycle and microcycle. For example, planning at the level of the macrocycle must consider the key dates in the competition season. Planning at microcycle level concerns not only structuring individual sessions to meet the goals of particular phases of the training mesocycle, but also scheduling the training week to account for the respective demands of competitive matches, different training sessions and technical and/or tactical practices. Scheduling each training microcycle also requires consideration of potential negative interaction between conflicting forms of training – for example aerobic conditioning and strength/power training.

Periodisation schemes

A variety of periodisation models have been described in the literature. A brief outline of the different categories of periodisation schemes that are employed in various sports is presented here.

Linear periodisation

The classic 'linear' format for training periodisation is characterised by gradual increases in training intensity between successive mesocycles, with simultaneous reductions in training volumes. This progression culminates in a competition cycle, which is scheduled to coincide with one or more major competitions in the calendar and designed to allow the athlete to arrive at these competitions in peak physical condition (Wathen *et al.* 2000). Reverse periodisation approaches have also been employed which feature the opposite pattern – that is, high intensity and low volume employed at the outset, with progressive decrease in intensity and increase in volume thereafter, culminating in low intensity and high training volume. The reverse linear periodisation approach is, however, consistently found to produce inferior results to standard linear periodisation and other approaches (Prestes *et al.* 2009; Rhea *et al.* 2002).

With the classical linear periodisation format there is considerable variation in training prescription between consecutive phases in the training year, but little or no variation within each training block. Hence it is suggested that this approach may not provide sufficient variation in the training stimulus for athletes with extensive training experience. Modifications to the traditional linear periodisation approach have been employed that feature condensed training mesocycles, which serves to provide more frequent variation of training parameters. One example is the eight-week condensed linear model described by Allerheiligen and colleagues (2003) featuring condensed two-week mesocycles performed in series. A recent study successfully implemented another modified and condensed linear periodisation scheme that employed weekly alterations in training parameters, following the classical diverging pattern of progressively increasing intensity with concurrent reductions in volume (Prestes *et al.* 2009).

Block periodisation

This modified approach to periodisation was proposed as a solution to perceived shortcomings of the traditional linear approach in the context of the demands of modern high-performance sport, and in particular the challenges posed by the mixture of different forms of training performed by athletes in many sports (Issurin 2010). The rationale for block periodisation is based on the contention that different forms of training will produce conflicting physiological and endocrine responses, and as such attempting to perform 'mixed training' in combination for a prolonged period would elicit excessive fatigue and provide a suboptimal training stimulus over time. This contention has been challenged by other authors (Kiely 2010).

The proposed solution that is encompassed by the block periodisation approach is to adopt a more 'unidirectional' training emphasis within each training mesocycle. Specifically, the different forms of training performed concurrently by the athlete at any time should be restricted to only a minimal number. This approach essentially proposes a short (one- to three-week) concentrated block featuring a high volume of targeted training aimed at developing only one or two selected abilities, which is typically followed by a taper to prepare the athlete for an identified competition and a period of active recovery prior to the next intensive training cycle (Issurin 2010).

Nonlinear periodisation

Nonlinear or 'undulating' periodisation schemes involve variation in intensity and volume within a training microcycle, in addition to variation between mesocycles (Wathen *et al.* 2000). Nonlinear undulating periodisation is suggested to be more appropriate for highly trained athletes due to the greater level of training variation (both within and between training cycles) afforded by this approach (Monteiro *et al.* 2009). This approach is also devised to keep the athlete close to their peak for multiple competitions spanning an extended period. The variation between workouts within each microcycle also allows for multiple training goals to be addressed simultaneously (Zatsiorsky and Kraemer 2006).

Both daily and weekly undulating periodisation schemes are described in the literature and employed in the field (Buford *et al.* 2007). Daily undulating periodisation involves variation on a daily basis so that the training stimulus provided by each session within the training week is markedly different (Rhea *et al.* 2003). Weekly undulating periodisation involves large fluctuations in training intensity prescribed between consecutive weeks; however, the programming of sessions within each week remains consistent. For those with less training experience there is some evidence that the large fluctuations in training intensity that feature in the weekly undulating periodisation approach may limit the effectiveness of this approach due to the muscle soreness caused (Apel *et al.* 2011). In this case, the traditional linear approach appears to be more effective and might therefore be more suitable for younger or less experienced players, depending on their training history.

Summated mesocycles approach

Variations of the summated mesocycles method have been successfully applied in both rugby union and rugby league football (Baker 1998). This format involves a step-like increase in volume load (the product of training volume multiplied by training intensity) followed by a pronounced taper. Classically, the summated microcycles format operates around a four-week cycle, with the final week of the four-week cycle acting as an unloading week with considerably decreased volume load. This is designed to accommodate the time course of physiological processes underlying training adaptations and fatigue effects (Plisk and Stone 2003). These 'mini-cycles' are repeated in series at greater or lesser relative intensities. This basic pattern can therefore be employed sequentially to create a wave-like pattern in lifting intensity and training volume.

Use of periodisation in professional team sports

Strength and conditioning coaches working in a multitude of team sports at various levels report adopting a periodised approach to their programme design. The use of periodisation was indicated by the vast majority of Division One collegiate strength and conditioning coaches in the United States responding to a survey of their methods (Durell *et al.* 2003). Similar surveys of professional North American team sports reported comparable use of periodised training design (Ebben and Blackard 2001; Ebben *et al.* 2004, 2005; Simenz *et al.* 2005). These included National Basketball Association (90 per cent of respondents using periodised programmes) (Simenz *et al.* 2005), National Hockey League (91.3 per cent using periodisation) (Ebben *et al.* 2004), and Major League baseball (83.4 per cent) (Ebben *et al.* 2005).

National Football League coaches reported by far the lowest use of periodisation models (69 per cent) (Ebben and Blackard 2001). This may be a result of the contact nature of the sport. On the issue of training periodisation, one coach was quoted as saying 'Weight training in football is different than any other sport. When you have them healthy, (you) train them' (Ebben and Blackard 2001). The fact that the data collection for this study was notably earlier (1997–98) than the other respective surveys may also have played a part. This may in turn explain the relatively greater use of 'high-intensity training' methods (19 per cent) by the coaches in the sample (Ebben and Blackard 2001), which was enjoying relative popularity at the time.

Such difficulties as injuries and residual fatigue underline the unique challenges of designing periodised programmes for team sports athletes, particularly in the case of contact sports. Despite these considerations, training variation remains vitally important for team sports athletes. This is important to alleviate the monotony that can otherwise affect compliance throughout a long season of training and competition (Wathen *et al.* 2000). Taking player motivation aside, it is counterproductive and even harmful to train in the same way for extended periods. Short-term training studies consistently show training programmes that incorporate periodised training variation elicit superior results

(Stone *et al.* 2000b; Willoughby 1993). Solutions to these complications must therefore be sought to enable periodised training to be incorporated into athletes' physical preparation in a given sport.

Challenges and practical solutions for periodised team sports training

Extended season of competition

A major obstacle for coaches working in seasonal team sports is the frequent matches and extended competition period involved. The classical periodisation models for planned training variation were developed for the competitive season in track and field athletics (Plisk and Stone 2003). As a result, the classical linear periodised format features extended training cycles, designed to progressively prepare the athlete for one or two major championships in the year (Wathen *et al.* 2000).

The playing season for sports such as soccer and rugby union can span in excess of 35 weeks, particularly in Europe. If coaches were to follow the classic model, training would taper considerably for the duration of the competition phase. This is clearly counterproductive for most team sports (Baker 1998; Hoffman and Kang 2003). It has been identified that following such restrictive competition phase repetition schemes may lead to excessive losses in lean body mass during the season, which is unfavourable for most power sports (Allerheiligen 2003). Given this requirement to continue regular training over many months, achieving the necessary training variation represents a sizeable challenge.

It is vital that strength training is maintained in-season to prevent significant losses in strength, power and lean body mass (Allerheiligen 2003; Baker 1998). Periodisation schemes for in-season training will necessarily differ from those applied during off-season and pre-season training cycles. This will be discussed in greater detail later in the chapter.

Multiple training goals

Team sports require several disparate training goals. These can include, but are not limited to: hypertrophy, maximum strength, explosive power, metabolic conditioning and injury prevention (Gamble 2004b). Multiple and often conflicting training goals must therefore be addressed in the course of the training plan. In view of this, there is a need for planned variations in the training programme to systematically shift the emphasis to promote these different training effects at different points in the players' preparation.

Due to the need to maintain different neuromuscular and metabolic training goals as well as cater for technical and tactical practice, some periodisation strategies may not be appropriate for a given sport. An example of a periodisation scheme that appears less suited to the multiple training goals associated with many team sports is the conjugate periodisation model (Plisk and Stone 2003). This is an advanced approach that aims to exploit fitness and fatigue after-effects by consecutive overload cycles, alternately stressing one motor quality (for example, strength) for a period then switching to overload another motor quality (such as speed) for the subsequent training cycle (Plisk and Stone 2003). Two main training goals are hence typically coupled in this approach. During the overload phase for the other motor quality in the couple (strength), a low volume maintenance programme is undertaken for the motor quality not being emphasised (speed) (Plisk and Stone 2003). These overload cycles are alternated in series. The greater number of training goals required by many team sports than the two motor qualities typically addressed in this periodisation format would obviously make the application of this approach problematic.

It has been suggested that undulating, 'non-linear', periodised approaches are more viable when planning the training year for team sports (Wathen et al. 2000). The rationale for this is that such periodisation strategies allow for more variation in both training intensity and volume, both within and between training cycles. As such multiple training goals can be emphasised in each training microcycle (Zatsiorsky and Kraemer 2006). However, at some phases of the training year, in particular the off-season and pre-season, sequential approaches similar to the classical linear periodisation model may still have merit. This is explored further in a later section.

Interaction between different forms of training

When programming strength training, coaches must also take account of the interaction of the different forms of training that are undertaken concurrently within the training week by team sports players (Gamble 2004b). From this viewpoint, the physical activity involved in technical and/or tactical sessions and team practices should also be considered. Specifically, a major consideration is the high volume of metabolic conditioning undertaken alongside strength training and power and speed development in many team sports. It has been documented that a prior bout of endurance exercise in the training day is shown to impair an athlete's ability to perform strength training (Kraemer et al. 1995; Leveritt and Abernethy 1999). After performing a conditioning session, players are reportedly not able to complete the same number of repetitions with a given load that they are capable of without having previously performed endurance exercise (Leveritt and Abernethy 1999).

These interference effects are also associated with conflicting hormonal responses to strength versus endurance training, which may blunt the response to strength and power training. When strength training is performed in the same day following endurance training, training outcomes with respect to power indices in particular are shown to be affected (Kraemer et al. 1995). It therefore appears that strength and power training outcomes that are associated with greater neuromuscular co-ordination demands may be most susceptible to such interference effects.

Time constraints imposed by concurrent technical and tactical training

Given the time constraints imposed by the high volumes of team practices and other skill training common to all professional team sports, the time-efficiency of physical preparation is paramount. As the playing season approaches, focus inevitably shifts to tactical aspects – with a greater number of team practices to prepare for the forthcoming fixtures (Hedrick 2002; Wathen et al. 2000). During the season, the need to maximise the effectiveness of what limited training time is available is greater still.

The issue of limited training time may be addressed by optimising the time-efficiency of the training that is performed. A useful strategy is to incorporate different elements in order to combine practice and physiological training aspects in a single session. Particularly in-season, speed development and agility work can be included in team practice sessions (Wathen *et al.* 2000). Similarly, plyometric work can be incorporated into strength training sessions – for instance by employing complex training methods.

A good example of combined physiological and technical training is the use of game-related methods for metabolic conditioning (Gamble 2007b). The skill element involved encourages coaches to continue metabolic conditioning via the use of conditioning games when the training emphasis shifts to skills practice and game strategy (Gamble 2004a). Continuing metabolic conditioning in this form during the playing season is likely to allow cardiorespiratory endurance to be better maintained in-season.

Impact of physical stresses from games

When planning training during competition periods, allowances will inevitably need to be made for players' recovery after each match. Particularly in the days following games, this need to allow the players' bodies to recover is likely to limit the intensity and volume of physical training they are able to perform. As such there is the potential for the high volumes of physically demanding practice sessions and competitive games during the season to result in players losing muscle mass during the playing season (Allerheiligen 2003).

In the case of contact sports in particular, consideration must also be given to the physical stresses that result from violent bodily contact with opponents and the playing surface during both practices and matches. As a consequence muscle tissue damage incurred particularly during the playing season may compromise the quantity and content of strength training that players are able to undertake, potentially to the extent that strength and power levels may be diminished over time (Hoffman and Kang 2003).

Scheduling of training in-season and during late pre-season when competitive matches are being played should take appropriate measures to tailor training sessions to the players' physical status. In the day(s) immediately following the game, strength training will necessarily be limited to light recovery workouts, implemented alongside acute recovery practices. Similarly, the strength and conditioning coach should be prepared to modify the workout scheduled for a given day in the event that a player reports to training suffering from excessive residual fatigue or with a diagnosed acute injury that will impair their ability to perform the particular session set on that day (Plisk and Stone 2003).

Practical application of periodised training for a team sports season

As discussed earlier in the chapter, the degree of variation in training loads and volumes will depend on the age and experience of the player. Elite players are capable of tolerating higher training stress – hence training intensity and volume may remain close to their upper ranges for a large part of the training year (Wathen *et al.* 2000). Furthermore, elite athletes will tend to require a greater degree of variation to optimise the effectiveness of their training (Plisk and Stone 2003; Stone *et al.* 2000b).

In this section sample mesocycles will be described to illustrate the periodisation strategies proposed for each phase of the training year for a generic team sports athlete. The rationale behind the approaches used for each of the respective training cycles is outlined below. Specific programme variables, such as the length of each phase and exercise selection, will vary according to the length of the playing season and demands of the particular sport. A sample periodised plan is also presented in Tables 11.1 to 11.4.

Off-season

For the purposes of clarity, the 'off-season' phase for team sports will be defined as the period prior to the start of structured technical and tactical practices. Whether the strength and conditioning specialist actually has the luxury of a supervised off-season period when the players report back after the post-season break tends to depend on the willingness of the coaching staff to delay the start of practices to allow them to do so. As a consequence of the length of the playing season, particularly in European soccer and rugby football leagues, this is often not the case.

Due to the long season of competition, it is vitally important to allow a period of active rest following the end of the playing season (Wathen *et al.* 2000). That said, the length of the active rest period should be restricted to avoid players entering off-season training in a detrained state. Similarly, in view of the length of time players are engaged in supervised training it may make sense to allow players to undertake the early initial part of off-season training in an unsupervised setting. This will undoubtedly have a psychological benefit in sports with an extended playing season by limiting the monotony of the training ground environment.

Programming during the off-season will resemble the classical 'general preparation phase'. As such, training parameters during this time of year will be characterised by relatively higher volume and frequency of training conducted at lower intensity, and exercise selection will emphasise general training modes for overall development. Accordingly, general strength exercises that might be considered non-specific do still have merit during this phase of the athlete's preparation (Siff 2002). One aspect of this is that from the point of view of training variation, lifts which are considered sport-specific should not be used exhaustively throughout the duration of the training year (Wathen *et al.* 2000). The other determining factor is that the training goals for this point in the training year should be building a foundation of athleticism prior to concentrating on sport-specific development in later phases.

As such, the starting point when prescribing off-season strength training should be the results of the player's musculoskeletal and movement screening which should be undertaken when players report back to training at the beginning of the new training year. Exercise selection can then address any deficiencies identified and focus upon developing strength and motor abilities for fundamental athletic movements, such as variations of the squat, lunge and step up. Likewise, upper-body development during this phase will emphasise generic pushing and pulling lifts and raises in various planes of movement.

Pre-season

As alluded to previously, 'pre-season' for team sports will be deemed to be the period of supervised training prior to the start of the playing season when technical and tactical practices are concurrently scheduled. Accordingly, during this phase physiological training must be planned in the context of the other training and practices players are required to perform. From this point of view, it is therefore vital that scheduling of training is carried out in collaboration with the coaching staff.

Table 11.1 Representative off-season training mesocycle

	Training modes	*Periodisation of intensity, volume, frequency*
Strength training	'General strength development' training modes (refer to Chapter 5) Corrective exercises to address any issues identified during screening	Linear
Speed-strength training	N/A	N/A
Plyometric training	N/A	N/A
Metabolic conditioning	Aerobic interval training (refer to Chapter 4) Combination of cross training modes and running conditioning	Linear
Speed training	N/A	N/A
Change of direction training and agility development	N/A	N/A

The traditional linear format for training periodisation still merits application during the pre-season phase of training for team sports. Depending on the length of the pre-season in the particular sport, the initial part of pre-season may be a continuation of the general preparation phase begun during the off-season period. The remainder of the pre-season period will resemble the 'special preparation phase' in the classic model. Broadly there will be a progressive increase in training intensity prescribed and correspondingly decreasing volume over the period. Training goals will show a sequential shift from hypertrophy and/ or strength-endurance to strength, culminating in a power-oriented phase prior to the start of the playing season.

A suggested amendment to the classic linear model during the pre-season preparation phase for team sports athletes is to shorten the duration of the respective cycles (Hedrick 2002). The relative emphasis in terms of length and nature of each mesocycle will be determined by the requirements of the sport (Hedrick 2002). For example, in a sport that is reliant on lean body mass, the higher volume hypertrophy-oriented cycles will be relatively longer and will feature more prominently. Conversely, sports in which excessive hypertrophy is counterproductive will favour strength and particularly power cycles.

Equally, the block periodisation approach (Issurin 2010) described in a previous section may also be a viable alternative for the pre-season training period. The pre-season may be divided into blocks of varying length, depending on what is most appropriate given the time available. In accordance with this approach, only two or three training goals will be prioritised within each training block. The selection of training goals emphasised in successive training blocks should be sequenced appropriately in order to take advantage of the residual and cumulative effects of preceding training cycles (Issurin 2010). For example, heavy resistance strength training performed earlier in the pre-season period will have a favourable effect on training outcomes when specialised power and speed development is undertaken in later training cycles.

A further suggested manipulation is to incorporate day-to-day variation, by varying prescribed RM loads during each respective training week. This allows variation on multiple levels – both within and between microcycles. Such an approach has been suggested to favour optimal training responses (Stone *et al.* 2000b). As such the periodisation of training intensity and volume during pre-season might comprise elements of both linear and undulating periodisation, featuring weekly variation in intensity and volume within an overall trend for progressively increasing intensity and decreasing volume over the wider period.

Selection of strength training modes will similarly follow the sequential progression in training goals during each respective phase from general strength during the initial stages to power development and sport-specific strength at the culmination of the pre-season training period (Wathen *et al.* 2000). Strength training exercise selection will thus feature progressive introduction of speed-strength training modes and increasingly sport-specific exercises as the player advances through pre-season training cycles.

Table 11.2 Representative pre-season training mesocycle

	Training modes	*Periodisation of intensity, volume, frequency*
Strength training	Progression from general strength development in early preseason to special preparation phase strength development training modes (refer to Chapter 5) Corrective exercises to address any issues identified during screening	Linear
Speed-strength training	Introduction of bilateral ballistic resistance training modes and basic Olympic-style lifts at the midpoint of pre-season (refer to Chapter 6)	Linear
Plyometric training	Introduction of bilateral slow SSC training modes mid-preseason followed by progression to unilateral slow SSC training modes (refer to Chapter 6)	Linear
Metabolic conditioning	Progression aerobic interval to anaerobic interval training modes to repeated sprint conditioning late pre-season (refer to Chapter 4) Combination of conditioning modes including skill-based games and conditioning drills at appropriate intensities	Linear
Speed training	Introduction of technique development drills and instruction/development of acceleration mechanics mid-preseason, followed by progression to higher velocity sprint repetitions and acceleration drills (refer to Chapter 7)	Linear
Change of direction training and agility development	Introduction of movement skills training mid-pre-season, followed by progression to reactive agility drills (refer to Chapter 7)	Linear

In-season

Undulating 'non-linear' periodisation models are typically suggested for in-season training (Wathen *et al.* 2000). The rationale is that this approach may be better suited to maintain the athlete close to their peak throughout an extended season of regular competitions. The variation in training prescription within each training microcycle under this format will also allow the strength and conditioning specialist to concurrently account for the multiple training goals that are a common feature of team sports during the playing season (Zatsiorsky and Kraemer 2006).

Alternative approaches to periodisation for the competition season are however available. It has been highlighted that performing extended training blocks characteristic of classical linear periodisation models in-season may not be sufficient to maintain lean body mass in power sports athletes, such as American football players (Allerheiligen 2003). Another approach advocated for team sports players that are reliant on strength and power involves a condensed linear periodisation format, featuring two-week training blocks performed in series. It is suggested that this eight-week sequence can be repeated throughout the length of the playing season (Allerheiligen 2003). A similar 'condensed linear' approach involving weekly progression of training parameters may also be employed in the same way (Prestes *et al.* 2009).

Another framework for in-season periodised training is the 'summated microcycles' approach described in a previous section (Plisk and Stone 2003). This approach may also be adapted in order to tailor respective microcycles to the fixture list, by modifying the length of each summated cycle. Important matches and games against particularly strong opponents represent natural times to taper in-season training. Periods with many games concentrated into a short space of time likewise require reduced training frequency. Both these instances will necessitate an unloading week, in order to allow players to enter these matches in peak condition. Hence, depending on the timing of these games the summated microcycle may range from two to four weeks in length, always concluding with an unloading week. Microcycles may therefore feature a 1:1, 2:1 or 3:1 ratio of loading:unloading weeks. How these variations of in-season microcycles are sequenced into the in-season plan will depend on the fixture list and density of games in different periods within the season.

It has been identified that average training intensity should be maintained above 80 per cent 1-RM, in order to maintain strength levels during the course of a playing season (Hoffman and Kang 2003). Similarly, two days per week training frequency is often recommended for training during the competitive phase (Wathen *et al.* 2000). High loads (at or above 80 per cent 1-RM, or at or above 8–RM) are thus implemented two days per week for multi-joint lifts. This loading scheme is shown to maintain, or even increase, strength levels throughout the playing season in American football (Hoffman and Kang 2003).

In accordance with this, the majority of strength and conditioning coaches in professional leagues typically report strength training twice per week in-season (Ebben and Blackard 2001; Ebben *et al.* 2004, 2005; Simenz *et al.* 2005). However, these recommendations for in-season training need not be excessively restrictive. A range of training frequencies and training parameters are possible that will maintain average training frequency and intensity within the ranges recommended. Players may train between one and three times per week at various times in the season. Likewise, a variety of intensity prescriptions may be used at different phases, while still maintaining average training intensity above 80 per cent 1-RM throughout the season.

Conversely there will generally be opportunities during the season for more intensive strength training – such as during fixtures in lesser competitions, or mid-season breaks for international matches. In sports with an extended competitive season, such as is seen in European soccer and rugby leagues, this may be necessary to maintain physiological adaptations. This will tend to be the case particularly in collision sports that are reliant upon high levels of lean body mass, strength and power. At appropriate times mid-season, short overload microcycles may therefore be implemented, followed by a taper and/or active recovery. For these 'shock blocks' during the in-season period the strength and conditioning specialist can therefore adopt an approach similar to the block periodisation model (Issurin 2010).

Scheduling considerations for the weekly microcycle

During the period when players are not required to participate in competitive matches, scheduling of weekly training during pre-season should aim to take account of fitness and fatigue effects. As such, the sessions that require the greatest neuromuscular co-ordination while the athletes are fresh will be placed early in the week, whereas the more fatiguing

Table 11.3 Representative in-season training mesocycle

	Training modes	*Periodisation of intensity, volume, frequency*
Strength training	Progression from special preparation phase strength development to transfer training modes (refer to Chapter 5)	Summated mesocycles
Speed-strength training	Progression to advanced Olympic-style lifts, unilateral ballistic resistance training modes and introduction of co-ordination training modes (refer to Chapter 6)	Modified linear
Plyometric training	Progression from unilateral slow SSC training modes to fast SSC training modes (refer to Chapter 6)	Modified linear
Metabolic conditioning	Cycling of aerobic interval training, anaerobic interval training and repeated sprint conditioning (refer to Chapter 4) Combination of conditioning games, skill-based conditioning drills, and movement-specific high-intensity conditioning drills, depending on respective block	Blocked periodisation
Speed training	Progression to game-related acceleration and speed work (refer to Chapter 7)	Weekly undulating periodisation
Change of direction training and agility development	Progression to more challenging and context-specific reactive agility drills and partner drills (refer to Chapter 7)	Daily undulating periodisation

Table 11.4 Representative 'peaking' training mesocycle

	Training modes	*Periodisation of intensity, volume, frequency*
Strength training	Transfer training modes (refer to Chapter 5)	Summated mesocycles
Speed-strength training	Unilateral ballistic resistance training modes and resisted sprint training modes (refer to Chapter 6)	Summated mesocycles
Plyometric training	Predominantly unilateral fast SSC training modes (refer to Chapter 6)	Summated mesocycles
Metabolic conditioning	Repeated sprint conditioning and speed-endurance training (refer to Chapter 4) Movement-specific high-intensity conditioning drills	Daily undulating periodisation
Speed training	High-intensity game-related acceleration and speed work (refer to Chapter 7)	Daily undulating periodisation
Change of direction training and agility development	High-intensity game-specific reactive agility and partner drills (refer to Chapter 7)	Daily undulating periodisation

workouts are performed at the end of the week to allow the athlete the weekend to recover (Chiu and Barnes 2003).

Conversely, weekly scheduling of workouts in-season is dictated by the dual need to allow the player to recover from the previous match and avoid excessive residual fatigue at the end of the week in preparation for the next game. This is true of all the variations of the in-season training cycles. Similarly, the strength and conditioning specialist must be prepared on any given day to revise the schedule and modify the session plan as is appropriate to the current status of the player.

The sequencing of the training day appears key to minimising the degree to which strength and power development are compromised by concurrent metabolic conditioning work (Leveritt and Abernethy 1999). It has been established that when strength (or speed-strength) training is prioritised in the training day, and performed before conditioning, these interference effects can be reduced (Leveritt and Abernethy 1999). Sequencing training in this way is shown to optimise strength training responses of professional rugby league players, to the extent that strength and power measures can be maintained during the course of a lengthy (29-week) in-season period (Baker 2001). Younger (college-aged) players can even increase strength and power scores during the playing season by adopting this approach (Baker 2001).

Summary and conclusions

There are currently too few studies of sufficient length to make categorical assertions regarding the superiority of one approach to periodisation over another – particularly given the paucity of periodisation studies featuring athlete subjects (Fleck 1999; Cissik *et al.* 2008). Furthermore, such debates may be redundant – by definition periodisation concerns variation of training. As a result it seems unlikely that a single periodised training scheme exists that will elicit optimum results when applied for extended periods. Rather it seems probable that a range of periodisation strategies implemented in combination will produce the best results throughout players' long-term training (Plisk and Stone 2003).

Some evidence for this assertion was observed in the superior strength gains during initial stages of training in strength-trained subjects with a daily undulating periodised (DUP) model, in comparison to a linear periodisation group (Rhea et al. 2002). This was attributed to the novelty of the DUP scheme for the subjects, whose previous training had been characterised by linear periodisation (Rhea et al. 2002). Equally the attenuated training response and reports of training strain in the latter part of the study period in the DUP group indicates that the continued use of this scheme in isolation may similarly be unproductive (Rhea et al. 2002).

Hence, the best approach would appear to involve strategically combining methods, implementing periodisation schemes in each training mesocycle throughout the training year according to the needs of the respective phase of players' preparation (Plisk and Stone 2003). Periods in the off-season and pre-season without competitive games will undoubtedly allow different approaches to periodised training from those that will be conducive for adequate recovery when matches are scheduled.

12

PHYSICAL PREPARATION FOR YOUTH SPORTS

Introduction

Youth training requires a specific and quite different approach to design and implementation of physical preparation. As famously stated by Tudor Bompa, young people cannot merely be considered 'mini adults' (Bompa 2000). The physiological makeup of children and adolescents is markedly different from that of mature adults (Naughton *et al.* 2000) – it follows that the parameters applied to training design should reflect these differences.

The young athlete's neural, hormonal and cardiovascular systems develop with advances in biological age, leading to corresponding changes in neuromuscular and athletic performance (Quatman *et al.* 2006). Rates of development of a number of physiological and physical performance parameters measured in young team sports athletes are shown to peak at approximately the same time as they attain peak height velocity (Philippaerts *et al.* 2006). The age at which this occurs is highly individual; 'typical' ages are around 11.5 years for females (Barber-Westin *et al.* 2006) and for males in the range of 13.8–14.2 years (Philippaerts *et al.* 2006). However, this does vary considerably – levels of biological and physiological maturation can be markedly different between young athletes of the same chronological age (Bompa 2000; Kraemer and Fleck 2005).

What constitutes appropriate strength training and metabolic conditioning for young team sports players is therefore determined by, and is specific to, the individual player's stage of physical development. The phase of growth and maturation also influences the mechanism of training effects – such as whether improvements are predominantly mediated by neural factors, or if morphological and physiological adaptations play the greater role (Stratton *et al.* 2004). The emotional and psychological maturity of the individual is another important factor to be considered when designing and implementing training for youth sports players (Kraemer and Fleck 2005; Stratton *et al.* 2004).

Another area of training for young athletes that has received less attention is neuromuscular training, including specific instruction and practice of fundamental movement mechanics. Neuromuscular and postural control as well as movement biomechanics for jumping, landing, running and changing direction can all be developed in the young team sports player as a means to improve athleticism. Such development of fundamental movement skills may also help reduce injury risk by equipping the young player to be better able to react to challenges in the game environment.

Necessity of physical preparation for young team sports players

Major public health concerns are the sedentary behaviours and declining levels of physical activity of youth worldwide (Hills *et al.* 2007). As a result of modern sedentary lifestyles, young people are also often not physically prepared for the rigours of youth sports (Faigenbaum and Schram 2004; Kraemer and Fleck 2005). Accordingly, the increase in participation in organised youth sports in North America has been accompanied by a dramatic rise in sport-related injuries (Goldberg *et al.* 2007; Kraemer and Fleck 2005). It has not been documented whether this increase in the number of injuries has been proportional to the increased numbers participating, or whether there has been a relative increase in the rate of injury among these young players.

Whatever the case, approximately one-third of young athletes participating in organised sports in the United States sustain injuries requiring medical attention (Barber-Westin *et al.* 2005). Incidence of medical treatment for sports injuries peaks between the ages of 5 and 14 years and then progressively declines thereafter (Adirim and Cheng 2003). The ankle and knee are the most frequent sites of injury reported in these young athletes (Adirim and Cheng 2003; Barber-Westin *et al.* 2005). Youth sports players also appear to be at greater risk of low back pain and acute lumbar spine injury, particularly during adolescence (Kujala *et al.* 1996).

Inadequate physical preparation is believed to play a role in the majority of sport-related injuries in young athletes (Kraemer and Fleck 2005). Conditions of muscle fatigue do place athletes at greater risk of injury: tired players in the latter stages of a game are more likely to sustain injury than when they are fresh. Likewise, players are more likely to be injured early in the season when their fitness levels are not up to standard (Thacker *et al.* 2003). Injuries incurred during youth sports are a commonly cited reason for ceasing to participate in sport as an adult (Mackay *et al.* 2004). This has negative health implications given the established links between physical inactivity, obesity and chronic disease in adulthood (Hills *et al.* 2007). From this perspective, prevention of injury in youth sports assumes increased importance, beyond merely enhancing young players' sports performance (Mackay *et al.* 2004).

Physical preparation, which includes strength training in addition to training to develop cardiorespiratory fitness, is therefore an established and integral part of strategies employed to prevent sports injuries, including those in children and youth sports (Mackay *et al.* 2004). Inadequate motor skills are another factor identified as increasing youth sports injury risk (Adirim and Cheng 2003). Again, these abilities may be developed via appropriate athletic preparation.

Addressing fundamental movement skill development

Pre-adolescents exhibit considerable potential for motor learning. Many authors state that complex motor skills are not mastered until ages 10–12 (Adirim and Cheng 2003; Barber-Westin *et al.* 2006). It is suggested that there is a prime window of opportunity for motor development prior to puberty. Teaching basic movement mechanics for running, decelerating and changing direction should form a fundamental part of training for all young players. Performing complex whole-body training exercises is advocated to enhance co-ordination and athleticism. Such training also develops kinaesthetic awareness and proprioception, making the young player better able to retain their balance under pressure from opponents and adjust to uneven terrain. Improving these functional abilities might therefore have a protective effect, helping to guard against injury (Faigenbaum and Schram 2004).

It has been identified that prepubescent athletes have a tendency to exhibit neuromuscular control deficits relating to aberrant lower alignment during various tasks (Barber-Westin *et al.* 2005). This is indicative of impaired ability to control lower limb joint motion, and as such is associated with increased injury risk (Ford *et al.* 2003). Training to specifically improve lower limb neuromuscular control would therefore appear important in order to correct the potentially injurious lower limb alignment when it is observed in these prepubescent team sports players. Young females in particular show these traits throughout their development (Barber-Westin *et al.* 2005). Recent studies show that post-pubescent male athletes may also continue to exhibit valgus lower limb alignment during drop landing tasks, despite markedly increased lower limb strength levels (Barber-Westin *et al.* 2006; Noyes *et al.* 2005). It follows that appropriate screening and neuromuscular training should not be neglected with adolescent male team sports players.

In prepubescent players such neuromuscular control issues and injurious lower limb alignment are offset by their lower body mass and movement velocity (Barber-Westin *et al.* 2006). In contrast, adolescent players are much heavier and generate greater forces and movement speeds – markedly increasing imposed stresses as a result of their greater inertia and momentum (Barber-Westin *et al.* 2006). The consequences of any deficits in neuromuscular control in adolescent players are therefore greatly magnified.

Supporting growth, development and body composition

Regular physical activity in combination with proper nutrition exerts a major influence upon growth and development in children and adolescents. It is suggested that there is a threshold level of physical activity which, in combination with proper nutrition, is required in order that young players achieve their genetic potential in terms of growth and maturation (Hills *et al.* 2007). A structured programme of physical preparation offers a means to ensure that this is achieved, particularly at critical periods in the young player's growth and maturation.

From this perspective, appropriate physical preparation assumes increased importance to a young player's athletic development given the apparent lack of habitual physical activity elsewhere in their lifestyle. The absence of such a programme of physical preparation to help achieve a threshold level of physical activity may otherwise hinder young players' development during critical periods in their growth and maturation to the extent that they may not fulfil their genetic potential (Hills *et al.* 2007).

Furthermore, dedicated training for youth sports also appears vital to help these players maintain lean body composition in view of the declining physical activity and rising obesity among youth in general. This would appear to be particularly important during certain critical periods of growth and maturation. For example, during and following puberty females exhibit characteristic changes in body composition including gains in body fat mass, which can be unfavourable to performance and potentially to health (Naughton *et al.* 2000). Appropriate resistance training, in conjunction with aerobic exercise, has been proposed for losing body fat and for weight maintenance with young people – in much the same way as is recommended for adults (Faigenbaum and Schram 2004). In view of the increasing incidence of childhood obesity the potential of physical preparation which includes resistance training to favourably alter body composition is also advantageous from a health perspective (Hills *et al.* 2007).

Conversely, the potential for strength training to increase lean body mass is of relevance to players in collision sports from a selection and performance perspective. In sports such as rugby and American football, physical size is a determining factor for participation at higher levels (Olds 2001). Young players are naturally predisposed to – and selected for – particular playing positions on the basis of their anthropometric (height and body mass) characteristics as well as their strength capabilities (Duthie *et al.* 2003). Without a background of systematic strength training, young players are unlikely to have undergone the requisite physical development for selection at the highest levels.

Influence of growth and maturation on the development of physical performance capabilities

The scope for improvements in different aspects of fitness and motor performance varies as the young athlete passes through different stages of physical maturation. Rates of development of a number of physiological parameters appear to peak at around the same time as peak height velocity (stage of maximal growth in height) in young team sports players (Philippaerts *et al.* 2006). The age that peak height velocity is attained varies considerably, but is reported to occur at around 11.5 years for females (Barber-Westin *et al.* 2006) and for males in the range of 13.8–14.2 years (Philippaerts *et al.* 2006).

During puberty spontaneous growth-related improvements in motor performance and physiological parameters occur. A longitudinal study of youth soccer players showed that these natural gains may plateau during the interval prior to the young athlete reaching peak height velocity – performance may even decline during this period, as occurs with 30m speed scores (Philippaerts *et al.* 2006). Once the player then reaches the age when peak height velocity is attained, several of these natural gains in physiological and motor performance scores appear to reach their peak rate of development. In the 12–18 months following peak height velocity, declining rates of growth-related improvements are observed in several parameters (Philippaerts *et al.* 2006). Hence, scores in motor performance (in the absence of training interventions) appear to plateau at the end of this phase of development in youth sports players.

Prepubescent athletes exhibit lower levels of mechanical efficiency compared to adolescents. Although this improves as the young athlete progresses through puberty, adolescent athletes still demonstrate lower mechanical efficiency than adults (Naughton *et al.* 2000). It follows that there is considerable scope for this aspect of performance to be improved via specific instruction and practice. Exercise economy has been identified as an area for development in young athletes (Naughton *et al.* 2000) – allowing the young player to sustain a higher relative work rate throughout the course of a match.

As males pass through puberty they undergo a 'neuromuscular spurt'. Accompanied by limb growth and favourable changes in body composition (increased muscle mass relative to fat mass), these natural gains in strength and neuromuscular performance bring about a natural improvement in male players' biomechanics during movement (Quatman *et al.* 2006). One observed aspect of this improvement is an enhanced ability to dissipate ground reaction forces upon landing. These landing impact forces in turn directly influence the loading absorbed through lower limb joints (Hewett *et al.* 1999).

This 'neuromuscular spurt' phenomenon does not occur in females. The lack of any marked improvement in neuromuscular power and control, in combination with limb growth and body mass gains, in fact results in reduced lower limb stability in adolescent females (Quatman *et al.* 2006). Specifically, rapid growth of in particular the lower limbs during puberty increases the lengths of levers of the lower limb, and this is compounded by concurrent increases in body mass, so that female players face greater difficulty controlling motion of the trunk and lower limbs during athletic tasks; this has consequences for loads placed on the knee joint (Myer *et al.* 2008). Female players characteristically exhibit a tendency for potentially injurious lower limb alignment and movement mechanics as adolescents (Barber-Westin *et al.* 2006; Quatman *et al.* 2006). In the absence of neuromuscular training, female players also often preferentially recruit the quadriceps over the hamstring muscles during activity: a phenomenon known as 'quadriceps dominance' (Ford *et al.* 2003). Such biomechanical factors and aberrant recruitment patterns are implicated in the gender differences in rates of ACL injury post-puberty, which is not seen before this stage of development. Various studies report adolescent female players suffer 2–10 times greater incidence of ACL injury compared to male players, depending on the sport (Goldberg *et al.* 2007).

Changes in both musculoskeletal and cardiorespiratory systems during and following puberty have major implications for metabolic conditioning (Naughton *et al.* 2000). There are marked differences between prepubescent and adolescent players in terms of their responses to anaerobic and aerobic exercise (McManus and Armstrong 2008). Both children and adolescents exhibit gains in cardiorespiratory fitness with aerobic training (Naughton *et al.* 2000). Significant gains can be made particularly during puberty in young players as they reach peak height velocity (around 14 years of age in boys, 12 years in girls), partly due to aforementioned maturation effects (Philippaerts *et al.* 2006). Overall gains in aerobic fitness (for example, VO_2peak) reported in response to metabolic conditioning with young athletes are, however, suggested to be less than those observed with adults (Matos and Winsely 2007).

Prior to puberty the glycolytic metabolic system is less well developed and this is reflected in young athletes' metabolic responses to exercise, with oxidative metabolism dominating (Boisseau and Delamarche 2000). This may in part reflect differences in muscle fibre profiles pre- and post-puberty. Prepubescent athletes are reported to have a greater proportion of type I fibres compared to untrained adults; whereas this is not evident in adolescent athletes (Boisseau and Delamarche 2000). During puberty the capacity of young players for anaerobic (glycolytic) metabolism progressively increases (Naughton *et al.* 2000). The rate of maturation-related improvements in anaerobic enzyme content and activity during puberty appears to peak around the time the young athlete's growth curve attains peak height velocity (Philippaerts *et al.* 2006).

'Overuse' injury incidence in youth sports

When organising participation of adolescents in physical training and organised sports, it is important to recognise that young people are still growing (Bompa 2000; Kraemer and Fleck 2005). Coaches must consider the fact that the bones, muscles and connective tissues of the young athlete are not yet fully developed. As such, high volumes of repetitive practice may render the young player susceptible to overuse injury. This dictates that there is a need not only for age-appropriate practice and competition schedules but also for young players' physical preparation to be designed to reflect their specific stage of growth and maturation.

Biomechanical factors seem to play a role in the incidence of overuse injuries with youth sports participation. The rapid changes in the size and length of limbs during growth spurts alter the mechanics of athletic movements (Hawkins and Metheny 2001). As young players grow, this actually increases the forces and mechanical stresses involved in sports movements. When the young player is undergoing a growth spurt particular care should be taken, in view of the combined strain associated with rapid growth and physical stresses during competition and practices (Naughton *et al.* 2000). During this time, the immature skeleton may be more susceptible to injury than at later stages in the player's development – lumbar spine injuries particularly appear to increase in young adolescent athletes (Kujala *et al.* 1996). Growing cartilage is similarly more prone to injury in comparison to when the player reaches physical maturity, which can also be a factor in some overuse injuries (Adirim and Cheng 2003).

Given time, muscles and connective tissues respond to accommodate these growth-related changes; however, there is a time lag before this adaptation takes place (Hawkins and Metheny 2001). Under normal circumstances connective tissues remain within their failure limits during this lag phase. However, during puberty in males particularly there is a rapid increase in body mass and strength. As tendon and ligament strength respond relatively more slowly than muscle, these structures are placed closer to their failure limits in young players during and immediately following periods of rapid growth (Hawkins and Metheny 2001). Repeatedly performing a given sports movement during this sensitive phase in the young player's development can lead to overuse injury.

The point of attachment of tendon to bone (the apophysis) is an area particularly prone to overuse injury in the growing player (Adirim and Cheng 2003). Microtrauma injury – apophysitis – commonly occurs at the heel (Sever's disease) and the elbow ('Little League elbow') in younger children (ages 7–10). A similar condition – 'Osgood–Schlatter disease' – occurs at the insertion of the patella tendon and is often seen in young people aged 11–15 years (Adirim and Cheng 2003).

In certain youth sports, there is a risk of overuse injuries simply due to the strains involved in repetitive performance of a particular sports skill movement during practices and games – such as in throwing sports. In the United States it has been estimated that these overuse injuries make up approximately one-half of all sport-related injuries requiring medical treatment (Hawkins and Metheny 2001). In an effort to combat this, some governing bodies suggest limits for the number of repetitions of particular sports movements (such as the number of throws) that should be performed by the young player during a practice session (Hawkins and Metheny 2001).

A long-term perspective on youth training

It is critical when training young athletes to remain mindful of the processes of growth and maturation and how these will interact with the training stress placed upon the young athlete. Relative age and stage of growth and maturation are key factors when designing an appropriate training plan for young team sports players; this may vary widely between players competing at the same age group. Young athletes are often stratified into 'early developers' and 'late developers' in terms of the relative chronological age at which biological, physiological and neuromuscular performance changes occur. Two young players at the same 'chronological' age can therefore differ considerably in terms of their relative stage of biological and physiological maturation (Bompa 2000; Kraemer and Fleck 2005).

These considerations would clearly seem to necessitate a different approach in terms of training prescription for young and developing athletes, in relation to what is optimal for an adult. Training guidelines for young players should also take account of individual players' respective stage of growth and maturation (Gamble 2008). Unfortunately, the financial incentives for those who achieve success in sport, such as scholarships and professional contracts, often lead to excessive and inappropriate demands being placed on the young player, particularly those who have been identified as 'talented' or elite performers at age-grade level (Malina 2009). The growing awareness of 'sport-specific training methods' among coaches, parents and the young players themselves may similarly result in pressure to solely prescribe and perform training that mimics the chosen sport in which the young player participates.

The dangers of early specialisation

Authorities on the topic of long-term athlete development stress the need for variety in terms of not only training activities but also sports participation (Bompa 2000). Participating in multiple sports and athletic activities will provide young athletes with opportunities to develop a greater range of motor and cognitive skills that will ultimately benefit their performance in the sport in which they eventually choose to specialise (Malina 2009). It therefore appears that participating in multiple sports during the athlete's developmental years may in fact ultimately confer an advantage in performance terms relative to those who fall into early specialisation (Malina 2010).

Unfortunately, despite the benefits ascribed to varied sports participation, those who have been selected into elite or national-level programmes will in fact often participate much less in other sports (Malina 2010). One reason for this is that the practice and competition schedule no longer permits the athlete the time to do so. In many sports, for example soccer, those young athletes who show promise will typically be selected for representative teams in addition to their existing club and school team, so that they will often compete several times in a week.

Another reason that talented young athletes cease to participate in other sports is because to do so is in many cases actively discouraged by the coach in their primary sport (Malina 2009). Reports in the skill acquisition literature regarding the potential benefits of deliberate practice at an early age with respect to the long-term development of expert performance (Ericsson 2007) to some extent promote this early sport specialisation. Similarly, the 10-year or 10,000-hour rule in relation to experience and deliberate practice with respect to attaining mastery in a given discipline may encourage parents and coaches to attempt to get an 'early start' in the chosen sport with their child athlete (Malina 2010). Many professional sports teams and national governing bodies likewise increasingly begin their recruitment of junior athletes at a very young age.

As discussed in a previous section, the cumulative strains of high volumes of repetitious sports practice are identified as a major cause of overuse injury among young athletes (Valovich McLeod et al. 2011). This poses particular risk at sensitive phases in the athlete's growth and development (Hawkins and Metheny 2001). Early specialisation is a related causal factor in the scenario of excessive participation in practice and competition, which likewise predisposes young athletes to overuse injury (Malina 2010).

In addition to the physical strains of early sports specialisation, there are also psychological and psychosocial ill effects that must be considered (Malina 2009). This is likely a factor in the high rates of burnout observed in sports that promote early specialisation – for example, women's tennis. It is therefore advocated that the young player should only specialise in terms of sport and playing position as they advance into late adolescence – and much the same applies in terms of physical preparation.

A pyramid model for athletic development can be applied to youth training. Logically, training to build young athletes should begin at the foundation and build upwards. It follows that in developing 'structural integrity', mobility and stability should be the first priority when training young players. In turn these qualities underpin the player's ability to perform fundamental movements that are common to all sports. The young athletes' fundamental movement abilities will determine their ability to perform sport-specific movements. As such there is little point in trying to impose sport-specific strength or neuromuscular training upon deficient fundamental movement capabilities. It follows that training activities at this stage of the athlete's physical preparation should predominantly feature fundamental athletic movements alongside appropriate movement skills instruction and training (Myer et al. 2006a). Employing a greater variety of conditioning modes is advocated for young athletes, for example there should be greater emphasis on cross training modes, in contrast to what is undertaken with mature athletes (Bompa 2000; Gamble 2008).

Strength training for young team sports players

Safety and effectiveness of youth resistance training

The benefits of youth resistance training are well documented and are becoming universally accepted among health professionals, particularly in the US (Faigenbaum et al. 2009; Faigenbaum and Schram 2004) but also increasingly in the UK (Stratton et al. 2004). Fitness professional associations and health organisations are now in agreement that age-appropriate youth resistance training is safe and beneficial when performed under qualified supervision (Faigenbaum and Schram 2004; Kraemer and Fleck 2005; Stratton et al. 2004). However, public recognition of these benefits continues to lag behind, and misunderstanding and misconceptions remain.

Historically the concerns about youth resistance training stem from a perceived risk of damaging growth plates, which could potentially interfere with normal growth. In fact, such damage to growth plates has never been documented with strength training programmes for children that were administered and supervised by qualified personnel. Studies employing appropriate youth resistance training in fact report very low incidence of injuries of any type (Faigenbaum et al. 2009). Far from stunting growth, the contemporary evidence is that resistance training, in combination with proper nutrition, has the potential to enhance growth within genetic bounds at all stages of development (Faigenbaum *et al.* 2009).

The most frequent causes of injury when children and adolescents undertake resistance training are incorrect lifting technique, attempting to lift excessive loads, inappropriate use of equipment, and absence of qualified supervision (Faigenbaum *et al.* 2009). All of these factors can be reduced or eliminated with properly administered and supervised training (Stratton *et al.* 2004). Naturally, young players, as with any inexperienced lifters, should only engage in strength training programmes prepared by qualified coaches, with safe equipment, and supervised by qualified instructors. However, if these conditions are met, there are no safety grounds to preclude young players undertaking supervised strength training (Kraemer and Fleck 2005).

The reality is that children are exposed to far greater forces – and of longer duration – during sports and recreational physical activity than those encountered during strength training, even if they were to perform a maximal lift (Faigenbaum *et al.* 2009). Of all resistance training exercises, the Olympic lifts possibly impose the greatest forces upon the young musculoskeletal system. Even so, injury data suggest that Olympic weightlifting training and competition conducted under the supervision of qualified coaching is one of the safer athletic activities engaged in by young athletes (Hamill 1994).

Mechanisms for strength gains in prepubescent and adolescent athletes

Previously, the presumption had been that strength training prior to puberty was not viable or effective. However, it now appears that prepubescents exhibit significant scope for strength gains, far beyond those attributable to normal growth and maturation (Faigenbaum *et al.* 2009). Relative gains in strength documented with resistance training in prepubescent subjects are in fact of similar magnitude to those shown by adolescents (Faigenbaum *et al.* 2009).

That said, there are trends for greater absolute strength gains in adolescent subjects. Puberty triggers major physiological and hormonal changes (Naughton *et al.* 2000). Increases in circulating anabolic hormones during puberty impact considerably on how the young player responds to strength training. Lower levels of circulating anabolic hormones limit the contribution of hypertrophy (lean tissue growth) to strength gains (Faigenbaum *et al.* 2009). The changes to muscles that do occur appear to be more qualitative than quantitative. Neural effects thus appear to underpin many of the gains from resistance training in these younger participants.

Such neural adaptations are suggested to include improved recruitment and activation of the muscles mobilised during the training movement. Enhanced motor co-ordination, both within and between muscle groups, is also thought to contribute to strength gains following training. By the nature of these training adaptations, such strength gains would seem to be less permanent; prepubescent players will exhibit marked detraining effects once regular resistance training is discontinued (Faigenbaum *et al.* 2009). However, modest maintenance programmes (one or two days per week) do appear to be sufficient to sustain strength gains.

The greater hormonal response to resistance training in adolescents than at earlier stages of development leads to structural changes to the muscles and associated connective tissues (Faigenbaum *et al.* 2009). As a result, marked changes in terms of muscle hypertrophy and gains in fat-free mass are seen in this older age group. Such increases in muscle cross-sectional area and changes in muscle proteins therefore augment the gains in strength of neural origin that occur. This is the case especially among adolescent male players. However, the power per kilogram (body mass) that adolescents are capable of generating is still less than the corresponding values for adults (Naughton *et al.* 2000).

Strength training for performance enhancement in youth Sports

It is becoming recognised that young players can experience similar benefits from strength training to those observed with adults (Faigenbaum *et al.* 2009). All youth sports demand strength and power to varying degrees, in order to overcome the player's own body weight when moving and the resistance of opponents – particularly in contact sports. It follows that developing strength via resistance training should positively impact upon performance in the young player's sport (Stratton *et al.* 2004).

The effects of strength training in young players, which include increased strength and improved motor skills and co-ordination, have the potential to improve athleticism. Improvements in scores on motor performance measures are often observed following resistance training in children (Stratton *et al.* 2004). Positive changes have been noted in vertical jump, standing long jump, sprint times and agility run times (Faigenbaum *et al.* 2009).

The available data from the limited number of studies that have been published indicate that increases in flexibility can be made, particularly if the resistance training incorporates specific stretching, warm-up and cool-down (Stratton *et al.* 2004). This appears to refute concerns in some youth sports that resistance training will lead to the young athlete becoming muscle-bound and consequently decrease their flexibility and range of motion. Warm-up prior to training and team practices should comprise dynamic flexibility exercises; this form of stretching appears to offer most effective preparation for dynamic activity (Little and Williams 2006a).

Strength training for injury prevention

Participation in team sports does involve some inherent risk of injury. Although these injuries can never be entirely eliminated, appropriate training can help to reduce the number of injuries and severity of injuries that do occur. Young players are subject to additional risk due to physiological and developmental factors. The strains on connective tissues during growth and the changing properties of the growing tissues render these structures more prone to injury in the young player than is the case with adults (Adirim and Cheng 2003). Strengthening muscles and connective tissues via strength training offers a means to increase the forces they are capable of sustaining, helping to make the young player more resistant to soft tissue injury. In adolescents particularly, it is important to strengthen these connective tissues to accommodate the rapid gains in strength and body mass that occur during puberty (Adirim and Cheng 2003).

Strengthening muscles around upper-limb and lower-limb joints via appropriate training similarly offers a means to increase the active stability provided to these joints, which can serve a protective function (Stratton *et al.* 2004). Strength training was shown to improve neuromuscular control indices during jumping and landing in female adolescent athletes (Lephart *et al.* 2005). Such development of motor control and co-ordination helps to improve postural balance, dynamic stabilisation and active joint stability – all of which are beneficial in reducing incidence of lower limb injury.

In the case of young female players, lower limb strength development in general and hamstring strengthening in particular should be a major area of emphasis (Barber-Westin *et al.* 2006). Measures of hamstring strength are reported to plateau very early in female athletes' physical development – with older age groups (13–17 years) showing no significant gains on this measure compared to 11-year-old females (Barber-Westin *et al.* 2006). The hamstrings compress the knee joint and oppose anterior shear forces during weight-bearing closed-chain movements – as a result of these functions the hamstring is described as an 'ACL agonist' (Hewett *et al.* 1999). The relative weakness of the hamstrings of female players is of clinical relevance given the two to ten times greater rates of non-contact knee ligament injury in adolescent female athletes, compared with males (Goldberg *et al.* 2007).

Prepubescent athletes are shown to have a greater tendency than older populations to exhibit asymmetrical lower limb performance, based on scores with single-leg hopping functional tests (Barber-Westin *et al.* 2005). In the absence of intervention such imbalances may persist post-puberty in both males and females (Barber-Westin *et al.* 2006). Appropriate strength training offers a means to help correct such right–left imbalances in lower limb function, particularly in combination with plyometric or dynamic balance training (Myer *et al.* 2006a). This role of strength training in correcting side-to-side strength imbalances is crucial for young players at all stages of development. Strength and flexibility imbalances are identified as major risk factors for injury (Knapik *et al.* 1991). Strength imbalances can have negative consequences for both limbs: over-reliance may place excessive strain on the stronger limb; whereas the weaker limb is less able to actively counter injurious forces (Ford *et al.* 2003).

Studies show that young players who have strength training experience tend to sustain fewer injuries (Faigenbaum and Schram 2004). Incidence of injury in strength-trained youngsters is approximately one-third that of young athletes without any strength training experience (Bompa 2000). As well as serving to reduce overall incidence of injury, strength training can also help to reduce the severity of injuries. Following injury, strength-trained young players also respond better to rehabilitation (Faigenbaum and Schram 2004). Hence strength training can assist the young player in making a more rapid return to training and competition (Kraemer and Fleck 2005).

For these reasons, strength training is recommended in a 'preconditioning' role for young people before they start to compete in organised youth sports (Bompa 2000). Young players who are better conditioned and less prone to injury due to appropriate physical preparation – including strength training – are more likely to continue to participate in youth sports. In this way strength training can help reduce drop-out rates, which in turn can help keep youngsters healthy in later life (Faigenbaum and Schram 2004).

Aside from the benefits of general strength training, targeted strength training involving particular exercises may also be used to guard against certain injuries that commonly occur in sports. This targeted injury prevention role for strength training is often overlooked, particularly in young athletes. Too often exercises to strengthen areas that are prone to injury are only prescribed once an injury has already occurred. Unfortunately, there are currently an insufficient number of prospective studies in the literature involving youth sports players to provide evidence-based training guidelines regarding effective training for injury prevention (Mackay *et al.* 2004).

Training to develop bone health and connective tissue

In much the same way as for adults, it is established that physical activity has positive links to bone mineral density and connective tissue integrity in young people (Greene and Naughton 2006; Stratton *et al.* 2004). Although genetics is a determining factor, the major stimulus for accumulation of bone mass and mineral content is mechanical loading (Greene and Naughton 2006). The cross-sectional area and architecture of connective tissues are also trainable; appropriate strength training can therefore also be applied to develop strength and size of tendons and ligaments (Conroy and Earle 2000).

Mechanical loads must exceed a threshold in order to trigger adaptive responses (Conroy and Earle 2000). In accordance with this, both high-force weight-bearing and strength-type activities appear most suitable to elicit bone and connective tissue adaptations. Dynamic skeletal loading – that is, loading during movement – appears to be relatively more osteogenic than the same loads applied under static conditions (Greene and Naughton 2006). It follows that relatively high mechanical loading occurring during dynamic training activities should result in the greatest bone adaptation.

Recommended exercises generally involve weight bearing – so that the young player's own body weight provides additional loading (Conroy and Earle 2000). Athletic activities that involve high ground reaction forces are associated with increased bone mineral content and density (Greene and Naughton 2006). Sprinting, jumping and other lower-body plyometric exercises are identified as good training activities for developing bone strength as they offer high ground reaction forces and impact loading. Young athletes in all running-based sports and athletic events can benefit from these training modes. However, the volume of such training (for example, total foot contacts for plyometric training) must be monitored in order to avoid excessive strains and potential overuse injury.

Applying resistance via strength training is another means to generate the mechanical stresses required for an osteogenic response (Greene and Naughton 2006). This particular role of strength training for young athletes has been termed 'anatomical adaptation' (Bompa 2000). Associated positive effects include increased strength of supporting connective tissues and passive joint stability, as well as increased bone density and tensile strength (Faigenbaum and Schram 2004). In the same way as weight-bearing activities are recommended, 'structural' multi-joint strength training lifts (for example, variations of the squat, lunge and step up) offer a means to elicit whole-body skeletal adaptations. The strength and conditioning specialist can also harness site-specific gains in strength and cross-sectional area of bone and connective tissues associated with the muscles recruited during particular strength training exercises (Conroy and Earle 2000). Specifically, strength training exercises can be used to strengthen bones and connective tissues at particular sites that tend to be exposed to strain in the particular sport – such as the shoulder girdle in contact sports.

Immediately prior to and during puberty appears to be a key phase that offers a window of opportunity for skeletal adaptations (Greene and Naughton 2006). It is suggested that osteogenic training activities can therefore be used to amplify the skeletal growth and growth-related gains in lean body mass that occur naturally during these stages. Studies have shown that post-puberty females may be less responsive to skeletal adaptation – this suggests that there is an earlier and narrower window of opportunity for developing bone and associated connective tissues with female players (Greene and Naughton 2006).

Increases in bone density brought about by strength training are of relevance to female players from a longer-term health perspective. Females have a higher incidence of osteoporosis in comparison to males during late adulthood. During adolescence the growing skeleton seems to be particularly responsive to training (Greene and Naughton 2006). For this reason, young players (females in particular) are recommended to perform dynamic weight-bearing exercise and appropriate strength training during childhood and adolescence (Conroy and Earle 2000; Kraemer and Fleck 2005). Increasing the female player's bone mineral content at this stage of development is likely to have a favourable impact on their risk profile for osteoporosis in later life.

Metabolic conditioning

Responsiveness of young athletes to different forms of metabolic conditioning

Data from early studies in the literature suggested that prior to puberty young athletes might be less responsive to aerobic training. More recent studies have not found this to be the case, so some authors suggest that the equivocal findings were merely a result of the training provided being insufficiently taxing to elicit a significant response (McManus and Armstrong 2008). It now appears that a variety of endurance training modes and protocols produce gains in aerobic capacity with prepubescent subjects (Baquet *et al.* 2002, 2010; McManus *et al.* 2005).

As discussed in a previous section, prepubescent athletes exhibit a lower capacity for glycolytic metabolism. In view of this, it had previously been suggested that prepubescents are not amenable to performing anaerobic forms of training, such as interval conditioning. Guidelines in the literature have therefore advocated that these forms of metabolic conditioning should be avoided at this stage of development. However, over recent years a growing body of data have accumulated that challenge this assertion (McManus and Armstrong 2008). These studies find that while the nature of the metabolic responses of prepubescent athletes to high-intensity interval training may differ, they remain highly capable of performing this form of exercise and demonstrate a propensity to adapt very positively to high-intensity interval training (McManus and Armstrong 2008).

Mechanisms of training adaptations

There is a lack of data from young athletes, in part due to ethical reasons, which preclude invasive methods of assessment being undertaken with children. In particular, it is not yet clear to what extent central cardiorespiratory adaptations or peripheral adaptations are responsible for the improvements in endurance seen in prepubescent, pubertal and adolescent athletes in response to different training interventions (Baquet *et al.* 2010). It has been speculated by Baquet and colleagues (2010) that the relative contribution of central versus peripheral adaptations might differ according to the mode, format and intensity of conditioning employed.

It is also likely that different mechanisms may be attributed to the training responses observed following high-intensity anaerobic conditioning with prepubescent versus adolescent athletes. For example, the limited capacity of prepubescent athletes for glycolytic metabolism results in reduced levels of lactate production during this form of exercise. Lower muscle lactate concentrations are reported with prepubescent athletes, and the drop in muscle pH is correspondingly less due to the reduced levels of H^+ ions released with lactate production via glycolysis (Boisseau and Delamarche 2000). It follows that this is likely to limit specific training adaptations associated with buffering H^+ ions and clearing lactate that are seen following puberty in response to anaerobic training.

Aerobic conditioning

The training parameters for metabolic conditioning may vary according to the respective stages of growth and maturation, particularly in terms of overall volume and duration. Prior to puberty it is likewise suggested that the rate of progression in terms of duration or distances covered should be gradual and relatively conservative for younger athletes (Bompa 2000). Both these perspectives point to a less regimented approach than that used with older groups of players. In this way conditioning not only remains enjoyable but also the young player can self-regulate work intensity.

The selection of training modes employed should also alter as the player grows and matures. A wider variety of activities and cross training modes is advocated for prepubescent players (Bompa 2000; Kraemer and Fleck 2005). It is recommended that endurance training activities employed with prepubescent players should be selected to avoid monotony and aim to incorporate a fun element (Bompa 2000; Kraemer and Fleck 2005). As the young player matures, training guidelines change to reflect corresponding changes in physical capabilities: training modes will become more specific to the sport and the intensity of conditioning activities may likewise increase.

Running-based interval conditioning has been used successfully to improve the aerobic capacities of young team sports players (Buchheit et al. 2009). Skill- and sport-related movement drills can also be adapted for conditioning purposes (Bompa 2000; Hoff 2005). Ball games with simplified rules are another good choice for conditioning activities with these young players (Buchheit et al. 2009). As the young player moves into adolescence, there will be an increasing demand for the training modes used for metabolic conditioning to become more specific to the sport.

Anaerobic conditioning modes

During puberty young athletes' capacity for anaerobic metabolism increases (Philippaerts et al. 2006). However, each individual player's tolerance for training will differ according to their stage of development. This can vary widely in a group of players of the same chronological age (Bompa 2000; Kraemer and Fleck 2005). This must be considered particularly when training players of an age where they may be undergoing puberty.

Adolescence is identified as the time for specialisation in young players' physical preparation (Bompa 2000; Naughton et al. 2000). Physiological changes during puberty increase young players' capacity for, and responsiveness to, anaerobic training (Naughton et al. 2000). This form of conditioning is a requirement of the majority of team sports; it therefore follows that anaerobic training should feature increasingly in adolescent players' physical preparation.

Various modes of interval training are shown to be effective in improving measures of endurance fitness and performance indices with team sports players (Helgerud et al. 2001; Hoff et al. 2002). High-intensity interval hill running was shown to elicit significant improvements, including lactate threshold, in young soccer players, which importantly also carried over to measures of soccer performance during matches (Helgerud et al. 2001). A soccer-specific protocol running through a set course involving dribbling a ball alternated with backwards and forwards shuttle sprints through cones is also reported to elicit sufficiently high intensities (93 per cent HRmax or 91 per cent VO$_2$max) for developing anaerobic capacity (Hoff et al. 2002).

Summary

The need for different aspects of physical preparation – including strength training, metabolic conditioning and also neuromuscular training – has been described for a range of sports and for young athletes at different stages of maturation. The efficacy of each of these different components of physical preparation for athletes in general, and young team sports players in particular, is becoming increasingly well established. The nature of responses to each of these forms of training at different stages of growth and maturation has also been elucidated, albeit further research is necessary to provide a clearer picture.

Any training programme should be geared to the physical and emotional maturity of the individuals in the group. Due to the paucity of well-controlled studies in the literature, there is a shortage of conclusive recommendations regarding training design for young populations at different stages of maturation (Naughton et al. 2000). That said, guidelines have been published that differentiate between chronological age and, more importantly, biological age (Bompa 2000; Faigenbaum et al. 2009; Kraemer and Fleck 2005). Fundamentally, the primary emphasis of training for young team sports players is on balanced physical development and building a foundation of athleticism. Only once this is undertaken and physical maturation has taken place should the focus then progressively shift to specialised preparation for the particular sport and playing position.

Training recommendations for young players

As discussed, rates of growth and maturation within a group of young athletes can vary widely. When training young team sports players it is therefore difficult to define phases of development within a squad of players. For the purposes of this section, guidelines will be divided into: 'prepubescent' – the stage of development prior to exhibiting physical signs indicating the onset of puberty; 'early puberty' – defined as the phase between the onset of puberty and attaining peak height velocity; and 'adolescence' – the period following peak height velocity being attained and advancing into adulthood.

The divisions between stages are necessarily vague: the average age at which peak height velocity is attained (marking the transition between 'early puberty' and 'adolescence' as defined above) is around 12 years of age for girls and 14 years for boys (Malina et al. 2004) but there is considerable variability in this. Observing changes in physical characteristics, assessing neuromuscular performance, and monitoring seated and standing heights at regular intervals will help in determining the progression between stages. The latter – standing and seated heights – are the most helpful objective measure to track with young players when used to plot velocity curves (gain in height per unit of time) for each player (Baxter-Jones and Sherar 2006). Seated height is helpful as trunk length tends to lag behind leg growth. Ultimately it is dependent on the coach to use their experience and observations of each player's performance during training over time as the deciding factor that determines how and when to progress training for each individual player.

Within these guidelines, consideration must also be given to the training age of the young player entering a programme of physical preparation. Prior training experience – of strength training particularly – will influence individual decisions regarding training prescription. For example, one player who falls into the 'early puberty' category based on age and physical characteristics who enters the programme with a background of two years strength training may be ready for more complex training exercises more than another player who is significantly older but has no prior strength training experience. Regardless of the age or stage of growth and maturation of the player, initial training prescription will reflect the primary objective of developing competency performing fundamental movements and addressing any functional deficits. Only once this has been undertaken should the focus then shift to performance-related training goals and more advanced training.

Prepubescent players

Neuromuscular and movement skills training

Neuromuscular training should be initiated early in young players' physical preparation. This is important to help correct the valgus lower limb alignment during athletic movements that is common in prepubescent athletes of both genders (Barber-Westin et al. 2005). This form of training also has a role to play improving the movement efficiency that has been identified as lacking among these young players (Naughton et al. 2000).

The starting point for proven short-term neuromuscular training programmes appropriate for young team sports players is instruction of athletic position and safe movement mechanics (Hewett et al. 1999). This fundamentals phase of established neuromuscular training protocols can be implemented with young players during this stage of development. This includes instruction and practice of jumping, landing and change of direction movements as discrete skills. Neuromuscular movement skill training with young athletes may be effectively augmented by postural balance and dynamic stabilisation exercises (Myer et al. 2006). The emphasis with all neuromuscular training exercises should be sound posture and correct lower limb alignment for prepubescent players of both genders.

Metabolic conditioning

It follows that the lower capacity of prepubescents for anaerobic exercise should be reflected in the training employed with these players. The majority of training at this stage of development should be aerobic in nature. However, the training modes used to achieve this may be skill-based to reduce training monotony and include elements of fun and competition.

Skill- or game-related movement drills can be adapted for use as conditioning activities. For example, an obstacle course can be constructed involving different movements and ball skills, perhaps running relays between teams of athletes (Bompa 2000). Alternatively, ball games with simplified rules may be used – the numbers on each team and playing area can be manipulated to alter exercise intensity. This less structured approach allows the young player to self-regulate work intensity according to their individual tolerance.

Strength training

In general, if a child is ready for participation in organised sports, they are likely ready to undergo instruction and resistance training. However, for young players with known or suspected medical conditions, medical clearance should be sought prior to participation in resistance training, as with other sports (Faigenbaum *et al.* 2009). The specific design of training for young team sports players should be reflective of their stage of psychological and emotional development, in order to engender motivation and facilitate compliance (Stratton *et al.* 2004).

When coaching prepubescent players, it is important that training should be enjoyable and give the young player an immediate sense of fun and discovery-based learning (Stratton *et al.* 2004). In practical terms, the choice of training exercises and loads used should be conducive to allow this approach to be safely implemented. For example, bodyweight resistance exercises are more appropriate when training more complex whole-body movements.

A meta-analysis of training studies featuring children and adolescents of varying ages has identified repetition schemes from 6–15 repetitions and 50–100 per cent of 1–RM to be effective for resistance training with young athletes (Falk and Tenenbaum 1996). In general, resistance training volumes of two to three sets and frequency of training of two to three days per week appear to be most effective. When young players are introduced to strength training, light loads and high repetition schemes (12–15 repetitions) are most appropriate (Faigenbaum *et al.* 2009). During this early stage of training progression should be achieved by increasing number of sets performed and number of exercises in the workout. The relative loading and number of training days employed can then be increased at a later stage.

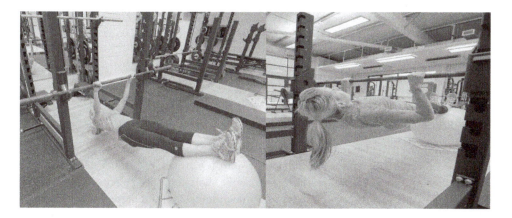

Figure 12.1 Swiss ball suspended row

Table 12.1 Training guidelines: prepubescent players

	Training modes	*Intensity*	*Volume, frequency*
Strength training	Combination of unilateral and bilateral general strength-training exercises	8–15-RM	1–3 sets; 2–3 sessions per week (non-consecutive days)
Metabolic conditioning	Combination of cross-training, conditioning games and skill-based conditioning activities	Self-regulated	Duration should be progressed before intensity
Neuromuscular training	Instruction and practice of fundamental movement skills; single-leg balance exercises (stable surface)	Self-paced, low intensity (full recovery between drills)	Short high-quality sessions (minimising fatigue effects); up to 2 sessions per week

Adequate rest and recovery are key components of successful youth resistance training. Younger players and those in the early stages of their physical preparation will require more recovery time between training days. Training on non-consecutive days is therefore recommended for prepubescent players, in order to maximise the effectiveness of training and reduce the risk of injury (Faigenbaum and Schram 2004).

Given that many of the benefits of strength training prior to puberty stem from improved co-ordination, balance and proprioception, it follows that exercise modes that favour development of these aspects should be emphasised when training prepubescent players. Body weight resistance exercises and free weights offer advantages from this point of view, in comparison to fixed resistance machines, although these exercises may require closer supervision. Another consideration if choosing to use resistance machines with young players is that the apparatus must be fitted to the dimensions of the young person. Some apparatus cannot be adjusted sufficiently to be suitable for use (Faigenbaum *et al.* 2009).

Exercise selection should feature a combination of unilateral and bilateral exercises appropriate to the young player's capabilities. The inclusion of unilateral exercises in prepubescent players' training is important in order to promote balanced development between limbs (Kraemer and Fleck 2005). These exercises do not allow the young player to compensate with their stronger limb as can happen with bilateral exercises. Bilateral exercises should also feature in the young player's programme at this stage of maturation as a means to develop strength from a more stable base of support.

Early puberty

Neuromuscular and movement skills training

Puberty is characterised in males particularly by a progressive improvement in neuromuscular abilities – this is known as the neuromuscular spurt (Quatman *et al.* 2006). However, prior to attainment of peak height velocity there may be short-term decrements in some aspects of neuromuscular performance. It follows that neuromuscular training should be progressed during this phase of the young player's development in a way that is responsive to his or her individual rate of neuromuscular development and sensitive to any short-term changes.

Training to reduce the potentially injurious loading that occurs with poor neuromuscular control of lower limb alignment assumes increased importance given the gains in body mass that occur during puberty (which in turn increases the loading and stresses imposed on joints and connective tissues). In female players, this form of training is advocated as a means to artificially create a 'neuromuscular spurt' similar to that which occurs naturally in males during this phase of maturation (Quatman *et al.* 2006). Neuromuscular training is a priority for female players to tackle the higher rates of lower limb injury (in comparison to males) that become apparent from this stage of maturation onwards (Lephart *et al.* 2005).

Neuromuscular training during this stage will continue to feature dynamic balance and stabilisation work. These exercises have numerous progressions, which can be implemented as appropriate with advances in maturation and neuromuscular performance.

Metabolic conditioning

During and following puberty, metabolic training responses become increasingly specific to the type of metabolic training employed. It follows that the training modes used must account for this and increasingly reflect the demands of the sport and playing position from this stage of maturation onwards. Cross training activities will tend to feature less during the playing season (however, these remain an important training tool particularly for off-season training).

Depending on individual tolerance, intensity of metabolic conditioning will likewise be progressively increased during this stage – in order to reflect the higher intensities of exertion experienced during competitive games. Conditioning games can be manipulated (reducing number of players each side, modifying size of playing area, and so on) to become more demanding. The rest intervals used between conditioning drills may also be decreased – again within individual tolerance.

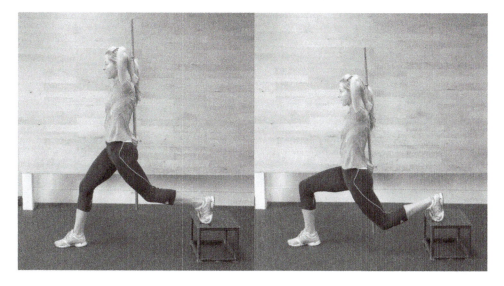

Figure 12.2 In-line single-leg squat

Strength training

Adequate rest and recovery continue to be an integral aspect when scheduling strength training during puberty. Given the concomitant strains of growth and maturation during this stage, recovery time is crucial between training days. Strength training on non-consecutive days therefore continues to be advocated during puberty (Faigenbaum and Schram 2004).

Exercise selection will also reflect the need for balanced development and improving strength for fundamental movements. General strength exercises and unilateral exercises should feature prominently during puberty. With advances in training experience, structural multi-joint lifts (variations of the squat and deadlift) can be introduced. In the case of experienced young lifters, Olympic-style lifts can also be integrated into the strength-training programme as appropriate; under qualified supervision this form of training carries no greater risk for young players than other athletic activities (Hamill 1994). Olympic lifts and their variations should be taught initially using a light implement such as a broom handle or empty barbell, with the emphasis on the quality of the lifting movement.

Whatever the exercise, the focus throughout should be on proper lifting form, with loading limited until the young player has mastered lifting technique. The coach should also be vigilant for temporary reductions in co-ordination and performance that may occur as the young player approaches peak height velocity, and be prepared to modify exercise selection and loading accordingly. Likewise, loading should be restricted from the point of view of attenuating the stresses on skeletal and connective tissue structures during phases of rapid growth (Naughton *et al.* 2000). Loading of the lumbar spine particularly should be carefully monitored in recognition of the higher risk of lumbar spine injury at this phase of development (Kujala *et al.* 1996).

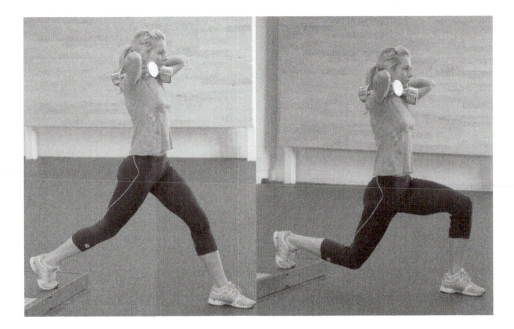

Figure 12.3 Dumbbell split squat

Table 12.2 Training guidelines: early puberty

	Training modes	Intensity	Volume, frequency
Strength training	More complex strength-training exercises – greater emphasis on unilateral exercises and introduction Olympic lifting movements	6–12-RM	Max of 3 sets (not including warm-up set); 2–4★ sessions per week (non-consecutive days)
Metabolic conditioning	Predominantly interval-based conditioning – including (more demanding) conditioning games and skill-based conditioning activities	Higher intensity – still largely self-regulated to allow for individual differences in tolerance	2–3 sessions per week (non-consecutive days)
Neuromuscular training	Progression of movement skill development; single-leg balance (unstable surface) and dynamic stabilisation exercises	Self-paced, progression in intensity (full recovery)	2–3 sessions per week (non-consecutive days)

★ Number of sessions will depend on how the strength training programme is structured – specifically whether it is a split routine; whatever scheme is used, each body part should only be trained a maximum of twice per week.

In the absence of corrective training, significant asymmetries are observed both before and following puberty (Barber-Westin *et al.* 2006). From both function and injury-prevention perspectives it is vital that any differences in performance between dominant and non-dominant limbs are addressed during this stage via strength training. Practical recommendations include manipulating the number of repetitions and sets performed with each limb for single-limb strength exercises (Cook 2003b). For example, the young player may perform three repetitions on their weaker side for every two on their dominant side (keeping the load constant).

For female players targeted hamstring strength training should begin during this stage – ideally in conjunction with neuromuscular training to help increase hamstring recruitment during dynamic activity (Hewett *et al.* 1999). This is important to offset the quadriceps dominance that can increase strain on the ACL in female athletes (Ford *et al.* 2003).

Adolescent players

Neuromuscular and movement skills training

The fundamental movement skills phase characteristic of earlier neuromuscular training will be progressed during this stage of development to more demanding jumping exercises and more sport-specific change of direction drills. For all exercises the emphasis should remain on posture, sound movement mechanics and correct lower limb alignment, particularly during landing and change of direction movements (Myer *et al.* 2006).

As the player matures and their neuromuscular performance develops, further advances in training may include single-leg plyometric-type jumping and landing exercises in various directions, and unanticipated change of direction movement drills. Postural balance and dynamic stabilisation exercises can similarly be progressed during this stage by incorporating various training devices to increase demand for balance and proprioception (Myer *et al.* 2006a; Yaggie and Campbell 2006).

Metabolic conditioning

Aerobic endurance remains a training priority for adolescent players. A continuing emphasis on appropriate metabolic conditioning would appear to be vital for female players particularly, in order to counter the decline in aerobic endurance that is otherwise observed in females after the onset of puberty (Naughton *et al.* 2000).

In many team sports, adolescent players will require repeated sprint conditioning to elicit appropriate anaerobic training effects (Naughton *et al.* 2000). Various modes of high-intensity interval conditioning can be effective – including hill running (Helgerud *et al.* 2001) and high-intensity sport skill conditioning drills (Hoff 2005; Hoff *et al.* 2002). By manipulating numbers on each team, playing rules and playing area, skill-based conditioning games can also elicit sufficiently high exercise intensities for repeated sprint conditioning (Gamble 2004b; Hoff *et al.* 2002; Little and Williams 2006b).

Where it is appropriate to the sport, speed-endurance work may be introduced into speed and agility work undertaken by players – providing that the adolescent player is technically proficient. Prior to this stage in development, any speed and agility training undertaken by players would exclusively be categorised as neuromuscular training, with emphasis on movement mechanics and complete recovery between repetitions.

As this is a stage of increasing specialisation in training, the training modes used for individual training should be increasingly mode-specific. Given this, by the time the young athlete reaches late adolescence it is probable that cross training modes will only be emphasised during the off-season. By selecting appropriate work bouts and rest–recovery intervals it is possible for high-intensity interval training to elicit significant aerobic and anaerobic endurance gains (Tabata *et al.* 1997). Over time it follows that the maturing player's aerobic endurance development may be predominantly achieved via high intensity training (Little and Williams 2006b), particularly during the playing season. However, these repetition schemes will, by definition, be highly demanding and as such should be progressively introduced during late adolescence. Skill-based conditioning games aimed at aerobic endurance development employed in squad training should likewise become more specific to the sport.

Strength training

Adolescent athletes are more conducive to a more adult longer-term approach with regard to physical preparation undertaken in a more structured training setting (Stratton *et al.* 2004). The starting point for any strength training will depend on the adolescent player's training history. If appropriate strength development has occurred prior to and/or during puberty, then strength training may be progressed to include a more advanced and sport-specific exercise selection. However, if significant deficits are noted, the starting point will be developing strength for fundamental movements and addressing imbalances. In this case, initial exercise selection will be more reflective of generic strength training for improved athleticism.

Assuming physical preparation has been undertaken prior to this stage of maturation, training design should be increasingly based upon a comprehensive needs analysis of the sport and playing position. As with adults, exercise specificity influences young players' responses to strength training. Exercise selection should therefore be progressively sport-specific, within the constraints of the skill level and training experience of the young player.

Sport-specific exercise selection will vary according to the sport and playing position. Typically, multi-joint lifts for speed-strength development (Olympic-style lifts, barbell jump squats, and so on) that incorporate triple extension of hips, knees and ankles will feature in the adolescent player's programme – given this is the principle biomechanical action common to many dynamic movements in team sports (Gamble 2004a). Likewise, unilateral support exercises should necessarily comprise a significant portion of the young team sport athlete's training – on the basis that the majority of game-related movements are executed supported partly or fully on one or other leg (McCurdy and Conner 2003). The reader is referred to Chapters 3 and 5 for guidelines on strength training and speed-strength training exercise prescription.

Exercise selection from an injury prevention viewpoint should be based upon injury data for the sport, and for the playing position where available. Specifically, targeted strength-training exercises should be included in adolescent players' training to address areas identified as being prone to injury in the sport (and playing position) – see Chapter 9 for this topic. In the case of contact sports, hypertrophy may be an important programme goal for adolescent players, to varying degrees depending on their playing position. The shoulders should be an area for specific strengthening and hypertrophy, as this is the site for impact forces during collisions with other players (Gamble 2004a).

Table 12.3 Training guidelines: adolescent players

	Training modes	*Intensity*	*Volume, frequency*
Strength training	Increasing sport-specific emphasis: unilateral exercises, Olympic and multi-joint strength training exercises	4–12-RM	3–5 sets; 3–5* sessions per week
Metabolic conditioning	Anaerobic interval-based conditioning – including (more demanding) conditioning games and skill-based conditioning activities	Higher intensity; shorter recovery durations to develop anaerobic capacity	2–4 sessions per week (non-consecutive days)
Neuromuscular training	Progression of speed and decision-making components of movement skills; progression of single-leg balance and dynamic stabilisation (featuring unstable support training devices)	Increased intensity, progressive introduction of speed-endurance development	2–3 sessions per week (non-consecutive days)

* Number of sessions will depend on how the strength training programme is structured – specifically whether it is a split routine; whatever scheme is used, each body part should only be trained a maximum of three times per week.

APPENDIX: PRACTICAL EXAMPLES OF TRAINING DESIGN

Designing the programme: needs analysis

The basis for any training programme in any sport is a thorough needs analysis. This process comprises two parts. The first task of a needs analysis is objectively to define the demands and requirements of the sport and playing position. The second aspect concerns the specific requirements of the player, which will depend on the relative strengths of the individual as well as their training and injury history.

Needs analysis for the sport comprises the biomechanics, bioenergetics and injury profile of the sport and playing position. The biomechanics of a given team sport can be qualitatively assessed by observing the predominant movements and forms of locomotion involved during competitive play. Bioenergetics refers to the relative contribution from different energy systems during games. Time–motion and physiological data can be used to offer insight into bioenergetics of the sport and playing position, if available (Chapter 4). In the absence of relevant data from matches, elite players' physiological test profiles can offer an insight into the relative contribution and importance of different aspects (Chapter 2). Injury data for the sport and playing position will similarly indicate the types of injuries players may be exposed to during competition (Chapter 9), which will help to guide training prescription (Chapter 10).

Needs analysis pertaining to the individual predominantly concerns their training history, current assessment of strengths and weaknesses, and the player's injury history. Training history will influence exercise selection, training progression and choice of periodisation scheme (Chapter 11). Relevant test data for the player can be used to identify their strengths and areas that require attention (Chapter 2), which will influence training design in terms of the areas that require particular emphasis. The player's injury history will determine the areas that require ongoing rehabilitation and will similarly guide exercise selection to help prevent re-injury (Chapter 10).

Example 1: Female team sport – women's basketball

Off-season/early pre-season training cycle

Strength training	Frequency: 4 per week: 2 whole-body 1 upper-body 1 shoulder maintenance Intensity: 7–10RM (all lifts) Volume: 3–5 sets Workout format: Heavy resistance circuit Rest: Short rest (<60sec) between lifts Core work (~2 mins) between (circuit) sets	**Example whole-body workout** *8–RM; 3 Sets* Front squat Incline dumbbell bench press Dumbbell step up with hip flexion One-arm dumbbell row Dumbbell split squat Single-leg good morning
Metabolic conditioning	Long aerobic interval training Combination of cross-training modes and running conditioning	
Movement skills training	Instruction of fundamental movement skills. Self-paced. No read/reaction element.	

Late pre-season training cycle

Strength training	Frequency: 3 per week: 2 whole-body 1 shoulder maintenance Intensity: 5–7RM multi-joint lifts 8RM assistance lifts Volume: 3–4 sets Workout format: 2 × 3-lift complexes Rest: Short rest (<60sec) between lifts Core work (~2 mins) between (complex) sets	**Example whole-body workout** *6–RM; 3 Sets* Jump squat (2 × 3-rep 'clusters') Single-arm cable row Front racked backward lunge Push press (3 × 2-rep 'clusters') Front racked barbell step up Single-leg barbell straight-legged deadlift
Metabolic conditioning	Progression aerobic interval to anaerobic interval training modes to repeated sprint conditioning late pre-season Combination of conditioning modes including skill-based games and conditioning drills at appropriate intensities	
Movement skills training **Speed and agility development**	Progression of technique development drills and instruction/development of acceleration mechanics mid-pre-season, followed by introduction to higher velocity acceleration drills. Progression of change of direction movement skill drills, including simple reaction tasks, followed by gradual introduction of 'read–react' agility drills.	

In-season training cycle

Strength training	Frequency: 3 per week 2 whole-body 1 shoulder maintenance Intensity: 4–6RM (all lifts) Volume: 3–4 sets Workout format: 2 × 3-lift complexes Rest: Complete (self-selected) rest between consecutive lifts Core work (~2 mins) between (complex) sets	**Example whole-body workout** *5–RM; 3 sets* Power clean One-arm incline dumbbell bench press Box-to-box drop jump Loaded split bounds (3 × 2-rep 'clusters') Single-leg single-arm dumbbell row Front racked barbell lateral step up
Metabolic conditioning		Cycling of aerobic interval training, anaerobic interval training and repeated sprint conditioning Combination of conditioning games, skill-based conditioning drills, and movement-specific high-intensity conditioning drills, depending on respective block
Speed and agility development		Progression to more challenging and context-specific reactive agility drills and partner drills

Peaking (in-season) training cycle

Strength training	Frequency: 2 per week 1 whole-body 1 shoulder maintenance Intensity: 4–5RM (all lifts) Volume: 2 sets Workout format: 2 × 3-lift complexes (whole body); circuit (shoulder workout) Rest: Complete rest between consecutive lifts Core work (~2 mins) between (complex) sets	**Example whole-body workout** *4–RM; 3 sets* Split jerk Cable resisted alternate knee/shoulder flexion Unilateral horizontal bounds Barbell bound step up Ballistic push up (lower legs supported on domed device) Compass bounds landing on domed device
Metabolic conditioning		Repeated sprint conditioning Movement-specific high-intensity conditioning drills
Speed and agility development		High-intensity game-related acceleration drills and game-related specific reactive agility and partner drills

Example 2: Contact sport – rugby union football

Off-season training cycle

<table>
<tr><td rowspan="2">Strength training</td><td>Frequency: 3 per week:
2 whole-body
1 upper-body

Intensity: 10–12RM (all lifts)

Volume: 3–5 sets

Workout format:
Heavy resistance circuit

Rest:
Short rest (<60sec) between lifts
Core work (~2 mins) between (circuit) sets</td><td>Example whole-body workout
10–RM; 3 sets</td></tr>
<tr><td>Barbell overhead squat
Seated cable row
Seated dumbbell shoulder press
Machine leg press
Bench press
Dumbbell single-leg calf raise</td></tr>
<tr><td colspan="2">Metabolic conditioning</td><td>Long aerobic interval training
Predominantly cross-training modes</td></tr>
<tr><td colspan="2">Movement skills training
Speed and agility development</td><td>N/A</td></tr>
</table>

Early-mid pre-season training cycle

<table>
<tr><td rowspan="2">Strength training</td><td>Frequency: 4 per week:
2 whole-body
1 upper-body
1 shoulder maintenance

Intensity: 7–10RM multi-joint lifts
8RM assistance lifts

Volume: 3–4 sets

Workout format:
Heavy resistance circuit

Rest: Short rest (<60sec) between lifts
Core work (~2 mins) between (complex) sets</td><td>Example whole-body workout
8–RM; 3 sets</td></tr>
<tr><td>Barbell snatch pull (6 reps)
Bent-over barbell row
Deadlift
Incline dumbbell bench press
Barbell step up
Single-leg barbell straight-legged deadlift</td></tr>
<tr><td colspan="2">Metabolic conditioning</td><td>Aerobic interval and progressive introduction of anaerobic interval training modes
Combination of conditioning modes including running conditioning at individually prescribed velocities, skill-based conditioning games and conditioning drills</td></tr>
<tr><td colspan="2">Movement skills training
Speed and agility development</td><td>Sprint technique development drills and instruction/development of acceleration mechanics, progression to higher velocity acceleration and speed drills
Change of direction movement skill drills, progression to reactive conditions and simple 'read/react' agility drills</td></tr>
</table>

Early in-season training cycle

Strength training	Frequency: 3 per week 2 whole-body 1 shoulder maintenance Intensity: 4–6RM (all lifts) Volume: 3–4 sets Workout format: 2 × 3–lift complexes Rest: Complete (self-selected) rest between consecutive lifts Core work (~2 mins) between (complex) sets	**Example whole-body workout** *5–RM; 3 sets* Stop clean Wide-grip chins Box-to-box drop jump Jump squat (6 reps – 2 × 3-rep 'clusters') Ballistic push up Barbell cross-over lateral step up
Metabolic conditioning	Cycling of aerobic interval training, anaerobic interval training and repeated sprint conditioning Combination of conditioning games, skill-based conditioning drills, and movement-specific high-intensity conditioning drills, depending on respective block	
Speed and agility development	Reactive acceleration and speed development drills Progression to more challenging and context-specific reactive agility drills and partner drills	

Peaking (in-season) training cycle

Strength training	Frequency: 2 per week 1 whole-body 1 shoulder maintenance Intensity: 4–5RM (all lifts) Volume: 3 sets Workout format: 2 × 3-lift complexes (whole body); Circuit (shoulder workout) Rest: Complete rest between consecutive lifts Core work (~2 mins) between (complex) sets	**Example whole-body workout** *4–RM; 3 sets* Stop split clean Single-arm single-leg dumbbell row Unilateral horizontal bounds (forwards, quarter-turn, half-turn) Barbell bound step up Alternate arm medicine ball ballistic push up Dumbbell clockwork lunge
Metabolic conditioning	Repeated sprint conditioning High-intensity small-sided conditioning games	
Speed and agility development	High-intensity game-related acceleration drills and game-related specific reactive agility and partner drills	

Example 3: Striking and/or throwing team sport–baseball

Early pre-season training cycle

Strength training	Frequency: 4 per week: 2 whole-body 1 upper-body 1 shoulder maintenance Intensity: 7–10RM (all lifts) Volume: 3–5 sets Workout format: Heavy resistance circuit Rest: Short rest (<60sec) between lifts Core work (~2 mins) between (circuit) sets	**Example whole-body workout** *8–RM; 3 sets* Parallel back squat Incline dumbbell bench press Barbell step up One-arm dumbbell row Barbell single-leg squat ('pitcher's squat') Single-leg good morning
Metabolic conditioning	Short aerobic interval training Combination of cross-training modes and running conditioning	
Speed and agility development	Instruction and technique development drills	

Mid-late pre-season training cycle

Strength training	Frequency: 3 per week: 2 whole-body 1 shoulder maintenance Intensity: 5–7RM multi-joint lifts 8RM assistance lifts Volume: 3–4 sets Workout format: 2 × 3-lift complexes Rest: Short rest (<60sec) between lifts Core work (~2 mins) between (complex) sets	**Example whole-body workout** *6–RM; 3 sets* Jump squat Single-arm cable row Barbell forward lunge Power clean One-arm dumbbell incline bench press Barbell lateral step up
Metabolic conditioning	Progression aerobic interval to anaerobic interval training modes late pre-season Combination of conditioning modes including skill-based conditioning games and conditioning drills at appropriate intensities	
Speed and agility development	Progression of technique development drills and instruction/development of acceleration mechanics mid-pre-season, followed by introduction to higher velocity acceleration drills. Progression of change of direction movement skill drills, including simple reaction tasks	

Early in-season training cycle

Strength training	*Frequency:* 2–3 per week 1–2 whole-body 1 shoulder maintenance *Intensity:* 4–6RM (all lifts) *Volume:* 3–4 sets Workout format: 2 × 3-lift complexes *Rest:* Self-selected rest between consecutive lifts Core work (~2 mins) between (complex) sets	**Example shoulder workout** *6–RM; 3 sets* Prone dumbbell external rotation Standing one arm dumbbell shoulder press Cable diagonal pulley Prone dumbbell lateral raise Supine alternating leg dumbbell pull-over Alternate-arm cable reverse fly
Metabolic conditioning	Cycling of anaerobic interval training and repeated sprint conditioning Combination of high-intensity running conditioning drills and movement-specific high-intensity conditioning drills	
Speed and agility development	Reactive acceleration drills Maximum speed development Progression to more challenging change of direction tasks and context-specific read-and-react drills	

Mid-season training cycle

Strength training	*Frequency:* 2 per week 1 whole-body 1 shoulder maintenance *Intensity:* 4–5RM (all lifts) *Volume:* 2 sets *Workout format:* 2 × 3-lift complexes (whole body); Circuit (shoulder workout) *Rest:* Complete rest between consecutive lifts Core work (~2 mins) between (complex) sets	**Example whole-body eorkout** *4–RM; 3 sets* Stop split clean Cable resisted alternate knee/shoulder flexion Unilateral horizontal bounds High box lateral bounds Single-arm cable fly Dumbbell clockwork lunge
Metabolic conditioning	Repeated sprint conditioning Movement-specific high-intensity conditioning drills	
Speed and agility development	Reactive specific acceleration and drills and speed development over game-related distances Game-specific read-and-react agility drills	

REFERENCES

Aagaard, P., E.B. Simonsen, J.L. Andersen, P. Magnusson and P. Dyhre-Poulsen (2002) Neural Adaptation to Resistance Training: Changes in Evoked V-Wave and H-Reflex Responses, *Journal of Applied Physiology*, 92: 2309–18

Aagaard, P., J.L. Andersen, P. Dyhre-Poulson, A-M. Leffers, A. Wagner, S.P. Magnusson, J. Halkjaer-Kristensen and E.B. Simonsen (2001) A Mechanism for Increased Contractile Strength of Human Pennate Muscle in Response to Strength Training: Changes in Muscle Architecture, *Journal of Physiology*, 534(2): 621–3

Abernethy, P., G. Wilson and P. Logan (1995) Strength and Power Assessment: Issues, Controversies and Challenges, *Sports Medicine*, 19(6): 410–17

Adirim, T.A. and T.L. Cheng (2003) Overview of Injuries in the Young Athlete, *Sports Medicine*, 33(1): 75–81

Agel, J., R. Dick, B. Nelson, S.W. Marshall and T.P. Dompier (2007a) Descriptive Epidemiology of Collegiate Women's Ice Hockey Injuries: National Collegiate Athletic Association Injury Surveillance System, 2000–2001 through 2003–2004, *Journal of Athletic Training*, 42(2): 249–54

Agel, J., D.E. Olson, R. Dick, E.A. Arendt, S.W. Marshall and R.S. Sikka (2007b) Descriptive Epidemiology of Collegiate Women's Basketball Injuries: National Collegiate Athletic Association Injury Surveillance System, 1988–1989 through 2003–2004, *Journal of Athletic Training*, 42(2): 202–10

Agel, J., R.M. Palmieri-Smith, R. Dick, E.M. Wojtys and S.W. Marshall (2007c) Descriptive Epidemiology of Collegiate Women's Volleyball Injuries: National Collegiate Athletic Association Injury Surveillance System, 1988–1989 through 2003–2004, *Journal of Athletic Training*, 42(2): 295–302

Agel, J., E.A. Arendt and B. Bershadsky (2005) Anterior Cruciate Ligament Injury in National Collegiate Athletic Association Basketball and Soccer: A 13-Year Review, *American Journal of Sports Medicine*, 33(4): 524–31

Aguinaldo, A.L., J. Buttermore and H. Chambers (2007) Effects of Upper Trunk Rotation on Shoulder Joint Torque Among Baseball Pitchers of Various Levels, *Journal of Applied Biomechanics*, 23: 42–51

Albright, J.P., J.W. Powell, A. Martindale, R. Black, E. Crowley, P. Schmidt, J. Monroe, D. Locy, T. Aggler, W.R. Davis, G. Salvaterra, D. Miller, D. Helwig, S. Soboroff, J. Nivens, J. Carpenter, J. Kovan, E. Arndt, H. Sweeney, J. Lombardo, W.J. Sebastianelli, M. Krauss and G. Landry (2004) Injury Patterns in Big Ten Conference Football, *American Journal of Sports Medicine*, 32(6): 1394–404

Alcaraz, P.E., J. Perez-Gomez, M. Chavarrias and A.J. Blazevich (2011) Similarity in Adaptations to High-Resistance Circuit vs. Traditional Strength Training in Resistance-Trained Men, *Journal of Strength and Conditioning Research*, 25(9): 2519–27

Alcaraz, P.E., J. Sanchez-Lorentz and A.J. Blazevich (2008) Physical Performance and Cardiovascular Responses to an Acute Bout of Heavy Resistance Circuit Training versus Traditional Strength Training, *Journal of Strength and Conditioning Research*, 22(3): 667–71

Allerheiligen, B. (2003) In-Season Strength Training for Power Athletes, *Strength and Conditioning Journal*, 25(3): 23–8

American College Of Sports Medicine (1998) The Recommended Quantity and Quality of Exercise for Developing and Maintaining Cardiorespiratory and Muscular Fitness and Flexibility in Healthy Adults: Position Stand, *Medicine and Science in Sports and Exercise*, 30: 975–91

Anderson, K. and D.G. Behm (2005) The Impact of Instability Resistance Training on Balance and Stability, *Sports Medicine*, 35(1): 43–53

Apel, J.M., R.M., Lacey and R.T. Kell (2011) A Comparison of Traditional and Weekly Undulating Periodized Strength Training Programs with Total Volume and Intensity Equated, *Journal of Strength and Conditioning Research*, 25(3): 694–703

Arnason, A., T.E. Andersen, I. Holme, L. Engebretsen and R. Bahr (2008) Prevention of Hamstring Strains in Elite Soccer: An Intervention Study, *Scandinavian Journal of Sports Medicine*, 18: 40–8

Arnason, A., S.B. Sigurdsson, A. Gudmundsson, I. Holme, L. Engebretsen and R. Bahr (2004) Risk Factors for Injuries in Football, *American Journal of Sports Medicine*, 32(1)Suppl: S5–S16

Aughey, R. (2011) Application of GPS Technologies to Field Sports, *International Journal of Sports Physiology and Performance*, 6: 295–310

Axler, C.T. and S.M. McGill (1997) Low Back Loads over a Variety of Abdominal Exercises: Searching for the Safest Abdominal Challenge, *Medicine and Science in Sports and Exercise*, 29(6): 804–11

Aziz, A.R., M.Y.H. Chia, K.C. The (2005) Measured Maximal Oxygen Uptake in a Multi-stage Shuttle Test and Treadmill-run Test in Trained Athletes, *Journal of Sports Medicine and Physical Fitness*, 45: 306–14

Baechle T.R., R.W. Earle and D. Wathen (2000) Resistance Training. In: *Essentials of Strength Training and Conditioning* (2nd Edition). Baechle T.R. and R.W. Earle (Eds), Champaign, IL: Human Kinetics

Bahr, R. and T. Krosshaug (2005) Understanding Injury Mechanisms: A Key Component of Preventing Injuries in Sport, *British Journal of Sports Medicine*, 39: 324–9

Baker, D. (2003) Acute Effects of Alternating Heavy and Light Resistances on Power Output during Upper-Body Complex Power Training, *Journal of Strength and Conditioning Research*, 17(3): 493–7

Baker, D. (2002) Differences in Strength and Power Among Junior-High, Senior-High, College-Aged and Elite Professional Rugby League Players, *Journal of Strength and Conditioning Research*, 16(4): 581–5

Baker, D. (2001a) Acute and Long Term Power Responses to Power Training: Observations on the Training of an Elite Power Athlete, *Strength and Conditioning Journal*, 23(1): 47–56

Baker, D. (2001b) Comparison of Upper-Body Strength and Power between Professional and College-aged Rugby League Players, *Journal of Strength and Conditioning Research*, 15(1): 30–5

Baker, D. (2001c) The Effects of an In-Season of Concurrent Training on the Maintenance of Maximal Strength and Power in Professional and College-aged Rugby League Football Players, *Journal of Strength and Conditioning Research*, 15(2): 172–7

Baker, D. (2001d) A Series of Studies on the Training of High-Intensity Muscle Power in Rugby League Football Players, *Journal of Strength and Conditioning Research*, 15(2): 198–209

Baker, D. (1998) Applying the In-Season Periodization of Strength and Power Training to Football, *Strength and Conditioning*, 20(2): 18–27

Baker, D. (1996) Improving Vertical Jump Performance through General, Special and Specific Strength Training: A Brief Review, *Journal of Strength and Conditioning Research*, 10(2): 131–6

Baker, D. and R.U. Newton (2005) Methods to Increase the Effectiveness of Maximal Power Training for the Upper Body, *Strength and Conditioning Journal*, 27(6): 24–32

Baker, D. and S. Nance (1999a) The Relation between Strength and Power in Professional Rugby League Players, *Journal of Strength and Conditioning Research*, 13(3): 224–9

Baker, D. and S. Nance (1999b) The Relation between Running Speed and Measures of Strength and Power in Professional Rugby League Players, *Journal of Strength and Conditioning Research*, 13(3): 230–5

Baker, D., S. Nance and M. Moore (2001) The Load that Maximises the Average Mechanical Power Output during Explosive Bench Press Throws in Highly Trained Athletes, *Journal of Strength and Conditioning Research*, 15(1): 20–4

Baker, D., G. Wilson and B. Carlyon (1994) Generality versus Specificity: A Comparison of Dynamic and Isometric Measures of Strength and Speed-Strength, *European Journal of Applied Physiology*, 68: 350–5

Balsom, P.D., J.Y. Seger, B. Sjodin and B. Ekblom (1992) Maximal-Intensity Intermittent Exercise: Effect of Recovery Duration, *International Journal of Sports Medicine*, 13(7): 528–33

Bangsbo, J., F.M. Iaia and P. Krustrup (2008) The Yo-Yo Intermittent Recovery Test: A Useful Tool for Evaluation of Physical Performance in Intermittent Sports, *Sports Medicine*, 38(1): 37–51

Bangsbo. J., L. Norregaard and F. Thorso (1991) Activity Profile of Competition Soccer, *Canadian Journal of Sports Sciences*, 16(2): 110–16

Baquet, G., F.-X. Gamelin, P. Mucci, D. Thevenet, E. van Praagh and S. Berthoin (2010) Continuous vs. Interval Aerobic Training in 8- to 11-Year-Old Children, *Journal of Strength and Conditioning Research*, 24(5): 1381–8

Baquet, G., E. van Praagh and S. Berthoin (2003) Endurance Training and Aerobic Fitness in Young People, *Sports Medicine*, 33(15): 1127–43

Baquet, G., S. Berthoin, G. Dupont, N. Blondel, C. Fabre and E. van Praagh (2002) Effects of High Intensity Intermittent Training on Peak VO_2 in Prepubertal Children, *International Journal of Sports Medicine*, 23: 439–44

Barber-Westin, S.D., F.R. Noyes and M. Galloway (2006) Jump-Land Characteristics and Muscle Strength Development in Young Athletes, *American Journal of Sports Medicine*, 34(3): 375–84

Barber-Westin, S.D., M. Galloway, F.R. Noyes, G. Corbett and C. Walsh (2005) Assessment of Lower Limb Neuromuscular Control in Prepubescent Athletes, *American Journal of Sports Medicine*, 33(12): 1853–60

Barfield, J.-P., R.J. Johnson, P. Russo and D.C. Cobler (2007) Reliability and Validity of the Performance Index Evaluation among Men's and Women's College Basketball Players, *Journal of Strength and Conditioning Research*, 21(2): 643–5

Barr, K.P., M. Griggs and T. Cadby (2005) Lumbar Stabilization: Core Concepts and Current Literature, Part One, *American Journal of Physical Medicine and Rehabilitation*, 84: 473–80

Bathgate, A., J.P. Best, G. Craig and M. Jamieson (2002) A Prospective Study of Injuries to Elite Australian Rugby Union Players, *British Journal of Sports Medicine*, 36: 265–9

Baxter-Jones, A.D.G. and L.B. Sherar (2006) Growth and Maturation. In: *Paediatric Exercise Physiology*. N. Armstrong, Ed. Edinburgh: Elsevier Health Sciences

Behm, D.G. (1995) Neuromuscular Implications and Applications of Resistance Training, *Journal of Strength and Conditioning Research*, 9(4): 264–74

Behm, D.G. and D.G. Sale (1993) Intended rather than Actual Movement Velocity Determines Velocity-Specific Training Response, *Journal of Applied Physiology*, 74(1): 359–68

Behm, D.G., A.M. Leonard, W.B. Young, W.A.C. Bonsey and S.N. Mackinnon (2005) Trunk Muscle Electromyographic Activity with Unstable and Unilateral Exercises, *Journal of Strength and Conditioning Research*, 19(1): 193–201

Behnke, R.S. (2001) *Kinetic Anatomy*. Champaign, IL: Human Kinetics

Bell, G.J., G.D. Snydmiller, D.S. Davies and H.A. Quinney (1997) Relationship between Aerobic Fitness and Metabolic Recovery From Intermittent Exercise in Endurance Athletes, *Canadian Journal of Applied Physiology*, 22(1): 78–85

Bellew, J.W. and S. Dunn (2002) Ankle Rehabilitation: A Reintroduction of the Peroneus Longus, *Strength and Conditioning Journal*, 24(4): 61–3

Beneka, A., N. Aggeloussis, K. Giannakopoulos and G. Godolias (2006) Identifying and Treating Rotator Cuff Imbalances, *Strength and Conditioning Journal*, 28(2): 92–5

Besier, T.F., D.G. Lloyd, T.R. Ackland and J.L. Cochrane (2001) Anticipatory Effects on Knee Joint Loading during Running and Cutting Maneuvers, *Medicine and Science in Sports and Exercise*, 33(7): 1176–81

Best, J.P., A.S. McIntosh and T.N. Savage (2005) Rugby World Cup 2003 Injury Surveillance Project, *British Journal of Sports Medicine*, 39: 812–17

Beunen, G. and M. Thomis (2006) Gene Driven Power Athletes? Genetic Variation in Muscular Strength and Power, *British Journal of Sports Medicine*, 40: 822–3

Beynnon, B.D., P.M. Vacek, D. Murphy, D. Alosa and D. Paller (2005) First-time Inversion Ankle Ligament Trauma: The Effects of Sex, Level of Competition and Sport on the Incidence of Injury, *American Journal of Sports Medicine*, 33(10): 1485–91

Billat, V.L. (2001a) Interval Training for Performance: A Scientific and Empirical Practice. Special Recommendations for Middle- and Long-Distance Running. Part I: Aerobic Interval Training, *Sports Medicine*, 31(1): 13–31

Billat, V.L. (2001b) Interval Training for Performance: A Scientific and Empirical Practice. Special Recommendations for Middle- and Long-Distance Running. Part II: Anaerobic Interval Training, *Sports Medicine*. 31(2): 75–90

Billat, V.L., P. Sirvent, G. Py, J-P. Koralsztein and J. Mercier (2003) The Concept of Maximal Lactate Steady State, *Sports Medicine*, 33(6): 407–26

Bishop, D., O. Girard and A. Mendez-Villanueva (2011) Repeated Sprint Ability – Part II: Recommendations for Training, *Sports Medicine*, 41(9): 741–56

Bishop, D., J. Edge and C. Goodman (2004) Muscle Buffer Capacity and Aerobic Fitness are Associated with Repeated Sprint Ability in Women, *European Journal of Applied Physiology*, 92: 540–7

Bishop, D., J. Edge, C. Thomas and J. Mercier (2008) Effects of High-Intensity Training on Muscle Lactate Transporters and Postexercise Recovery of Muscle Lactate and Hydrogen Ions in Women, *American Journal of Physiology. Regulatory, Integrative and Comparative Physiology*, 295: R1991–8

Bishop, D., M. Spencer, R. Duffield and S. Lawrence (2001) The Validity of a Repeated Sprint Ability Test, *Journal of Science and Medicine in Sport*, 4(1): 19–29

Bloomfield, J., R. Polman, P. O'Donoghue and L. McNaughton (2007) Effective Speed and Agility Conditioning Methodology for Random Intermittent Dynamic Type Sports, *Journal of Strength and Conditioning Research*, 21(4): 1093–100

Boddington, M.K., M.I. Lambert, A. St Clair Gibson and T.D. Noakes (2001) Reliability of a 5-m Multiple Sprint Shuttle Test, *Journal of Sports Sciences*, 19: 223–8

Bogdanis, G.C., M.E. Nevill, L.H. Boobis and H.K.A. Lakomy (1996a) Contribution of Phosphocreatine and Aerobic Metabolism to Energy Supply during Repeated Sprint Exercise, *Journal of Applied Physiology*, 80(3): 876–84

Bogdanis, G.C., M.E. Nevill, H.K.A. Lakomy, C.M. Graham and G. Louis (1996b) Effects of Active Recovery on Power Output during Repeated Maximal Sprint Cycling, *European Journal of Applied Physiology*, 74: 461–9

Boisseau, N. and P. Delamarche (2000) Metabolic and Hormonal Responses to Exercise in Children and Adolescents, *Sports Medicine*, 30(6): 405–22

Boling, M.C., D.A. Padua and R.A. Creighton (2009) Concentric and Eccentric Torque of the Hip Musculature in Individuals with and without Patellofemoral Pain, *Journal of Athletic Training*, 44(1): 7–13

Bompa, T. (2000) *Total Training for Young Champions*, Champaign, IL: Human Kinetics

Bondarchuk, A. (2007) A Brief Overview of Transfer of Training, In: *Transfer of Training in Sports*, Grand Rapids, MI: Ultimate Athlete Concepts

Borghuis, J., A.L. Hof and K.A.P.M. Lemmink (2008) The Importance of Sensory-Motor Control in Providing Core Stability: Implications for Measurement and Testing, *Sports Medicine*, 38(11): 893–916

Borowski, L.A., E.E. Yard, S.K. Fields and R.D. Comstock (2008) The Epidemiology of US High School Basketball Injuries, 2005–2007, *American Journal of Sports Medicine*, 36(12): 2328–35

Bosquet, L. L. Leger and P. Legros (2002) Methods to Determine Aerobic Endurance, *Sports Medicine*, 32(11): 675–700

Bouchard, C. (2011) Genomic Predictors of Trainability, *Experimental Physiology*, 97(3): 347–52

Boyle. P.M., C.A. Mahoney and W.F.M. Wallace (1994) The Competitive Demands of Elite Male Field Hockey, *Journal of Sports Medicine and Physical Fitness*, 34(3): 235–41

Bradley, P.S., P.D. Olsen and M.D. Portas (2007) The Effect of Static, Ballistic and Proprioceptive Neuromuscular Facilitation Stretching on Vertical Jump Performance, *Journal of Strength and Conditioning Research*, 21(1): 223–6

Brechue, W.F., J.L. Mayhew and F.C. Piper (2010) Characteristics of Sprint Performance in College Football Players, *Journal of Strength and Conditioning Research*, 24(5): 1169–78

Bressel, E., J.C. Yonker, J. Kras and E.M. Heath (2007) Comparison of Static and Dynamic Balance in Female Collegiate Soccer, Basketball and Gymnastics Athletes, *Journal of Athletic Training*, 42(1): 42–6

Brockett, C.L., D.L. Morgan and U. Proske (2004) Predicting Hamstring Strain Injury in Elite Athletes, *Medicine and Science in Sports and Exercise*, 36(3): 379–87

Brockett, C.L., D.L. Morgan and U. Proske (2001) Human Hamstring Muscles Adapt to Eccentric Exercise by Changing Optimum Length, *Medicine and Science in Sports and Exercise*, 33(5): 783–90

Brooks, G.A. (2009) Cell-Cell and Intracellular Lactate Shuttles, *Journal of Physiology*, 587: 5591–600

Brooks, J.H.M., C.W. Fuller, S.P.T. Kemp and D.B. Reddin (2006) Incidence, Risk and Prevention of Hamstring Muscle Injuries in Professional Rugby Union, *American Journal of Sports Medicine*, 34(8): 1297–306

Brooks, J.H.M., C.W. Fuller, S.P.T. Kemp and D.B. Reddin (2005a) Epidemiology of Injuries in English Professional Rugby Union: Part 1 Match Injuries, *British Journal of Sports Medicine*, 39: 757–66

Brooks, J.H.M., C.W. Fuller, S.P.T. Kemp and D.B. Reddin (2005b) Epidemiology of Injuries in English Professional Rugby Union: Part 2 Training Injuries, *British Journal of Sports Medicine*, 39: 767–75

Brown, C.N. and R. Mynark (2007) Balance Deficits in Recreational Athletes with Chronic Ankle Instability, *Journal of Athletic Training*, 42(3): 367–73

Brown, L.E. and M. Greenwood (2005) Periodization Essentials and Innovations in Resistance Training Protocols, *Strength and Conditioning Journal*, 27(4): 80–5

Brown, T.D. (2006) Getting to the Core of the Matter, *Strength and Conditioning Journal*, 28(2): 50–3

Brown, T.D. and J.D. Vescovi (2003) Efficient Arms for Efficient Agility, *Strength and Conditioning Journal*, 25(4): 7–11

Brown, T.D., J.D. Vescovi and J.L. Vanheest (2004) Assessment of Linear Sprinting Performance: A Theoretical Paradigm, *Journal of Sports Science and Medicine*, 3: 203–10

Brughelli, M., J. Cronin, G. Levin and A. Chaouachi (2008) Understanding Change of Direction Ability in Sport: A Review of Resistance Training Studies, *Sports Medicine*, 38(12): 1045–63

Brummitt, J. and E. Meira (2006) Scapula Stabilization Rehab Exercise Prescription, *Strength and Conditioning Journal*, 28(3): 62–5

Buchheit, M. (2010) Improving Repeated Sprint Ability in Young Elite Soccer Players: Repeated Shuttle Sprints vs. Explosive Strength Training, *Journal of Strength and Conditioning Research*, 24(10): 2715–22

Buchheit, M. (2008) The 30–15 Intermittent Fitness Test: Accuracy for Individualising Interval Training of Young Intermittent Sport Players, *Journal of Strength and Conditioning Research*, 22(2): 365–74

Buchheit, M. and P. Ufland (2011) Effect of Training on Performance and Muscle Reoxygenation Rate during Repeated-Sprint Running, *European Journal of Applied Physiology*, 111: 293–301

Buchheit, M., C.R. Abbiss, J.J. Peiffer and P.B. Laursen (2012) Performance and Physiological Responses during a Sprint Interval Training Session: Relationship with Muscle Oxygenation and Pulmonary Oxygen Uptake Kinetics, *European Journal of Applied Physiology*, 112(2): 767–79

Buchheit, M., B. Haydar, K. Hader, P. Ufland and S. Ahmaidi (2011a) Assessing Running Economy during Field Running with Changes of Direction: Application to 20m Shuttle Runs, *International Journal of Sports Physiology and Performance*, 6: 380–95

Buchheit, M., B. Lefebvre, P.B. Laursen and S. Ahmaidi (2011b) Reliability, Usefulness and Validity of the 30–15 Intermittent Ice Test in Young Elite Ice Hockey Players, *Journal of Strength and Conditioning Research*, 25(5): 1457–64

Buchheit, M., D. Bishop, B. Haydar, F.Y. Nakamura and S. Ahmaidi (2010a) Physiological Responses to Shuttle Repeated-Sprint Running, *International Journal of Sports Medicine*, 31: 402–9

Buchheit, M., A. Mendez-Villanueva, M. Quod, T. Quesnel and S. Ahmaidi (2010b) Improving Acceleration and Repeated Sprint Ability in Well-Trained Adolescent Handball Players: Speed versus Sprint Interval Training, *International Journal of Sports Physiology and Performance*, 5: 152–64

Buchheit, M., A. Mendez-Villanueva, B.M. Simpson and P.C. Bourdon (2010c) Match Running Performance and Fitness in Youth Soccer, *International Journal of Sports Medicine*, 31: 818–25

Buchheit, M., P.B. Laursen, J. Kuhnle, D. Ruch, C. Renaud and S. Ahmaidi (2009) Game-Based Training in Youth Elite Handball Players, *International Journal of Sports Medicine*, 30: 251–8

Buford, T.W., S.J. Rossi, D.B., Smith and A.J. Warren (2007) A Comparison of Periodization Models During Nine Weeks with Equated Volume and Intensity for Strength, *Journal of Strength and Conditioning Research*, 21(4): 1245–50

Burgomaster, K.A., K.R. Howarth, S.M. Phillips, M. Rakobowchuk, M.J. Macdonald, S.L. McGee, and M.J. Gibala (2008) Similar Metabolic Adaptations during Exercise after Low Volume Sprint Interval and Traditional Endurance Training in Humans, *Journal of Physiology*, 586(1): 151-60

Burr, J.F., V.K, Jamnik, S. Dogra and N. Gledhill (2007) Evaluation of Jump Protocols to Assess Leg Power and Predict Hockey Playing Potential, *Journal of Strength and Conditioning Research*, 21(4): 1139–45

Carey, D.G., M.M. Drake, G.J. Pliego and R.L. Raymond (2007) Do Hockey Players Need Aerobic Fitness? Relation between VO_2max and Fatigue during High-Intensity Intermittent Ice Skating, *Journal of Strength and Conditioning Research*, 21(3): 963–6

Carroll, T.J., S. Riek and R.G. Carson (2001) Neural Adaptations to Resistance Training: Implications for Movement Control, *Sports Medicine*, 31(12): 829–40

Carter, J.M., W.C. Beam, S.G. McMahan, M.L. Barr, L.E. Brown (2006) The Effects of Stability Ball Training on Spinal Stability in Sedentary Individuals, *Journal of Strength and Conditioning Research*, 20(2): 429–35

Castagna, C., F.M. Impellizzeri, A. Chaouachi, N. Ben Abdelkrim and V. Manzi (2011) Physiological Responses to Ball-Drills in Regional Level Male Basketball Players, *Journal of Sports Sciences*, 29(12): 1329–36

Castagna, C., V. Manzi, F. Impellizzeri, M. Weston and J.C. Barbero Alvarez (2010) Relationship between Endurance Field Tests and Match Performance in Young Soccer Players, *Journal of Strength and Conditioning Research*, 24(12): 3227–33

Castagna, C., V. Manzi, S. D'Ottavio, G. Annino, E. Padua and D. Bishop (2007) Relation between Maximal Aerobic Power and Ability to Repeat Sprints in Young Basketball Players, *Journal of Strength and Conditioning Research*, 21(4): 1172–6

Castagna, C. F.M. Impellizeri, K. Chamari, D. Carlomagno and E. Rampinini (2006) Aerobic Fitness and Yo-Yo Continuous and Intermittent Test Performances in Soccer Players: A Correlation Study, *Journal of Strength and Conditioning Research*, 20(2): 320–5

Castagna, C., R. Belardinelli and G. Abt (2004) *Fifth World Congress of Science and Football Conference Communications:* The Oxygen Uptake and Heart Rate Response to Training with a Ball in Youth Soccer Players, *Journal of Sports Sciences*, 22(6): 532–3

Chappell, J.D., B. YU, D.T. Kirkendall and W.E. Garrett (2002) A Comparison of Knee Kinetics between Male and Female Recreational Athletes in Stop-Jump Tasks, *American Journal of Sports Medicine*, 30(2): 261–7

Chiu, L.Z.F. and J.L. Barnes (2003) The Fitness-Fatigue Model Revisited: Implications for Planning Short- and Long-Term Training, *Strength and Conditioning Journal*, 25(6): 42–51

Chiu, L.Z.F., A.C. Fry, L.W. Weiss, B.K. Schilling, L.E. Brown and S.L. Smith (2003) Postactivation Potentiation Response in Athletes and Recreationally Trained Individuals, *Journal of Strength and Conditioning Research*, 17(4): 671–7

Cholewicki, J. and S.M. McGill (1996) Mechanical Stability of the In Vivo Lumbar Spine: Implications for Injury and Chronic Low Back Pain, *Clinical Biomechanics*, 11(1): 1–15

Chtara, M., K. Chamari, M. Chaouachi, A. Chaouachi, D. Koubaa, Y. Feki, G.P. Millet and M. Amri (2005) Effects of Intra-Session Concurrent Endurance and Strength Training Sequence on Aerobic Performance and Capacity, *British Journal of Sports Medicine*, 39: 555–60,

Cissik, J., A. Hedrick and M. Barnes (2008) Challenges Applying the Research on Periodization, *Strength and Conditioning Journal*, 30(1): 45–51

Cissik, J.M. (2005) Means and Methods of Speed Training: Part II, *Strength and Conditioning Journal*, 27(1): 18–25

Cissik, J.M. (2002) Programming Abdominal Training, Part One, *Strength and Conditioning Journal*, 24(1): 9–15

Clark, R. (2009) The Effect of Training Status on Inter-Limb Joint Stiffness Regulation during Repeated Maximal Sprints, *Journal of Science and Medicine in Sport*, 12: 406–10

Conroy, B. and R.W. Earle (2000) Bone, Muscle and Connective Tissue Adaptations to Physical Activity, In: *Essentials of Strength Training and Conditioning* (2nd Edition). T.R. Baechle and R.W. Earle (Eds), Champaign, IL: Human Kinetics

Contreras, B., J. Cronin and B. Schoenfeld (2011) Barbell Hip Thrust, *Journal of Strength and Conditioning*, 33(5): 58–61

Cook, G. (2003a) Mobility and Stability Testing. In: *Athletic Body in Balance*. Champaign, IL: Human Kinetics

Cook, G. (2003b) Strength and Endurance Exercises. In: *Athletic Body in Balance*. Champaign, IL: Human Kinetics

Cormie, P., M.R. McGuigan and R.U. Newton (2011a) Developing Maximal Neuromuscular Power: Part 1 – Biological Basis of Maximal Power Production, *Sports Medicine*, 41(1): 17–38

Cormie, P., M.R. McGuigan and R.U. Newton (2011b) Developing Maximal Neuromuscular Power: Part 2 – Training Considerations for Improving Maximal Power Production, *Sports Medicine*, 41(2): 125–46

Cormie, P., M.R. McGuigan and R.U. Newton (2010a) Changes in the Eccentric Phase Contribution to Improved SSC Performance after Training, *Medicine and Science in Sports and Exercise*, 42(9): 1731–44

Cormie, P., M.R. McGuigan and R.U. Newton (2010b) Influence of Strength on the Magnitude and Mechanisms of Adaptation to Power Training, *Medicine and Science in Sports and Exercise*, 42(8): 1566–81

Cormie, P., R. Deane and J.M. McBride (2007a) Methodological Concerns for Determining Power Output in the Jump Squat, *Journal of Strength and Conditioning Research*, 21(2): 424–30

Cormie, P., J.M. McBride and G.O. McCaulley (2007b) Validation of Power Measurement Techniques in Dynamic Lower Body Resistance Exercises, *Journal of Applied Biomechanics*, 23: 103–18

Coutts, A.J. and R. Duffield (2010) Validity and Reliability of GPS Devices for Measuring Movement Demands of Team Sports, *Journal of Science and Medicine in Sport*, 13: 133–5

Coutts, A., P. Reaburn and G. Abt (2003) Heart Rate, Blood Lactate Concentration and Estimated Energy Expenditure in a Semi-Professional Rugby League Team during a Match: A Case Study, *Journal of Sports Sciences*. 21: 97–103

Cowan, S.M., K.M. Crossley and K.L. Bennel (2009) Altered Hip and Trunk Muscle Function in Individuals with Patellofemoral Pain, *British Journal of Sports Medicine*, 43: 584–8

Cowley, P.M. and T.C. Swensen (2008) Development and Reliability of Two Core Stability Field Tests, *Journal of Strength and Conditioning Research*, 22(2): 619–24

Craig, B.W. (2004) What is the Scientific Basis of Speed and Agility?, *Strength and Conditioning Journal*, 26(3): 13–14

Crewther, B.T., L.P. Kilduff, D.J. Cunningham, C. Cook, N. Owen and G.-Z. Yang (2011) Validating Two Systems for Estimating Force and Power, *International Journal of Sports Medicine*, 32: 254–8

Croisier, J.-L. (2004) Factors Associated with Recurrent Hamstring Injuries, *Sports Medicine*, 34(10): 681–95

Croisier, J.-L., S. Ganteaume, J. Binet, M. Genty and J.-M. Ferret (2008) Strength Imbalances and Prevention of Hamstring Injury in Professional Soccer Players: A Prospective Study, *American Journal of Sports Medicine*, 36(8): 1469–75

Croisier, J-L., B. Forthomme, M-H. Namurois, M. Vanderthommen and J.-M. Crielaard (2002) Hamstring Muscle Strain Recurrence and Strength Performance Disorders, *American Journal of Sports Medicine*, 30(2): 199–203

Cronin, J.B. and K.T. Hansen (2006) Resisted Sprint Training for the Acceleration Phase of Sprinting, *Strength and Conditioning Journal*, 28(4): 42–51

Cronin, J.B. and K.T. Hansen (2005) Strength and Power Predictors of Sports Speed, *Journal of Strength and Conditioning Research*, 19(2): 349–57

Cronin, J.B. and G. Sleivert (2005) Challenges in Understanding the Influence of Maximal Power Training on Improving Athletic Performance, *Sports Medicine*, 35(3): 215–34

Cronin, J.B., P.J. McNair and R.N. Marshall (2003) Force-Velocity Analysis of Strength-Training Techniques and Load: Implications for Training Strategy and Research, *Journal of Strength and Conditioning Research*, 17(1): 148–55

Cronin, J., P.J. McNair and R.N. Marshall (2001a) Developing Explosive Power: A Comparison of Technique and Training, *Journal of Science and Medicine in Sport*, 4(1): 59–70

Cronin, J., P.J. McNair and R.N. Marshall (2001b) Velocity Specificity, Combination Training and Sport Specific Tasks, *Journal of Science and Medicine in Sport*, 4(2): 168–78

Crossley, K.M., W.-J. Zhang, A.G. Schache, A. Bryant and S.M. Cowan (2011) Performance on the Single-Leg Squat Task Indicates Hip Abductor Muscle Function, *American Journal of Sports Medicine*, 39(4): 866–73

Crow, J.F., D. Buttifant, S.G. Kearny and C. Hrysomallis (2012) Low Load Exercises Targeting the Gluteal Muscle Group Acutely Enhance Explosive Power Output in Elite Athletes, *Journal of Strength and Conditioning Research*, 26(2): 438–42

Cusi, M.F., C.J. Juska-Butel, D. Garlick and G. Argyrous (2001) Lumbopelvic Stability and Injury Profile in Rugby Union Players, *New Zealand Journal of Sports Medicine*, 29(1): 14–18

Dallalana, R.J., J.H.M. Brooks, S.P.T. Kemp and A.M. Williams (2007) The Epidemiology of Knee Injuries in English Professional Rugby Union, *American Journal of Sports Medicine*, 35(5): 818–30

Danneels, L.A., G.G. Vanderstraeten, D.C. Cambier, E.E. Witvrouw, J. Bourgois, W. Dankaerts and H.J. De Cuyper (2001) Effects of Three Different Training Modalities on the Cross Sectional Area of the Lumbar Multifidus Muscle in Patients with Chronic Low Back Pain, *British Journal of Sports Medicine*, 35: 186–91

Dayne, A.M., J.M. McBride, J.L. Nuzzo, N.T. Triplett, J. Skinner and A. Burr (2011) Power Output in the Jump Squat in Adolescent Male Athletes, *Journal of Strength and Conditioning Research*, 25(3): 585–9

Deane, R.S., J.W. Chow, M.D. Tillman and K.A. Fournier (2005) Effects of Hip Flexor Training on Sprint, Shuttle Run and Vertical Jump Performance, *Journal of Strength and Conditioning Research*, 19(3): 615–21

Decker, M.J., J.M. Tokish, H.B. Ellis, M.R. Torry and R.J. Hawkins (2003) Subscapularis Muscle Activity during Selected Rehabilitation Exercises, *American Journal of Sports Medicine*, 31(1): 126–34

Delecluse, C. (1997) Influence of Strength Training on Sprint Running Performance: Current Findings and Implications for Training, *Sports Medicine*, 24(3): 147–56

Delecluse, C., H. van Coppenolle, E. Willems, M. van Leemputte, R. Diels and M. Goris (1995) Influence of High-Resistance and High-Velocity Training on Sprint Performance, *Medicine and Science in Sports and Exercise*, 27(8): 1203–9

Dellal, A., S. Hill-Haas, C. Lago-Penas and K. Chamari (2011) Small-Sided Games in Soccer: Amateur vs. Professional Players' Physiological Responses, Physical and Technical Activities, *Journal of Strength and Conditioning Research*, 25(9): 2371–81

Dellal, A., D. Keller, C. Carling, A. Chaouachi, D.P. Wong and K. Chamari (2010) Physiological Effects of Directional Changes in Intermittent Exercise in Soccer Players, *Journal of Strength and Conditioning Research*, 24(12): 3219–26

Dellal, A., K. Chamari, A. Pintus, O. Girard, T. Cotte and D. Keller (2008) Heart Rate Responses During Small-Sided Games and Short Intermittent Running Training in Elite Soccer Players: A Comparative Study, *Journal of Strength and Conditioning Research*, 22(5): 1449–57

DeRenne, C., B.P. Buxton, R.K. Hetzel and K. Ho (1994) Effects of Under and Overweighted Implement Training on Pitching Velocity, *Journal of Strength and Conditioning Research*, 8(4): 247–50

DeRenne, C., H. Kwok and A. Blitzblau (1990) Effects of Weighted Implement Training on Throwing Velocity, *Journal of Applied Sports Science Research*, 4(1): 16–19

Deutsch, M.U., G.J. Maw, D. Jenkins and P. Reaburn (1998) Heart Rate, Blood Lactate and Kinematic Data of Elite Colts (Under-19) Rugby Union Players during Competition, *Journal of Sports Sciences*, 16: 561–70

de Visser, H.M., M. Reijman, M.P. Heijboer and P.K. Bos (2012) Risk Factors for Recurrent Hamstring Injuries: A Systematic Review, *British Journal of Sports Medicine*, 46(2): 124–30

Dick, R., M.S. Ferrara, J. Agel, R. Courson, S.W. Marshall, M.J. Hanley and F. Reifsteck (2007a) Descriptive Epidemiology of Collegiate Men's Football Injuries: National Collegiate Athletic Association Injury Surveillance System, 1988–1989 through 2003–2004, *Journal of Athletic Training*, 42(2): 221–33

Dick, R., J. Hertel, J. Agel, J. Grossman and S.W. Marshall (2007b) Descriptive Epidemiology of Collegiate Men's Basketball Injuries: National Collegiate Athletic Association Injury Surveillance System, 1988–1989 through 2003–2004, *Journal of Athletic Training*, 42(2): 194–201

Distefano, L.J., J.T. Blackburn, S.W. Marshall, K.M. Guskiewicz, W.E. Garrett and D.A. Padua (2011) Effect of an Age-Specific Anterior Cruciate Injury Prevention Program on Lower Extremity Biomechanics in Children, *American Journal of Sports Medicine*, 39(5): 949–57

Divert, C., G. Mornieux, H. Baur, F. Mayer and A. Belli (2005) Mechanical Comparisons of Barefoot and Shod Running, *International Journal of Sports Medicine*, 26: 593–8

Drust, B., T. Reilly and N.T. Cable (2000) Physiological Responses to Laboratory-based Soccer-Specific Intermittent and Continuous Exercise, *Journal of Sports Sciences*, 18: 885–92

Drust, B., T. Reilly and E. Rienzi (1998) Analysis of Work Rate in Soccer, *Sports Exercise and Injury*, 4(4): 151–5

Dupont, G., A. McCall, F. Prieur, G. P. Millet and S. Berthoin (2010) Faster Oxygen Uptake Kinetics during Recovery is Related to Better Repeated Sprinting Ability, *European Journal of Applied Physiology*, 110(3): 627–34

Dupont, G., K. Akakpo and S. Berthoin (2004) The Effect of In-Season, High-Intensity Interval Training in Soccer Players, *Journal of Strength and Conditioning Research*, 18(3): 584–9

Durell, D.L., T.J. Puyol and J.T. Barnes (2003) A Survey of the Scientific Data and Training Methods Utilized by Collegiate Strength and Conditioning Coaches, *Journal of Strength and Conditioning Research*, 17(2): 368–73

Duthie, G., D. Pyne and S. Hooper (2003) Applied Physiology and Game Analysis of Rugby Union, *Sports Medicine*, 33(13): 973–91

Earle, R.W. and T.R. Baechle (2000) Resistance Training and Spotting Techniques. In *Essentials of Strength Training and Conditioning* (2nd Edition). Champaign, IL: Human Kinetics

Ebben, W.P. and D.O. Blackard (2001) Strength and Conditioning Practices of National Football League Strength and Conditioning Coaches, *Journal of Strength and Conditioning Research*, 15(1): 48–58

Ebben, W.P., C. Simenz and R.L. Jensen (2008) Evaluation of Plyometric Intensity Using Electromyography, *Journal of Strength and Conditioning Research*, 22(3): 861–8

Ebben, W.P., M.J. Hintz and C.J. Simenz (2005) Strength and Conditioning Practices of Major League Baseball Strength and Conditioning Coaches, *Journal of Strength and Conditioning Research*, 19(3): 538–46

Ebben, W.P., R.M. Carroll and C.J. Simenz (2004) Strength and Conditioning Practices of National Hockey League Strength and Conditioning Coaches, *Journal of Strength and Conditioning Research*, 18(4): 889–97

Edge, J., D. Bishop and C. Goodman (2006a) The Effects of Training Intensity on Muscle Buffer Capacity in Females, *European Journal of Applied Physiology*, 96: 97–105

Edge, J., D. Bishop, S. Hill-Haas, B. Dawson and C. Goodman (2006b) Comparison of Muscle Buffer Capacity and Repeated-Sprint Ability of Untrained, Endurance-Trained and Team-Sport Athletes, *European Journal of Applied Physiology*, 96: 225–34

Emery, C.A. and W.H. Meeuwisse (2010) The Effectiveness of a Neuromuscular Prevention Strategy to Reduce Injuries in Youth Soccer: A Cluster-Randomised Controlled Trial, *British Journal of Sports Medicine*, 44: 555–62

Emery, C.A. and W.H. Meeuwisse (2001) Risk Factors for Groin Injuries in Hockey, *Medicine and Science in Sports and Exercise*, 33(9): 1423–33

Engebretsen, A.H., G. Myklebust, I. Holme, L. Engebretsen and R. Bahr (2010) Intrinsic Risk Factors for Groin Injuries Among Male Soccer Players: A Prospective Cohort Study, *American Journal of Sports Medicine*, 38(10): 2051–7

Engebretsen, A.H., G. Myklebust, I. Holme, L. Engebretsen and R. Bahr (2008) Prevention of Injuries among Male Soccer Players: A Prospective, Randomised Intervention Study Targeting Players with Previous Injuries or Reduced Function, *American Journal of Sports Medicine*, 36(6): 1052–60

Enoka, R.M. (1997) Neural Adaptations with Chronic Physical Activity, *Journal of Biomechanics*, 30(5): 447–55

Ericsson, K. A. (2007) Deliberate Practice and the Modifiability of Body and Mind: Toward a Science of the Structure and Acquisition of Expert and Elite Performance, *International Journal of Sport Psychology*, 38: 4–34

Escamilla, R.F., K. Yamashiro, L. Paulos, and J.R. Andrews (2009) Shoulder Muscle Activity and Function in Common Shoulder Rehabilitation Exercises, *Sports Medicine*, 39(8): 663–85

Escamilla, R.F., S.W. Barrentine, G.S. Fleisig, N. Zheng, Y. Takada, D. Kingsley and J.R. Andrews (2007) Pitching Biomechanics as a Pitcher Approaches Muscular Fatigue during a Simulated Baseball Game, *American Journal of Sports Medicine*, 35(1): 23–33

Escamilla, R.F., K.P. Speer, G.S. Fleisig, S.W. Barrentine and J.R. Andrews (2000) Effects of Throwing Overweight and Underweight Baseballs on Throwing Velocity and Accuracy, *Sports Medicine*, 29(4): 259–72

Ettema, G., T. Glosen and R. van den Tillar (2008) Effect of Specific Resistance Training on Overarm Throwing Performance, *International Journal of Sports Physiology and Performance*, 3: 164–75

Evans, K., K.M. Refshauge and R. Adams (2007) Trunk Muscle Endurance Tests: Reliability and Gender Differences in Athletes, *Journal of Science and Medicine in Sport*, 10: 447–55

Fabrocini, B. and N. Mercaldo (2003) A Comparison between the Rotator Cuffs of the Shoulder and Hip, *Strength and Conditioning Journal*, 25(4): 63–8

Faigenbaum, A.D., W.J. Kraemer, C.J.R. Blimkie, I. Jeffreys, L.J. Micheli, M. Nikta and T.W. Rowland (2009) Youth Resistance Training: Updated Position Statement from the National Strength and Conditioning Association, *Journal of Strength and Conditioning Research*, 23(Suppl 5): S60–S79,

Faigenbaum, A.D. and J. Schram (2004) Can Resistance Training Reduce Injuries in Youth Sports, *Strength and Conditioning Journal*, 26(3): 16–21

Falk, B. and G. Tenenbaum (1996) The Effectiveness of Resistance Training in Children. A Meta-analysis, *Sports Medicine*, 22: 176–86

Farrow, D., W. Young, and L. Bruce, The Development of a Test of Reactive Agility for Netball: A New Methodology, *Journal of Science & Medicine in Sport*, 8(1): 52–60

Faude, O., A. Junge, W. Kindermann and J. Dvorak (2005) Injuries in Female Soccer Players: A Prospective Study in the German National League, *American Journal of Sports Medicine*, 33(11): 1694–700

Feltner, M.E., D.J. Fraschetti and R.J. Crisp (1999) Upper Extremity Augmentation of Lower Extremity Kinetics during Countermovement Vertical Jumps, *Journal of Sports Sciences*, 17: 449–66

Fenwick, C.M.J., S.H.M. Brown and S.M. McGill (2009) Comparison of Different Rowing Exercises: Trunk Muscle and Activation and Lumbar Spine Motion, Load and Stiffness, *Journal of Strength and Conditioning Research*, 23(5): 1408–17

Fleck, S.J. (1999) Periodized Strength Training: A Critical Review, *Journal of Strength and Conditioning Research*, 13(1): 82–9

Fleck, S.J. and W.J. Kraemer (1997) *Designing Resistance Training Programs* (2nd Edition). Champaign, IL: Human Kinetics

Flik, K., S. Lyman and R.G. Marx (2005) American Collegiate Men's Ice Hockey: An Analysis of Injuries, *American Journal of Sports Medicine*, 33(2): 183–7

Flouris, A.D., G.S. Metsios and Y. Koutedakis (2005) Enhancing the Efficacy of the 20m Multistage Shuttle Run Test, *British Journal of Sports Medicine*, 39: 166–70

Ford, K.R., G.D. Myer and T.E. Hewett (2010) Longitudinal Effects of Maturation on Lower Extremity Joint Stiffness in Adolescent Athletes, *American Journal of Sports Medicine*, 38(9): 1829–37

Ford, K.R., G.D. Myer, R.L. Smith, R.N. Byrnes, S.E. Dopirak and T.E. Hewett (2005) Use of an Overhead Goal Alters Vertical Jump Performance and Biomechanics, *Journal of Strength and Conditioning Research*, 19(2): 394–9

Ford, K.R., G.D. Myer and T.E. Hewett (2003) Valgus Knee Motion during Landing in High School Female and Male Basketball Players, *Medicine and Science in Sports and Exercise*, 35(10): 1745–50

Foster, C., L.L. Hector, R. Welsh, M. Schrager, M.A. Green and A.C. Snyder (1997) Effects of Specific versus Cross-Training on Running Performance, *European Journal of Applied Physiology*, 70: 367–72

Fouré, A., A. Nordez and C. Cornu (2010) Plyometric Training Effects on Achilles Tendon Stiffness and Dissipative Properties, *Journal of Applied Physiology*, 109: 849–54

Fredberg, U., L. Bolvig and N.T. Andersen (2008) Prophylactic Training in Asymptomatic Soccer Players with Ultrasonographic Abnormalities in Achilles and Patellar Tendons: The Danish Super League Study, *American Journal of Sports Medicine*, 36(3): 451–60

Frost, D.M., J. Cronin and R.U. Newton (2010) A Biomechanical Evaluation of Resistance: Fundamental Concepts for Training and Sports Performance, *Sports Medicine*, 40(4): 303–26

Frost, D.M., J.B. Cronin and D G. Levin (2008) Stepping Backward Can Improve Sprint Performance over Short Distances, *Journal of Strength and Conditioning Research*, 22(3): 918–22

Fry, A.C. (2004) The Role of Resistance Exercise Intensity on Muscle Fibre Adaptations, *Sports Medicine*, 34(10): 663–79

Fujii, K., Y. Yamada and S. Oda (2010) Skilled Basketball Players Rotate Their Shoulders More During Running while Dribbling, *Perceptual and Motor Skills*, 110(3): 983–4

Gabbe, B.J., K.L. Bennell and C.F. Finch (2006) Why are Older Australian Football Players at Greater Risk of Hamstring Injury?, *Journal of Science and Medicine in Sport*, 9: 327–33

Gabbett, T.J. (2008) Do Skill-based Conditioning Games Offer a Specific Training Stimulus for Junior Elite Volleyball Players, *Journal of Strength and Conditioning Research*, 22(2): 509–17

Gabbett, T.J. (2006) Skill-based Conditioning Games as an Alternative to Traditional Conditioning for Rugby League Players, *Journal of Strength and Conditioning Research*, 20(2): 309–15

Gabbett, T.J. (2004) Incidence of Injury in Junior and Senior Rugby League Players, *Sports Medicine*, 34(12): 849–59

Gabbett, T.J. (2002) Training Injuries in Rugby League: An Evaluation of Skill-Based Conditioning Games, *Journal of Strength and Conditioning Research*, 16(2): 236–41

Gabbett, T., and D. Benton (2009) Reactive Agility of Rugby League Players, *Journal of Science and Medicine in Sport*, 12: 212–14

Gaiga, M.C. and D. Docherty (1995) The Effect of an Aerobic Interval Training Program on Intermittent Anaerobic Performance, *Canadian Journal of Applied Physiology*, 20(4): 452–64

Gamble, P. (2011a) Introduction – What Defines Sports Speed and Agility?, In: *Training for Sports Speed and Agility – An Evidence-Based Approach*, Abingdon, UK: Routledge

Gamble, P.(2011b) Assessing Physical Parameters of Speed and Agility, In: *Training for Sports Speed and Agility – An Evidence-Based Approach*, Abingdon, UK: Routledge

Gamble, P. (2011c) Neuromuscular Training for Balance and Athleticism, In: *Training for Sports Speed and Agility – An Evidence-Based Approach*, Abingdon, UK: Routledge

Gamble, P. (2011d) Strength Training for Speed and Agility Development, In: *Training for Sports Speed and Agility – An Evidence-Based Approach*, Abingdon, UK: Routledge

Gamble, P. (2011e) Warm Up Methods and Mobility Training, In: *Training for Sports Speed and Agility – An Evidence-Based Approach*, Abingdon, UK: Routledge

Gamble, P. (2011f) Technical Aspects of Acceleration and Straight-line Speed Development, In: *Training for Sports Speed and Agility – An Evidence-Based Approach*, Abingdon, UK: Routledge

Gamble, P. (2011g) Developing Change of Direction Capabilities and Expression of Sports Agility, In: *Training for Sports Speed and Agility – An Evidence-Based Approach*, Abingdon, UK: Routledge

Gamble, P. (2008) Approaching Physical Preparation for Youth Team Sports Players, *Strength and Conditioning Journal*, 30(1): 29–42

Gamble, P. (2007a) An Integrated Approach to Training Core Stability, *Strength and Conditioning Journal*, 29(1): 58–68

Gamble, P. (2007b) Challenges and Game-related Solutions to Metabolic Conditioning for Team Sports Athletes, *Strength and Conditioning Journal*, 29(4): 60–5

Gamble, P. (2006) Implications and Applications of Training Specificity for Coaches and Athletes, *Strength and Conditioning Journal*, 28(3): 54–8

Gamble, P. (2005) Heavy Ball Complex Training for Development of Pass Velocity in Elite Academy-level Rugby Football Players, In: *Specificity in the Physical Preparation of Elite Rugby Union Football Players*, unpublished doctoral thesis.

Gamble, P. (2004a) A Skill-based Conditioning Games Approach to Metabolic Conditioning for Elite Rugby Football Players, *Journal of Strength and Conditioning Research*, 18(3): 491–7

Gamble, P. (2004b) Physical Preparation of Elite Level Rugby Union Football Players *Strength and Conditioning Journal*, 26(4): 10–23

Garhammer, J. (1993) A Review of Power Output Studies of Olympic and Powerlifting: Methodology, Performance Prediction and Evaluation Tests, *Journal of Strength and Conditioning Research*, 7(2): 76–89

Garraway, W.M., A.J. Lee, D.A.D. MacLeod, J.W. Telfer, I.J. Deary and G.D. Murray (1999) Factors Influencing Tackle Injuries in Rugby Union Football, *British Journal of Sports Medicine*, 33: 37–41

Giannakopoulos, K., A. Beneka, P. Malliou and G. Godolias (2004) Isolated vs. Complex Exercise in Strengthening the Rotator Cuff Muscle Group, *Journal of Strength and Conditioning Research*, 18(1): 144–8

Gibala, M.J. and S.L. McGee (2008) Metabolic Adaptations to Short-Term High-Intensity Interval Training: A Little Pain for a Lot of Gain?, *Exercise and Sports Sciences Reviews*, 36(2): 58–63

Gibala, M.J., J.P. Little, M. van Essen, G.P. Wilkin, K.A. Burgomaster, A. Safdar, S. Raha and M.A. Tarnopolsky (2006) Short-term Sprint Interval versus Traditional Endurance Training: Similar Initial Adaptations in Human Skeletal Muscle and Exercise Performance, *Journal of Physiology*, 575(3): 901–11

Gilchrist, J., B.R. Mandelbaum, H. Melancon, G.W. Ryan, H.J. Silvers, L.Y. Griffin, D.S. Watanabe, R.W. Dick and J. Dvorak (2008) A Randomized Controlled Trial to Prevent Noncontact Anterior Cruciate Ligament Injury in Female Collegiate Soccer Players, *American Journal of Sports Medicine*, 36(8): 1476–83

Gillet, E., D. Leroy, R. Thouvarecq, F. Megrot and J.-F. Stein (2010) Movement-Production Strategy in Tennis: A Case Study, *Journal of Strength and Conditioning Research*, 24(7): 1942–7

Gilman, M.B. and C.L. Wells (1993) The Use of Heart Rates to Monitor Exercise Intensity in Relation to Metabolic Variables, *Sports Medicine*, 14(6): 339–44

Girard, O., A. Mendez-Villanueva and D. Bishop (2011a) Repeated Sprint Ability – Part I: Factors Contributing to Fatigue, *Sports Medicine*, 41(8): 673–94

Girard, O., J.-P. Micallef and G.P. Millet (2011b) Changes in Spring-Mass Model Characteristics during Repeated Running Sprints, *European Journal of Applied Physiology*, 111(1): 125–34

Gisslen, K., C. Gyulai, K. Soderman and H. Alfredson (2005) High Prevalence of Jumper's Knee and Sonographic Changes in Swedish Elite Junior Volleyball Players Compared to Matched Controls, *British Journal of Sports Medicine*, 39: 298–301

Giza, E., K. Mithofer, L. Farrell, B. Zarins and T. Gill (2005) Injuries in Women's Professional Soccer, *British Journal of Sports Medicine*, 39: 212–16

Glaister, M., G. Howatson, J.R. Pattison and G. McInnes (2008) The Reliability and Validity of Fatigue Measures during Multiple-Sprint Work: An Issue Revisited, *Journal of Strength and Conditioning Research*, 22(5): 1597–601

Glaister, M. (2005) Multiple Sprint Work: Physiological Responses, Mechanisms for Fatigue and the Influence of Aerobic Fitness, *Sports Medicine*, 35(9): 757–77

Goldberg, A.S., L. Moroz, A. Smith and T. Ganley (2007) Injury Surveillance in Young Athletes: A Clinician's Guide to Sports Injury Literature, *Sports Medicine*, 37(3): 265–78

Graham, J.E., J. D. Boatwright, M.J. Hunskor and D.C. Howell (2003) Effect of Active vs. Passive Recovery on Repeat Suicide Run Time, *Journal of Strength and Conditioning Research*, 17(2): 338–41

Green, J.P., S.G. Grenier and S.M. McGill (2002) Low-Back Stiffness is Altered with Warm-Up and Bench Rest: Implications for Athletes, *Medicine and Science in Sports and Exercise*, 34(7): 1076–81

Greene, D.A. and G.A. Naughton (2006) Adaptive Skeletal Responses to Mechanical Loading during Adolescence, *Sports Medicine*, 36(9): 723–32

Griffiths, M. (2005) Putting on the Brakes: Deceleration Training, *Strength and Conditioning Journal*, 27(1): 57–8

Gullet, J.C., M.D. Tillman, G.M. Gutierrez, and J.W. Chow (2009) A Biomechanical Comparison of Back and Front Squats in Healthy Trained Individuals, *Journal of Strength and Conditioning Research*, 23(1): 284–92

Haff, G.G., R.T. Hobbs, E.E. Haff, W.A. Sands, K.C. Pierce and M.H. Stone (2008) Cluster Training: A Novel Method for Introducing Training Program Variation, *Strength and Conditioning Journal*, 30(1): 67–76

Haff, G.G., A. Whitley, L.B. McCoy, H.S. O'Bryant, J.L. Kilgore, E.E. Haff, K. Pierce and M.H. Stone (2003) Effects of Different Set Configurations on Barbell Velocity and Displacement During a Clean Pull, *Journal of Strength and Conditioning Research*, 17(1): 95–103

Hakkinen, K., P.V. Komi, M. Alen and H. Kauhanen (1987) EMG, Muscle Fibre and Force Production Characteristics During a One Year Training Period in Elite Weight-Lifters, *European Journal of Applied Physiology*, 56: 419–27

Hamill, B.P. (1994) Relative Safety of Weightlifting and Weight Training, *Journal of Strength and Conditioning Research*, 8(1): 53–7

Hamill, R.R., J.R. Beazell and J.M. Hart (2008) Neuromuscular Consequences of Low Back Pain and Core Dysfunction, *Clinics in Sports Medicine*, 27: 449–62

Hamilton, R.T., S.J. Shultz, R.J. Schmitz and D.H. Perrin (2008) Triple-Hop Distance as a Valid Predictor of Strength and Power, *Journal of Athletic Training*, 43(2): 144–51

Handford, C., K. Davids, S. Bennett and C. Button (1997) Skill Acquisition in Sport: Some Applications of an Evolving Practice Ecology, *Journal of Sports Sciences*, 15: 621–40

Hansen, K.T., J.B. Cronin and M.J. Newton (2011) The Effect of Cluster Loading on Force, Velocity and Power During Ballistic Jump Squat Training, *International Journal of Sports Physiology and Performance*, 6(4): 455–68

Hanson, A.M., D.A. Padua, J.T. Blackburn, W.E. Prentice and C.J. Hirth (2008) Muscle Activation during Side-Step Cutting Maneuvers in Male and Female Soccer Athletes, *Journal of Athletic Training*, 43(2): 133–43

Hardee, J.P., N.T. Triplett, A.C. Utter, K.A. Zwetsloot and J.M. McBride (2012) Effect of Inter-Repetition Rest on Power Output in the Power Clean, *Journal of Strength and Conditioning Research*, 26(4): 883–9.

Harman, E. and C. Pandorf (2000) Principles of Test Selection and Administration. In: Essentials of Strength Training and Conditioning (2nd Edition). T.R. Baechle and R.W. Earle (Eds) Champaign, IL: Human Kinetics

Harman, E., J. Garhammer and C. Pandorf (2000) Administration, Scoring and Interpretation of Selected Tests. In: *Essentials of Strength Training and Conditioning* (2nd Edition), Champaign, IL: Human Kinetics

Harris, G.R., M.H. Stone, H.S. O'Bryant, C.M. Proulx and R.L. Johnson (2000) Short-term Performance Effects of High Power, High Force, or Combined Weight-Training Methods, *Journal of Strength and Conditioning Research*, 14(1): 14–20

Harris, N.K., J.B. Cronin and W.G. Hopkins (2007) Power Outputs of a Machine Squat-Jump across a Spectrum of Loads, *Journal of Strength and Conditioning Research*, 21(4): 1260–4

Harris-Hayes, M., S.A. Sahrmann and L.R. van Dillen (2009) Relationship between the Hip and Low Back Pain in Athletes who Participate in Rotation-Related Sports, *Journal of Sports Rehabilitation*, 18(1): 60–75

Hawkins, D. and J. Metheny (2001) Overuse Injuries in Youth Sports: Biomechanical Considerations, *Medicine and Science in Sports and Exercise*, 33(10): 1701–7

Hawkins, R.D. and C.W. Fuller (1999) A Prospective Epidemiological Study of Injuries in Four English Professional Football Clubs, *British Journal of Sports Medicine*, 33: 196–203

Hawkins, R.D., M.A. Hulse, C. Wilkinson, A. Hodson and M. Gibson (2001) The Association Football Medical Research Programme: An Audit of Injuries in Professional Football, *British Journal of Sports Medicine*, 35: 43–7

Headey, J., J.H.M. Brooks and S.P.T. Kemp (2007) The Epidemiology of Shoulder Injuries in English Professional Rugby Union, *American Journal of Sports Medicine*, 35(9): 1537–43

Hedrick, A. (2002) Designing Effective Resistance Training Programs: A Practical Example, *Strength and Conditioning Journal*, 24(6): 7–15

Hedrick, A. (1999) Using Free Weights to Improve Lateral Movement Performance, *Strength and Conditioning Journal*, 21(5): 21–5

Hedrick, A. (1993) Literature Review: High Speed Resistance Training, *NSCA Journal*, 15(6): 22–30

Heiderscheidt, B.C., M.A. Sherry, A. Silder, E.S. Chumanov and D.G. Thelen (2010) Hamstring Strain Injuries: Recommendations for Diagnosis, Rehabilitation and Injury Prevention, *Journal of Sports and Orthopaedic Sports Physical Therapy*, 40(2): 67–81

Heidt, R.S., L.M. Sweeterman, R.L. Carlonas, J.A. Taub and F.X. Tekulve (2000) Avoidance of Soccer Injuries with Preseason Conditioning, *American Journal of Sports Medicine*, 28(5): 659–62

Helgerud, J., L.C. Engen, U. Wisloff and J. Hoff (2001) Aerobic Endurance Training Improves Soccer Performance, *Medicine and Science in Sports and Exercise*, 33(11): 1925–31

Hennessy, L. and J. Kilty (2001) Relationship of the Stretch-Shortening Cycle to Sprint Performance in Trained Female Athletes, *Journal of Strength and Conditioning Research*, 15(3): 326–31

Herman, D.C., P.S. Weinhold, K.M. Guskiewicz, W.E. Garrett, B. Yu and D.A. Padua (2008) The Effects of Strength Training on the Lower Extremity Biomechanics of Female Recreational Athletes during a Stop-Jump Task, *American Journal of Sports Medicine*, 36(4): 733–40

Hertel, J. (2008) Sensorimotor Deficits with Ankle Sprains and Chronic Ankle Instability, *Clinics in Sports Medicine*, 27: 353–70

Hetzler, R.K., C.D. Stickley, K.M. Lundquist and I.F. Kimura (2008) Reliability and Accuracy of Handheld Stopwatches Compared with Electronic Timing in Measuring Sprint Performance, *Journal of Strength and Conditioning Research*, 22(6): 1969–76

Hewett, T.E. and G.D. Myer (2011) The Mechanistic Connection between the Trunk, Hip, Knee and Anterior Cruciate Ligament Injury, *Exercise and Sports Science Reviews*, 39(4): 161–6

Hewett, T.E., J.S. Tong and B.P. Boden (2009) Video Analysis of Trunk and Knee Motion during Non-Contact Anterior Cruciate Ligament Injury in Female Athletes: Lateral Trunk and Knee Abduction Motion are Combined Components of the Injury Mechanism, *British Journal of Sports Medicine*, 43: 417–22

Hewett, T.E., G.D. Myer and K.R. Ford (2006a) Anterior Cruciate Injuries in Female Athletes, Part 1: Mechanisms and Risk Factors, *American Journal of Sports Medicine*, 34(2): 299–311

Hewett, T.E., K.R. Ford and G.D. Myer (2006b) Anterior Cruciate Injuries in Female Athletes, Part 2: A Meta-analysis of Neuromuscular Interventions Aimed at Injury Prevention, *American Journal of Sports Medicine*, 34(3): 490–8

Hewett, T.E., G.D. Myer and K.R. Ford (2005) Reducing Knee and Anterior Cruciate Ligament Injuries among Female Athletes, *Journal of Knee Surgery*, 18(1): 82–8

Hewett, T.E., T.N. Lindenfield, J.V. Riccobene and F.R. Noyes (1999) The Effect of Neuromuscular Training on the Incidence of Knee Injury in Female Athletes: A Prospective Study, *American Journal of Sports Medicine*, 27(6): 699–706

Hibbs, A.E., K.G. Thompson, D. French, A. Wrigley and I. Spears (2008) Optimising Performance by Improving Core Stability and Core Strength, *Sports Medicine*, 38(12): 995–1008

Hides, J.A., G.A. Jull and C.A. Richardson (2001) Long-term Effects of Specific Stabilizing Exercises for First-Episode Low Back Pain, *Spine*, 26: E243–8

Higashihara, A., T. Ono, J. Kubota, T. Okuwaki and T. Fukubayashi (2010) Functional Differences in the Activity of the Hamstring Muscles with Increasing Running Speed, *Journal of Sports Sciences*, 28(10): 1085–92

Hill-Haas, S.V., B. Dawson, F.M. Impellizzeri and A.J. Coutts (2011) Physiology of Small-Sided Games Training in Football: A Systematic Review, *Sports Medicine*, 41(3): 199–220

Hill-Haas, S.V., G. Rowsell, A.J. Coutts and B. Dawson (2008) The Reproducibility of Physiological Responses and Performance Profiles of Youth Soccer Players in Small-Sided Games, *International Journal of Sports Physiology and Performance*, 3: 393–6

Hills, A.P., N.A. King and T.P. Armstrong (2007) The Contribution of Physical Activity and Sedentary Behaviours to the Growth and Development of Children and Adolescents: Implications for Overweight and Obesity, *Sports Medicine*, 37(6): 533–45

Hoff, J. (2005) Training and Testing Physical Capacities for Elite Soccer Players, *Journal of Sports Sciences*, 23(6): 573–82

Hoff, J., U. Wisloff, L.C. Engen, O.J. Kemi and J. Helgerud (2002) Soccer Specific Aerobic Endurance Training, *British Journal of Sports Medicine*, 36(3), 218–21

Hoffman, J.R. and J. Kang (2003) Strength Changes During an In-Season Resistance Training Program for Football, *Journal of Strength and Conditioning Research*, 17(1): 109–14

Hoffman, J.R., N.A. Ratamess, J.J. Cooper, J. Kang, A. Chilakos and A.D. Faigenbaum (2005) Comparison of Loaded and Unloaded Jump Squat Training on Strength/Power Performance in College Football Players, *Journal of Strength and Conditioning Research*, 19(4): 810–15

Hoffman, J.R., J. Cooper, M. Wendell and J. Kang (2004) Comparison of Olympic vs Traditional Power Lifting Training Programs in Football Players, *Journal of Strength and Conditioning Research*, 18(1): 129–35

Hoffman, J.R., S. Epstein, M. Einbinder and Y. Weinstein (1999) The Influence of Aerobic Capacity on Anaerobic Performance and Recovery Indices in Basketball Players, *Journal of Strength and Conditioning Research*, 13(4): 407–11

Hoffman, J.R., G. Tenenbaum, C.M. Maresh and W.J. Kraemer (1996) Relationship between Athletic Performance Tests and Playing Time in Elite College Basketball Players, *Journal of Strength and Conditioning Research*, 10(2): 67–71

Hoffman, J.R., W.J. Kraemer, A.C. Fry, M. Deschenes and M. Kemp (1990) The Effect of Self-Selection for Frequency of Training in a Winter Conditioning Program for Football, *Journal of Applied Sports Science Research*, 4(3): 76–82

Holm, D.J., M. Stalbom, J.W.L. Keogh and J. Cronin (2008) Relationship between the Kinetics and Kinematics of a Unilateral Horizontal Drop Jump to Sprint Performance, *Journal of Strength and Conditioning Research*, 22(5): 1589–96

Holmberg, P.M. (2009) Agility Training for Experienced Athletes: A Dynamical Systems Approach, *Strength and Conditioning Journal*, 31(5): 73–8

Holmes, A. and E. Delahunt (2009) Treatment of Common Deficits Associated with Chronic Ankle Instability, *Sports Medicine*, 39(3): 207–24

Hopper, D.M., P. McNair and B.C. Elliott (1999) Landing in Netball: Effects of Taping and Bracing the Ankle, *British Journal of Sports Medicine*, 33: 409–13

Hori, N., R.U. Newton, W.A. Andrews, N. Kawamori, M.R. McGuigan and K. Nosaka (2008) Does Performance of Hang Power Clean Differentiate Performance of Jumping, Sprinting and Changing of Direction?, *Journal of Strength and Conditioning Research*, 22(2): 412–18

Hrysomallis, C. (2007) Relationship between Balance Ability, Training and Sports Injury Risk, *Sports Medicine*, 37(6): 547–56

Hsu, W-S., J.A. Fisk, Y.Yamamoto, R.E. Debski and S.L-Y. Woo (2006) Differences in Torsional Joint Stiffness of the Knee Between Genders: A Human Cadaveric Study, *American Journal of Sports Medicine*, 34(5): 765–70

Hume, P.A. and J.R. Steele (2000) A Preliminary Investigation of Injury Prevention Strategies in Netball: Are Players Heeding the Advice?, *Journal of Science & Medicine in Sport*, 3(4): 406–13

Hunter, J.P., R.N. Marshall and P.J. McNair (2005) Relationships between Ground Reaction Force Impulse and Kinematics of Sprint-Running Acceleration, *Journal of Applied Biomechanics*, 21: 31–43

Hydock, D. (2001) The Weightlifting Pull in Power Development, *Strength and Conditioning Journal*, 23(1): 32–37

Iaia, F.M. and J. Bangsbo (2010) Speed-Endurance Training is a Powerful Stimulus for Physiological Adaptations and Performance Improvements in Athletes, *Scandinavian Journal of Medicine and Science in Sports*, 20(Suppl 2): 11–23

Impellizzeri, F.M., E. Rampinini, C. Castagna, D. Bishop, D. Ferrari Bravo, A. Tibaudi and U. Wisloff (2008) Validity of a Repeated-Sprint Test for Football, *International Journal of Sports Medicine*, 29: 899–905

Impellizzeri, F.M., E. Rampinini and S.M. Marcora (2005) Physiological Assessment of Aerobic Training in Soccer, *Journal of Sports Sciences*, 23(6): 583–92

Imwalle, L.E., G.D. Myer, K.R. Ford and T.E. Hewett (2009) Relationship between Hip and Knee Kinematics in Athletic Women during Cutting Maneuvers: A Possible Link to Noncontact Anterior Cruciate Ligament Injury and Prevention, *Journal of Strength and Conditioning Research*, 23(8): 2223–30

Ingersoll, C.D., T.L. Grindstaff, B.G. Pietrosimone and J.M. Hart (2008) Neuromuscular Consequences of Anterior Cruciate Ligament Injury, *Clinics in Sports Medicine*, 27: 383–404

Issurin, V.B. (2010) New Horizons for the Methodology and Physiology of Training Periodization, *Sports Medicine*, 40(3): 189–206

Ives, J.C. and G.A. Shelley (2003) Psychophysics in Functional Strength and Power Training: Review and Implementation Framework, *Journal of Strength and Conditioning Research*, 17(1): 177–86

Jeffreys, I. (2006) Motor Learning – Applications for Agility, Part 1, *Strength and Conditioning Journal*, 28(5): 72–6

Jeffreys, I. (2004) The Use of Small-sided Games in the Metabolic Training of High School Soccer Players, *Strength and Conditioning Journal*, 26(5): 77–8

Jenkins, J.R. (2003) The Transverse Abdominis and Reconditioning the Lower Back, *Strength and Conditioning Journal*, 25(6): 60–6

Jones, A.M. and H. Carter (2000) The Effect of Endurance Training on Parameters of Aerobic Fitness, *Sports Medicine*, 29(6): 373–86

Jones, K., G. Hunter, G. Fleisig, R. Escamilla and L. Lemak (1999) The Effects of Compensatory Acceleration on Upper-Body Strength and Power in Collegiate Football Players, *Journal of Strength and Conditioning Research*, 13(2): 99–105

Jones, M.T., J.P. Ambegaonkar, B.C. Nindl, J.A. Smith and S.A. Headley (2012) Effects of Unilateral and Bilateral Lower-Body Heavy Resistance Exercise on Muscle Activity and Testosterone Responses, *Journal of Strength and Conditioning Research*, 26(4): 1094–100

Juker, D., S.M. McGill, P. Kropf and S. Thomas (1998) Quantitative Intramuscular Myoelectric Activity of Lumbar Portions of Psoas and the Abdominal Wall during a Wide Variety of Tasks, *Medicine and Science in Sports and Exercise*, 30(2): 301–10

Junge, A. and J. Dvorak (2004) Soccer Injuries: A Review on Incidence and Prevention, *Sports Medicine*, 34(13): 929–38

Jungers, W.L. (2010) Barefoot Running Strikes Back, *Nature*, 463: 433–4

Kaila, R. (2007) Influence of Modern Studded and Bladed Soccer Boots and Sidestep Cutting on Knee Loading during Match Play Conditions, *American Journal of Sports Medicine*, 35(9): 1528–36

Kaplan, L.D., D.C. Flanigan, J. Norwig, P. Jost and J. Bradley (2005) Prevalence and Variance of Shoulder Injuries in Elite Collegiate Football Players, *American Journal of Sports Medicine*, 33(8): 1142–6

Kawakami, Y., T. Muraoka, S. Ito, H. Kanehisa and T. Fukunaga (2002) *In Vivo* Muscle Fibre Behaviour during Counter-Movement Exercise in Humans Reveals a Significant Role for Tendon Elasticity, *Journal of Physiology*, 540(2): 635–46

Kawamori, N., A.J. Crum, P.A. Blumert, J.R. Kulik, J.T. Childers, J.A. Wood, M.H. Stone and G.G. Haff (2005) Influence of Different Relative Intensities on Power Output during the Hang Power Clean: Identification of the Optimal Load, *Journal of Strength and Conditioning Research*, 19(3): 698–708

Kettunen, J.A., M. Kvist, E. Alanen and U.M. Kujala (2002) Long-Term Prognosis for Jumper's Knee in Male Athletes, *American Journal of Sports Medicine*, 30(5): 689–92

Kibler, W.B., J. Press and A. Sciascia (2006) The Role of Core Stability in Athletic Function, *Sports Medicine*, 36(3): 189–98

Kidgell, D.J., D.M. Horvath, B.M. Jackson and P.J. Seymour (2007) Effect of Six Weeks of Dura Disc and Mini-Trampoline Balance Training on Postural Stability in Athletes with Functional Ankle Instability, *Journal of Strength and Conditioning Research*, 21(2): 466–9

Kiely, J. (2010) New Horizons of the Methodology and Physiology of Training Periodization. Block Periodization: New Horizon or False Dawn?, *Sports Medicine*, 40(9): 803–7

Kilduff, L.P., H.R. Bevan, M.I.C. Kingsley, N.J. Owen, M.A. Bennett, P.J. Bunce, A.M. Hore, J.R. Maw and D.J. Cunningham (2007) Postactivation Potentiation in Professional Rugby Players: Optimal Recovery, *Journal of Strength and Conditioning Research*, 21(4): 1134–8

Klavora, P., Vertical Jump Tests: A Critical Review (2000) *Strength and Conditioning Journal*, 22(5): 70–5

Knapik, J.J, Bauman, C.L., B.H. Jones, J.M. Harris and L. Vaughan (1991) Preseason Strength and Flexibility Imbalances Associated with Athletic Injuries in Female Collegiate Athletes, *American Journal of Sports Medicine*, 19: 76–81

Kofotolis, N. and E. Kellis (2007) Ankle Sprain Injuries: A 2-Year Prospective Cohort Study in Female Greek Professional Basketball Players, *Journal of Athletic Training*, 42(3): 388–94

Kollias, I., V. Panoutsakopoulos and G. Papaiakovou (2004) Comparing Jumping Ability among Athletes of Various Sports: Vertical Drop Jumping From 60 Centimeters, *Journal of Strength and Conditioning Research*, 18(3): 546–50

Kraemer, R. and K. Knobloch (2009) A Soccer-Specific Balance Training Program for Hamstring Muscle and Patellar and Achilles Tendon Injuries, *American Journal of Sports Medicine*, 37(7): 1384–93

Kraemer, W.J. (2000) Endocrine Responses to Resistance Exercise, In: *Essentials of Strength Training and Conditioning* (2nd Edition), Baechle T.R. and R.W. Earle (Eds) Champaign, IL: Human Kinetics

Kraemer, W.J. (1997) A Series of Studies – The Physiological Basis for Strength Training in American Football: Fact over Philosophy, *Journal of Strength and Conditioning Research*, 11(3): 131–42

Kraemer, W.J. and S.J. Fleck (2005) Strength Training for Young Athletes (2nd Edition). Champaign, IL: Human Kinetics

Kraemer, W.J. and N.A. Ratamess (2005) Hormonal Responses and Adaptations to Resistance Exercise and Training, *Sports Medicine*, 35(4): 339–61

Kraemer, W.J. and A.L. Gomez (2001) Establishing a Solid Fitness Base. In: *High-Performance Sports Conditioning*, B. Foran Ed. Champaign, IL: Human Kinetics

Kraemer, W.J., K. Adams, E. Cafarelli, G.A. Dudley, C. Dooly, M.S. Feigenbaum, S.J. Fleck, B. Franklin, A.C. FRY, J.R. Hoffman, R.U. Newton, J. Potteiger, M.H. Stone, N.A. Ratamess and T. Triplett-McBride (2002) American College of Sports Medicine Position Stand: Progression Models in Resistance Training for Healthy Adults, *Medicine and Science in Sports and Exercise*, 34(2): 364–80

Kraemer, W.J., J.F. Patton, S.E. Gordon, E.A. Harman, M.R. Deschenes, K. Reynolds, R.U. Newton, N.T. Triplett and J.E. Dziados (1995) Compatibility of High-intensity Strength and Endurance Training on Hormonal and Skeletal Muscle Adaptations, *Journal of Applied Physiology*, 78(3): 976–89

Kristensen, G.O., R. van den Tillar and G.J.C. Ettema (2006) Velocity Specificity in Early-Phase Sprint Training, *Journal of Strength and Conditioning Research*, 20(4): 833–7

Krustrup, P., M. Mohr, T. Amstrup, T. Rysgaard, L. Johansen, A. Steensberg, P.K. Pedersen and J. Bangsbo (2003) The Yo-Yo Intermittent Recovery Test: Physiological Response, Reliability and Validity, *Medicine and Science in Sports and Exercise*, 35(4): 697–705

Kubukeli, Z.N., T.D. Noakes and S.C. Dennis (2010) Training Techniques to Improve Endurance Exercise Performances, *Sports Medicine*, 32(8): 489–509

Kugler, F. and L. Janshen (2010) Body Position Determines Propulsive Forces in Accelerated Running, *Journal of Biomechanics*, 43: 343–8

Kujala, U.M., S. Taimela, M. Erkalinto, J.J. Salminen and J. Kaprio (1996) Low-back Pain in Adolescent Athletes, *Medicine and Science in Sports and Exercise*, 28(2): 165–70

Lachowetz, T., J. Evon and J. Pastiglione (1998) The Effect of an Upper Body Strength Program on Intercollegiate Baseball Throwing Velocity, *Journal of Strength and Conditioning Research*, 12(2): 116–19

Lajtai, G., C.W.A. Pfirmann, G. Aitzetmuller, C. Pirkl, C. Gerber and B. Jost (2009) The Shoulders of Professional Beach Volleyball Players: High Prevalence of Infraspinatus Muscle Atrophy, *American Journal of Sports Medicine*, 37(7): 1375–83

Lakomy, J. and D.T. Haydon (2004) The Effects of Enforced, Rapid Deceleration on Performance in a Multiple Sprint Test, *Journal of Strength and Conditioning Research*, 18(3): 579–83

Lamberts, R.P., J. Maskell, J. Borresen and M.I. Lambert (2011) Adapting Workload Improves the Measurement of Heart Rate Recovery, *International Journal of Sports Medicine*, 32: 698–702

Lambson, R.B., B.S. Barnhill and R.W. Higgins (1996) Football Cleat Design and Its Effect on Anterior Cruciate Ligament Injuries: A Three-Year Prospective Study, *American Journal of Sports Medicine*, 24(5): 705–6

Landry, S.C., K.A. McKean, C.L. Hubley-Kozey, W.D. Stanish and K.J. Deluzio (2997) Neuromuscular and Lower Limb Biomechanical Differences Exist between Male and Female Adolescent Soccer Players during an Unanticipated Side-cut Maneuver, *American Journal of Sports Medicine*, 35(11): 1888–900

Laursen, P.B. (2010) Training for Intense Exercise Performance; High-Intensity or High-Volume Training?, *Scandinavian Journal of Medicine and Science in Sports*, 20(2): 1–10

Laursen, P.B. and D.G. Jenkins (2002) The Scientific Basis for High-Intensity Interval Training: Optimising Training Programmes and Maximising Performance in Highly Trained Endurance Athletes, *Sports Medicine*, 32(1): 53–73

Lawson, B.R., T.M. Stephens II, D.E. DeVoe and R.F. Reiser II (2006) Lower-Extremity Bilateral Differences during Step-Close and No-Step Countermovement Jumps with Concern for Gender, *Journal of Strength and Conditioning Research*, 20(3): 608–19

Leetun, D.T., M.L. Ireland, J.D. Willson, B.T. Ballantyne and I.M. Davis (2011) Core Stability Measures as Risk Factors for Lower Extremity Injury in Athletes, *Medicine and Science in Sports and Exercise*, 36(6): 926–34

Legaz-Arrese, A., D. Munguia-Izquierdo, L.E. Carranza-Garcia and C.G. Torres-Davila (2011) Validity of the Wingate Anaerobic Test for the Evaluation of Elite Runners, *Journal of Strength and Conditioning Research*, 25(3): 819–24

Leger, L.A. and R. Boucher (1980) An Indirect Continuous Running Multistage Field Test: The Université de Montreal Track Test, *Canadian Journal of Applied Sports Sciences*, 5(2): 77–84

Leger, L.A., V. Seliger and L. Brassard (1979) Comparisons among VO$_2$max Values for Hockey Players and Runners, *Canadian Journal of Applied Sports Sciences*, 4: 18–21

Lehnhard, R.A., H.R. Lehnhard, R. Young and S.A. Butterfield (1996) Monitoring Injuries on a College Soccer Team: The Effect of Strength Training, *Journal of Strength and Conditioning Research*, 10(2): 115–19

Lemmink, K.A.P.M., C. Visscher, M.I. Lambert and R.P. Lamberts (2004) The Interval Shuttle Run Test for Intermittent Sport Players: Evaluation of Reliability, *Journal of Strength and Conditioning Research*, 18(4): 821–7

Lephart, S.M., J.P. ABT, C.M. Ferris, T.C. Sell, T. Nagai, J.B. Myers and J.J. Irrgang (2005) Neuromuscular and Biomechanical Characteristic Changes in High School Athletes: A Plyometric versus Basic Resistance Program, *British Journal of Sports Medicine*, 39: 932–8

Lephart, S.M., D.M. Pincivero and S.L. Rozzi (1998) Proprioception of the Ankle and Knee, *Sports Medicine*, 25(3): 149–55

Leveritt, M. and P.J. Abernethy (1999) Acute Effects of High-Intensity Endurance Exercise on Subsequent Resistance Activity, *Journal of Strength and Conditioning Research*, 13(1): 47–51

Lewis, C.L. and S.A. Sahrmann (2009) Muscle Activation and Movement Patterns during Prone Hip Extension Exercise in Women, *Journal of Athletic Training*, 44(3): 238–48

Lewis, C.L., S.A. Sahrmann and D.W. Moran (2009) Effect of Position and Alteration in Synergist Muscle Force Contribution on Hip Forces when Performing Hip Strengthening Exercises, *Clinical Biomechanics*, 24(1): 35–42

Lieberman, D.E., M. Venkadesan, W.A. Werbel, A.I. Daoud, S. D'Andrea, I.S. Davis, R. Ojiambo Mang'eni and Y. Pitsiladis (2010) Foot Strike Patterns and Collision Forces in Habitually Barefoot versus Shod Runners, *Nature*, 463: 531–5

Liemohn, W.P., T.A. Baumgartner and L.H. Gagnon (2005) Measuring Core Stability, *Journal of Strength and Conditioning Research*, 19(3): 583–6

Lintner, D., M. Mayol, O. Uzodinma, R. Jones and D. Labossiere (2007) Glenohumeral Internal Rotation Deficits in Professional Pitchers Enrolled in an Internal Rotation Stretching Program, *American Journal of Sports Medicine*, 35(4): 617–21

Little, T. and A.G. Williams (2007) Effects of Sprint Duration and Exercise:Rest Ratio on Repeated Sprint Performance and Physiological Responses in Professional Soccer Players, *Journal of Strength and Conditioning Research*, 21(2): 646–8

Little, T. and A.G. Williams (2006a) Effects of Differential Stretching Protocols during Warm-Ups on High-Speed Motor Performance in Professional Soccer Players, *Journal of Strength and Conditioning Research*, 20(1): 203–7

Little, T and A.G. Williams (2006b) Suitability of Soccer Training Drills for Endurance Training, *Journal of Strength and Conditioning Research*, 20(2): 316–19

Little, T. and A.G. Williams (2005) Specificity of Acceleration, Maximum Speed and Agility in Professional Soccer Players, *Journal of Strength and Conditioning Research*, 19(1): 76–8

Lockie, R.G., A.J. Murphy and C.D. Spinks (2003) Effects of Resisted Sled Towing on Sprint Kinematics in Field-Sport Athletes, *Journal of Strength and Conditioning Research*, 17(4): 760–7

Lynch, S.A. and P.A.F.H. Renstrom (1999) Groin Injuries in Sport: Treatment Strategies, *Sports Medicine*, 28(2): 137–44

Lyttle, A.D., G.J. Wilson and K.J. Ostrowski (1996) Enhancing Performance: Maximal Power versus Combined Weights and Plyometrics Training, *Journal of Strength and Conditioning Research*, 10(3): 173–9

Mackay, M., A. Scanlan, L. Olsen, D. Reid, M. Clark, K. McKim and P. Raina (2004) Looking for the Evidence: A Systematic Review of Prevention Strategies Addressing Sport and Recreational Injury among Children and Youth, *Journal of Science and Medicine in Sport*, 7(1): 58–73

McBride, J.M., T.L. Haines and T.J. Kirby (2011) Effect of Loading on Peak Power of the Bar, Body and System during Power Cleans, Squats and Jump Squats, *Journal of Sports Sciences*, 29(11): 1215–21

McBride, J.M., G.O. McCaulley and P. Cormie (2008) Influence of Preactivity and Eccentric Muscle Activity on Concentric Performance during Vertical Jumping, *Journal of Strength and Conditioning Research*, 22(3): 750–7

McBride, J.M., T. Triplett-McBride, A. Davie and R.U. Newton (1999) A Comparison of Strength and Power Characteristics between Power Lifters, Olympic Lifters and Sprinters, *Journal of Strength and Conditioning Research*, 13(1): 58–66

McConnell, T.R. (2001) Cardiorespiratory Assessment of Apparently Healthy Individuals. In: *ACSM's Resource Manual for Guidelines for Exercise Testing and Prescription* (4th Edition), J.L. Roitman Ed., Balimore, MD: Lippincott Williams & Wilkins

McCurdy, K. and C. Conner (2003) Unilateral Support Training Incorporating the Hip and Knee, *Strength and Conditioning Journal*, 25(2): 45–51

McCurdy, K.W., G.A. Langford, M.W. Doscher, L.P. Wiley and K.G. Mallard (2005) The Effects of Short-Term Unilateral and Bilateral Lower-Body Resistance Training on Measures of Strength and Power, *Journal of Strength and Conditioning Research*, 19(1): 9–15

McEvoy, K.P. and R.U. Newton (1998) Baseball Throwing Speed and Base Running Speed: The Effects of Ballistic Resistance Training, *Journal of Strength and Conditioning Research*, 12(4): 216–21

McGee, K.J. and L.N. Burkett (2003) The National Football League Combine: A Reliable Predictor of Draft Status, *Journal of Strength and Conditioning Research*, 17(1): 6–11

McGill, S.M. (2010) Core Training: Evidence Translating to Better Performance and Injury Prevention, *Strength and Conditioning Journal*, 32(3): 33–46

McGill, S.M. (2007a) Functional Anatomy of the Lumbar Spine, In: *Low Back Disorders: Evidence-based Prevention and Rehabilitation* (2nd Edition), Champaign, IL: Human Kinetics

McGill, S.M. (2007b) Normal and Injury Mechanics of the Lumbar Spine, In: *Low Back Disorders: Evidence-based Prevention and Rehabilitation* (2nd Edition), Champaign, IL: Human Kinetics

McGill, S.M. (2007c) Building Better Rehabilitation Programs for Low Back Injuries, In: *Low Back Disorders: Evidence-based Prevention and Rehabilitation* (2nd Edition), Champaign, IL: Human Kinetics

McGill, S.M. (2007d) Evaluating the Patient, In: *Low Back Disorders: Evidence-based Prevention and Rehabilitation* (2nd Edition), Champaign, IL: Human Kinetics

McGill, S.M. (2006a) Developing the Program. In: *Ultimate Back Fitness and Performance* (3rd Edition), Ontario, Canada: Wabuno

McGill, S.M. (2006b) Evaluating and Qualifying the Athlete/Client. In: *Ultimate Back Fitness and Performance* (3rd Edition), Ontario, Canada: Wabuno

McGill, S.M. (2006c) Fundamental Principles of Movement and Causes of Movement Error. In: *Ultimate Back Fitness and Performance* (3rd Edition), Ontario, Canada: Wabuno

McGill, S.M. (2006d) Laying the Foundation: Why We Need a Different Approach. In: *Ultimate Back Fitness and Performance* (3rd Edition), Ontario, Canada: Wabuno

McGill, S.M. (2006e) Stage 4: Developing Ultimate Strength. In: *Ultimate Back Fitness and Performance* (3rd Edition), Ontario, Canada: Wabuno

McGill, S.M. (2006f) Stage 1: Groove Motion/Motor Patterns and Corrective Exercise. In: *Ultimate Back Fitness and Performance* (3rd Edition), Ontario, Canada: Wabuno

McGill, S.M., J.D. Chaimberg, D.M. Frost and C.M.J. Fenwick (2010) Evidence of a Double Peak in Muscle Activation to Enhance Strike Speed and Force: An Example with Elite Mixed Martial Arts Fighters, *Journal of Strength and Conditioning Research*, 24(2): 348–57

McGuine, T.A. and J.S. Keene (2006) The Effect of a Balance Training Program on the Risk of Ankle Sprains in High School Athletes, *American Journal of Sports Medicine*, 34(7): 1103–11

McHugh, M.P., T.F. Tyler, M.R. Mirabella, M.J. Mullaney and S.J. Nicholas (2007) The Effectiveness of a Balance Training Intervention in Reducing the Incidence of Noncontact Ankle Sprains in High School Football Players, *American Journal of Sports Medicine*, 35(8): 1289–94

McHugh, M.P., T.F. Tyler, D.T. Tetro, M.J. Mullaney and S.J. Nicholas (2006) Risk Factors for Noncontact Ankle Sprains in High School Athletes: The Role of Hip Strength and Balance Ability, *American Journal of Sports Medicine*, 34(3): 464–70

McInnes, S.E., J.S. Carlson, C.J. Jones and M.J. McKenna (1995) The Physiological Load Imposed on Basketball Players during Competition, *Journal of Sports Sciences*, 13: 387–97

McKay, G.D., P.A. Goldie, W.R. Payne, B.W. Oakes (2001) Ankle Injuries in Basketball: Injury Rate and Risk Factors, *British Journal of Sports Medicine*, 35: 103–8

McKeon, P.O. and J. Hertel (2008) Systematic Review of Postural Control and Lateral Ankle Instability, Part I: Can Deficits be Detected with Instrumented Testing?, *Journal of Athletic Training*, 43(3): 293–301

McKeon, P.O. and C.G. Mattacola (2008) Interventions for the Prevention of First Time and Recurrent Ankle Sprains, *Clinics in Sports Medicine*, 27: 371–82

McKeon, P.O., C.D Ingersoll, D.C. Kerrigan, E. Saliba, B.C. Bennett and J. Hertel (2008) Balance Training Improves Function and Postural Control in Those with Chronic Ankle Instability, *Medicine and Science in Sports and Exercise*, 40(10): 1810–19

McLean, S.G., S.W. Lipfert and A.J. van den Bogert (2004) Effect of Gender and Defensive Opponent on the Biomechanics of Sidestep Cutting, *Medicine and Science in Sports and Exercise*, 36(6): 1008–16

McManus, A.M. and N. Armstrong (2008) The Elite Young Athlete, In: *Paediatric Exercise Science and Medicine*, N. Armstrong and M.V. Mechelen (Eds), Oxford, UK: Oxford University Press

McManus, A. and D.S. Cross (2004) Incidence of Injury in Elite Junior Rugby Union: A Prospective Descriptive Study, *Journal of Science and Medicine in Sport*, 7(4): 438–45

McManus, A.M., C.H. Cheng, M.P. Leung, T.C. Yung and D.J. Macfarlane (2005) Improving Aerobic Power in Primary School Boys: A Comparison of Continuous and Interval Training, *International Journal of Sports Medicine*, 26: 781–6

McMaster, D.T., N.D. Gill, J.B. Cronin and M.R. McGuigan (2011) Accelerometer Placement Greatly Affects Jump Kinematics and Kinetics, Poster Presentation, SPRINZ conference, Auckland

McMillan, K., J. Helgerud, S.J. Grant, J. Newell, J. Wilson, R. MacDonald and J. Hoff (2005a) Lactate Threshold Responses to a Season of Professional British Youth Soccer, *British Journal of Sports Medicine*, 39: 432–6

McMillan, K., J. Helgerud, R. MacDonald and J. Hoff (2005b) Physiological Adaptations to Soccer Specific Endurance Training in Professional Youth Soccer Players, *British Journal of Sports Medicine*, 39: 273–7

Maffey, L. and C. Emery (2007) What are the Risk Factors for Groin Strain Injury in Sport?: A Systematic Review of the Literature, *Sports Medicine*, 37(10): 881–94

Malina, R.M. (2010) Early Sport Specialization: Roots, Effectiveness, Risks, *Current Sports Medicine Reports*, 9(6): 364–71

Malina, R.M. (2009) Children and Adolescents in the Sport Culture: The Overwhelming Majority to the Select Few, *Journal of Exercise Science and Fitness*, 7(2) Suppl: S1–S10

Malina, R.M., C. Bouchard and O. Bar-Or (2004) Growth, Maturation and Physical Activity (2nd Edition). Champaign, IL: Human Kinetics

Malisoux, L. M. Francaux, H. Nielens and D. Theisen (2006) Stretch-shortening Cycle Exercises: An Effective Training Paradigm to Enhance Power Output of Human Single Muscle Fibers, *Journal of Applied Physiology*, 100: 771–9

Malliou, P.C., K. Giannakopoulos, A.G. Beneka, A. Gioftsidou and G. Godolias (2004) Effective Ways of Restoring Muscular Imbalances of the Rotator Cuff Muscle Group: A Comparative Study of Various Training Methods, *British Journal of Sports Medicine*, 38: 766–72

Mandelbaum, B.R., H.J. Silvers, D.S. Wanatabe, J.F. Knarr, S.D. Thomas, L.Y. Griffin, D.T. Kirkendall and W. Garrett (2005) Effectiveness of a Neuromuscular and Proprioceptive Training Program in Preventing Anterior Cruciate Ligament Injuries in Female Athletes: 2-Year Follow-up, *American Journal of Sports Medicine*, 33(7): 1003–10

Markovic, G. (2007) Does Plyometric Training Improve Vertical Jump Height? A Meta-Analytical Review, *British Journal of Sports Medicine*, 41: 349–55

Markovic, G., D. Dizdar, I, Jukic and M. Cardinale (2004) Reliability and Factorial Validity of Squat and Countermovement Jump Tests, *Journal of Strength and Conditioning Research*, 18(3): 551–5

Matavulj, D., M. Kukolj, D. Ugarkovic, J. Tihanyi and S. Jaric (2001) Effects of Plyometric Training on Jumping Performance in Junior Basketball Players, *Journal of Sports Medicine and Physical Fitness*, 41: 159–64

Matos, N. and R.J. Winsley (2007) Trainability of Young Athletes and Overtraining, *Journal of Sports Science and Medicine*, 6: 353–67

Matuszak, M.E., A.C. Fry, L.W. Weiss, T.R. Ireland and M.M. McKnight (2003) Effect of Rest Interval Length on Repeated 1 Repetition Maximum Back Squats, *Journal of Strength and Conditioning Research*, 17(4): 634–7

Maughan, R. and M. Gleeson (2004) The Games Player, In: *The Biochemical Basis of Sports Performance*, Oxford University Press

Meeuwisse, W.H., R. Sellmer and B.E. Hagel (2003) Rates and Risks of Injury during Intercollegiate Basketball, *American Journal of Sports Medicine*, 31(3): 379–85

Meir, R., R.U. Newton, E. Curtis, M. Fardell and B. Butler (2001) Physical Fitness Qualities of Professional Rugby League Football Players: Determination of Positional Differences, *Journal of Strength and Conditioning Research*, 15(4): 450–8

Mendiguchia, J., E. Alentorn-Gelli and M. Brughelli (2012) Hamstring Strain Injuries: Are We Heading in the Right Direction?, *British Journal of Sports Medicine*, 46(2): 81–5

Mendiguchia, J., K.R. Ford, C.E. Quatman, E. Alentorn-Geli and T.E. Hewett (2011) Sex Differences in Proximal Control of the Knee Joint, *Sports Medicine*, 41(7): 541–57

Merlau, S. (2005) Recovery Time Optimization to Facilitate Motor Learning during Sprint Intervals, *Strength and Conditioning Journal*, 27(2): 68–74

Mero, A. and P.V. Komi (1994) EMG, Force and Power Analysis of Sprint-Specific Strength Exercises, *Journal of Applied Biomechanics*, 10: 1–13

Metaxas, T.I., N.A. Koutlianos, E.J. Kouidi and A.P. Deligiannis (2005) Comparative Study of Field and Laboratory Tests for the Evaluation of Aerobic Capacity in Soccer Players, *Journal of Strength and Conditioning Research*, 19(1): 79–84

Meylan, C.M.P., K. Nosaka, J.P. Green and J.B. Cronin (2010) Variability and Influence of Eccentric Kinematics on Unilateral Vertical, Horizontal and Lateral Countermovement Jump Performance, *Journal of Strength and Conditioning Research*, 24(3): 840–5

Meylan, C., T. McMaster, J. Cronin, N.I. Mohammad, C. Rogers and M. Deklerk (2009) Single-leg Lateral, Horizontal and Vertical Jump Assessment: Reliability, Interrelationships and Ability to Predict Sprint and Change-of-Direction Performance, *Journal of Strength and Conditioning Research*, 23(4): 1140–7

Meylan, C., J. Cronin and K. Nosaka (2008) Isoinertial Assessment of Eccentric Muscular Strength, *Strength and Conditioning Journal*, 30(2): 56–64

Midgley, A.W., L.R. McNaughton and M. Wilkinson (2006) Is there an Optimal Training Intensity for Enhancing the Maximal Oxygen Uptake of Distance Runners. Empirical Research Findings, Current Opinions, Physiological Rationale and Practical Recommendations, *Sports Medicine*, 36(2): 117–32

Mihata, L.C., A.I. Beutler and B.P. Boden (2006) Comparing the Incidence of Anterior Cruciate Ligament Injury in Collegiate Lacrosse, Soccer and Basketball Players: Implications for Anterior Cruciate Ligament Mechanism and Prevention, *American Journal of Sports Medicine*, 34(6): 899–904

Mikkola, J.S., H.K. Rusko, A.T. Nummela, L.M. Paavolainen and K. Hakkinen (2007) Concurrent Endurance and Explosive Type Strength Training Increases Activation and Fast Force Production of Leg Extensor Muscles in Endurance Athletes, *Journal of Strength and Conditioning Research*, 21(2): 613–20

Millet, G.P., R.B. Candau, B. Barbier, T. Busso, J.D. Rouillon and J.C. Chatard (2002a) Modelling the Transfers of Training Effects on Performance in Elite Triathletes, *International Journal of Sports Medicine*, 23: 55–63

Millet, G.P., B. Jaouen, F. Borrani and R. Candau (2002b) Effects of Concurrent Endurance and Strength Training on Running Economy and VO_2 Kinetics, *Medicine and Science in Sports and Exercise*, 34(8): 1351–9

Mirkov, D., A. Nedeljkovic, M. Kukolj, D. Ugarkovic and S. Jaric (2008) Evaluation of the Reliability of Soccer-Specific Field Tests, *Journal of Strength and Conditioning Research*, 22(4): 1046–50

Mohammadi, F (2007) Comparison of Three Preventive Methods to Reduce the Recurrence of Ankle Inversion Sprains in Male Soccer Players, *American Journal of Sports Medicine*, 35(6): 922–6

Molsa, J., U. Kujala, P. Myllynen, I. Torstila and O. Airaksinen (2003) Injuries to the Upper Extremity in Ice Hockey: Analysis of a Series of 760 Injuries, *American Journal of Sports Medicine*, 31(5): 751–7

Monteiro, A.G., M.S. Aoki, A.L. Evangelista, D.A. Alveno, G.A. Monteiro, I.D.C. Picarro and C. Ugrinowitsch (2009) Nonlinear Periodization Maximises Strength Gains in Split Resistance Training Routines, *Journal of Strength and Conditioning Research*, 23(4): 1321–6

Montgomery, S. and M. Haak (1999) Management of Lumbar Injuries in Athletes, *Sports Medicine*, 27(2): 135–41

Moore, A. and A. Murphy (2003) Development of an Anaerobic Capacity Test for Field Sports Athletes, *Journal of Science and Medicine in Sport*, 6(3): 275–84

Morales, J. and S. Sobonya (1996) Use of Submaximal Repetition Tests for Predicting 1-RM Strength in Class Athletes, *Journal of Strength and Conditioning Research*, 10(3): 186–9

Morrissey, M.C., E.A. Harman and M.J. Johnson (1995) Resistance Training Modes: Specificity and Effectiveness, *Medicine and Science in Sports and Exercise*, 27(5), 648–60

Mullaney, M.J., M.P. McHugh, T.M. Conofrio and S.J. Nicholas (2005) Upper and Lower Extremity Muscle Fatigue after a Baseball Pitching Performance, *American Journal of Sports Medicine*, 33(1): 108–13

Muller, E, U. Benko, C. Raschner and H. Schwameder (2000) Specific Fitness Training and Testing in Competitive Sports, *Medicine and Science in Sports and Exercise*, 32(1): 216–20

Murphy, A.J. and G.J. Wilson (1997) The Ability of Tests of Muscular Function to Reflect Training-induced Changes in Performance, *Journal of Sports Sciences*, 15: 191–200

Murphy, D.F., D.A.J. Connolly and B.D. Beynnon (2003) Risk Factors for Lower Extremity Injury: A Review of the Literature, *British Journal of Sports Medicine*, 37: 13–29

Murray, D.P. and L.E. Brown (2006) Variable Velocity Training in the Periodized Model, *Strength and Conditioning Journal*, 28(1): 88–92

Myer, G.D., K.R. Ford, J. Khoury, P. Succop and T.E. Hewett (2010) Development and Validation of a Clinical-Based Prediction Tool to Identify Female Athletes at High Risk for Anterior Cruciate Ligament Injury, *American Journal of Sports Medicine*, 38(10): 2025–33

Myer, G.D., D.A. Chu, J.L. Brent and T.E. Hewett (2008) Trunk and Hip Control Neuromuscular Training for the Prevention of Knee Joint Injury, *Clinics in Sports Medicine*, 27: 425–48

Myer, G.D., K.R. Ford, J.L. Brent and T.E. Hewett (2006a) The Effect of Plyometric vs Dynamic Stabilisation and Balance Training on Power, Balance and Landing Force in Female Athletes, *Journal of Strength and Conditioning Research*, 20(2): 345–58

Myer, G.D., K.R. Ford, S.G. McLean and T.E. Hewett (2006b) The Effects of Plyometric Versus Dynamic Stabilisation Training on Lower Extremity Biomechanics, *American Journal of Sports Medicine*, 34(3): 445–55

Myer, G.D., K.R. Ford, J.P. Palumbo and T.E. Hewett (2005) Neuromuscular Training Improves Performance and Lower-Extremity Biomechanics in Female Athletes, *Journal of Strength and Conditioning Research*, 19(1): 51–60

Myers, C.A. and D. Hawkins (2010) Alterations to Movement Mechanics Can Greatly Reduce Anterior Cruciate Ligament Loading Without Reducing Performance, *Journal of Biomechanics*, 43: 2657–64

Myers, J.B. and S. Oyama (2008) Sensorimotor Factors Affecting Outcome Following Shoulder Injury, *Clinics in Sports Medicine*, 27: 481–90

Nadler, S.F., G.A. Malanga, L.A. Bartoli, J.H. Feinberg, M. Prybicien and M. Deprince (2002) Hip Muscle Imbalance and Low Back Pain in Athletes: Influence of Core Strengthening, *Medicine and Science in Sports and Exercise*, 34(1): 9–16

Nadler, S.F., G.A. Malanga, M. Deprince, T.P. Stitik and J.H. Feinberg (2000) The Relationship Between Lower Extremity Injury, Low Back Pain and Hip Muscle Strength in Male and Female Collegiate Athletes, *Clinical Journal of Sports Medicine*, 10: 89–97

Naughton, G., N.J. Farpour-Lambert, J. Carlson, M. Bradley and E. van Praagh (2000) Physiological Issues Surrounding the Performance of Adolescent Athletes, *Sports Medicine*, 30(5): 309–25

Nesser, T.W., K.C. Huxel, J.L. Tincher and T. Okada (2008) The Relationship between Core Stability and Performance in Division I Football Players, *Journal of Strength and Conditioning Research*, 22(6): 1750–4

Newton, R.U. and E. Dugan (2002) Application of Strength Diagnosis, *Strength and Conditioning Journal*, 24(5): 50–9

Newton, R.U. and W.J. Kraemer (1994) Developing Explosive Muscular Power: Implications for a Mixed Methods Training Strategy, *Strength and Conditioning*, 16: 20–31

Newton, R.U. and K.P. McEvoy (1994) Baseball Throwing Velocity: A Comparison of Medicine Ball Throwing and Weight Training, *Journal of Strength and Conditioning Research*, 8(3): 198–203

Newton, R.U., A. Gerber, S. Nimphius, J.K. Shim, B.K. Doan, M. Robertson, D.R. Pearson, B.W. Craig, K. Hakkinen and W.J. Kraemer (2006) Determination of Functional Strength Imbalance of the Lower Extremities, *Journal of Strength and Conditioning Research*, 20(4): 971–7

Newton, R.U., W.J. Kraemer and K. Hakkinen (1999) Effects of Ballistic Training on Preseason Preparation of Elite Volleyball Players, *Medicine and Science in Sports and Exercise*, 31(2): 323–30

Newton, R.U., A.J. Murphy, B.J. Humphries, G.J. Wilson, W.J. Kraemer and K. Hakkinen (1997) Influence of Load and Stretch Shortening Cycle on the Kinematics, Kinetics and Muscle Activation that Occurs during Explosive Upper-Body Movements, *European Journal of Applied Physiology*, 75: 333–42

Newton, R.U., W.J. Kraemer, K. Hakkinen, B.J. Humphries and A.J. Murphy (1996) Kinematics, Kinetics and Muscle Activation during Explosive Upper Body Movements, *Journal of Applied Biomechanics*, 12: 31–43

Nicholas, S.J. and T.F. Tyler (2002) Adductor Muscle Sprains in Sport, *Sports Medicine*, 32(5): 339–44

Niederbracht, Y., A.L. Shim, M.A. Sloniger, M. Paternostro-Bayles and T.H. Short (2008) Effects of a Shoulder Injury Prevention Strength Training Program on Eccentric External Rotator Muscle Strength and Glenohumeral Joint Imbalances in Female Overhead Activity Athletes, *Journal of Strength and Conditioning Research*, 22(1): 140–5

Nimphius, S., M.R. McGuigan and R.U. Newton (2010) Relationship between Strength, Power, Speed and Change of Direction Performance of Female Softball Players, *Journal of Strength and Conditioning Research*, 24(4): 885–95

Noyes, F.R., S.D. Barber-Westin, S.T. Smith and T. Campbell (2011) A Training Program to Improve Neuromuscular Indices in Female High School Volleyball Players, *Journal of Strength and Conditioning Research*, 25(8): 2151–60

Noyes, F.R. S.D. Barber-Westin, C. Fleckenstein, C. Walsh and J. West (2005) The Drop-Jump Screening Test: Differences in Lower Limb Control by Gender and Effect of Neuromuscular Training in Female Athletes, *American Journal of Sports Medicine*, 33(2): 197–207

Nummela, A., T. Keranen and L.O. Mikkelsson (2007) Factors Related to Top Running Speed and Economy, *International Journal of Sports Medicine*, 28: 655–61

Nuzzo, J.L., G.O. McCaulley, P. Cormie, M.J. Cavill and J.M. McBride (2008) Trunk Muscle Activity during Stability Ball and Free Weight Exercises, *Journal of Strength and Conditioning Research*, 22(1): 95–102

O'Connor, D.M. (2004) Groin Injuries in Professional Rugby League Players: A Prospective Study, *Journal of Sports Sciences*, 22: 629–36

Okada, T., K.C. Huxel and T.W. Nesser (2011) Relationship between Core Stability, Functional Movement and Performance, *Journal of Strength and Conditioning Research*, 25(1): 252–61

Olds, T. (2001) The Evolution of Physique in Male Rugby Union Players in the Twentieth Century, *Journal of Sports Sciences*, 19: 253–62

Oliver, G.D. and D.W. Keeley (2010) Gluteal Muscle Group Activation and its Relationship with Pelvis and Torso Kinematics in High-School Baseball Pitchers, *Journal of Strength and Conditioning Research*, 24(11): 3015–22

Oliver, J.L. (2009) Is a Fatigue Index a Worthwhile Measure of Repeated Sprint Ability?, *Journal of Science and Medicine in Sport*, 12: 20–3

Oliver, J.L., N. Armstrong and C.A. Williams (2009) Relationships between Brief and Prolonged Repeated Sprint Ability, *Journal of Science and Medicine in Sport*, 12: 238–43

Olsen, L., A. Scanlan, M. Mackay, S. Babul, D. Reid, M. Clark and P. Raina (2004) Strategies for Prevention of Soccer Related Injuries: A Systematic Review, *British Journal of Sports Medicine*, 38: 89–94

Opar, D.A., M.D. Williams and A.J. Shield (2010) Hamstring Strain Injuries: Factors that Lead to Injury and Re-Injury, *Sports Medicine*, 42(3): 209–26

Orchard, J. and H. Seward (2002) Epidemiology of Injuries in the Australian Football League, Seasons 1997–2000, *British Journal of Sports Medicine*, 36: 39–45

Orchard, J.P., P. Farhart, C. Leopold (2004) Lumbar Spine Region Pathology and Hamstring and Calf Injuries in Athletes: Is there a Connection? *British Journal of Sports Medicine*, 38: 502–4

Orchard, J., H. Seward, J. McGivern and S. Hood (2001) Intrinsic and Extrinsic Risk Factors for Anterior Cruciate Ligament Injury in Australian Footballers, *American Journal of Sports Medicine*, 29(2): 196–200

Osborne, M.D. and T.D. Rizzo, JR. (2003) Prevention and Treatment of Ankle Sprain in Athletes, *Sports Medicine*, 33(15): 1145–50

Paasuke, M., L. Saapar, J. Ereline, H. Gapeyeva, B. Requena and V. Oopik (2007) Postactivation Potentiation of Knee Extensor Muscles in Power- and Endurance-Trained and Untrained Women, *European Journal of Applied Physiology*, 101: 577–85

Paavolainen, L., K. Hakkinen, I. Hamalainen, A. Nummela and H. Rusko (1999) Explosive-strength Training Improves 5-km Running Time by Improving Running Economy and Muscle Power, *Journal of Applied Physiology*, 86(5): 1527–33

Padua, D.A., L.J. DiStefano, S.W. Marshall, A.I. Beutler, S.J. de la Motte and M.J. DiStefano (2012) Retention of Movement Pattern Changes after a Lower Extremity Injury Prevention Program is Affected by Program Duration, *American Journal of Sports Medicine*, 40(2): 300–6

Paradisis, G.P. and C.B. Cooke (2001) Kinematic and Postural Characteristics of Sprint Running on Sloping Surfaces, *Journal of Sports Sciences*, 19: 149–59

Parchman, C.J. and J.M. McBride (2011) Relationship between Functional Movement Screen and Athletic Performance, *Journal of Strength and Conditioning Research*, 25(12): 3378–84

Perrey, S., S. Racinais, K. Saimouaa and O. Girard (2010) Neural and Muscular Adjustments Following Repeated Running Sprints, *European Journal of Applied Physiology*, 109: 1027–36

Peterson, J. and P. Holmich (2005) Evidence-based Prevention of Hamstring Injuries, *British Journal of Sports Medicine*, 39: 319–23

Peterson, M.D., B.A. Alvar and M.R. Rhea (2006) The Contribution of Maximal Force Production to Explosive Movement among Young Collegiate Athletes, *Journal of Strength and Conditioning Research*, 20(4): 867–73

Peterson, M.D., M.R. Rhea and B.A. Alvar (2004) Maximising Strength Development in Athletes: A Meta-Analysis to Determine the Dose-Response Relationship, *Journal of Strength and Conditioning Research*, 18(2): 377–82

Pettit, R.W. and E.R. Bryson (2002) Training for Women's Basketball: A Biomechanical Emphasis for Preventing Anterior Cruciate Ligament Injury, *Strength and Conditioning Journal*, 24(5): 20–9

Philippaerts, R.M., R. Vaeyans, M. Janssens, B. Van Renterghem, D. Matthys, R. Craen, J. Bourgois, J. Vrijens, G. Beunen and R.M. Malina (2006) The Relationship between Peak Height Velocity and Physical Performance in Youth Soccer Players, *Journal of Sports Sciences*, 24(3): 221–30

Plisk, S.S (2000) Speed, Agility and Speed-Endurance Development, In: *Essentials of Strength Training and Conditioning* (2nd Edition), T.R. Baechle and R.W. Earle (Eds) Champaign, IL: Human Kinetics

Plisk, S.S. and M.H. Stone (2003) Periodization Strategies, *Strength and Conditioning Journal*, 25(6): 19–37

Plisk, S.S. and V. Gambetta (1997) Tactical Metabolic Training: Part 1, *Strength and Conditioning*, 19(2): 44–53

Pool-Goudzwaard, A.L., A. Vleeming, R. Stoeckart, C.J. Snijders and J.M.A. Mens (1998) Insufficient Lumbopelvic Stability: A Clinical, Anatomical and Biomechanical Approach to a Specific Low Back Pain, *Manual Therapy*, 3(1): 12–20

Popadic Gacesa, J.Z., O.F. Barak and N.G. Grujic (2009) Maximal Anaerobic Power Test in Athletes of Different Sport Disciplines, *Journal of Strength and Conditioning Research*, 23(3): 751–5

Potach, D.H. and D.A. Chu (2000) Plyometric Training. In: *Essentials of Strength Training and Conditioning* (2nd Editon). Baechle T.R. and R.W. Earle (Eds) Champaign, IL: Human Kinetics

Potteiger, J.A. and B.W. Evans (1995) Using Heart Rate and Ratings of Perceived Exertion to Monitor Intensity in Runners, *Journal of Sports Medicine and Physical Fitness*, 35(3): 181–6

Prestes, J., C. de Lima, A.B. Frollini, F.P. Donatto and M. Conte (2009) Comparison of Linear and Reverse Linear Periodization Effects on Maximal Strength and Body Composition, *Journal of Strength and Conditioning Research*, 23(1): 266–74

Pyne, D.B., P.U. Saunders, P.G. Montgomery, A.J. Hewitt and K. Sheehan (2008) Relationships between Repeated Sprint Testing, Speed and Endurance, *Journal of Strength and Conditioning Research*, 22(5): 1633–7

Quarrie, K.L. and B.D. Wilson (2000) Force Production in the Rugby Union Scrum, *Journal of Sports Sciences*, 18: 237–46

Quarrie, K.L., J.C. Alsop, A.E. Waller, Y.N. Bird, S.W. Marshall and D.J. Chalmers (2001) The New Zealand Rugby Injury and Performance Project VI. A Prospective Cohort Study of Risk Factors for Injury in Rugby Union Football, *British Journal of Sports Medicine*, 35: 157–66

Quarrie, K.L., P. Handcock, A.E. Waller, D.J. Chalmers, M.J. Toomey and B.D. Wilson (1995) The New Zealand Rugby Injury and Performance Project III Anthropometric and Physical Performance Characteristics of Players, *British Journal of Sports Medicine*, 29(4): 263–70

Quatman, C.E., K.R. Ford, G.D. Myer and T.E. Hewett (2006) Maturation Leads to Gender Differences in Landing Force and Vertical Jump Performance, *American Journal of Sports Medicine*, 34(5): 806–13

Rabita, G., A. Couturier and D. Lambertz (2008) Influence of Training Background on the Relationship between Plantarflexor Intrinsic Stiffness and Overall Musculoskeletal Stiffness During Hopping, *European Journal of Applied Physiology*, 103: 163–71

Rampinini, F., D. Bishop, S.M. Marcora, D. Ferrari Bravo, R. Sassi and F.M. Impelizzeri (2007a) Validity of Simple Field Tests as Indicators of Match-Related Physical Performance in Top-Level Professional Soccer Players, *International Journal of Sports Medicine*, 28: 228–35

Rampinini, F., F.M. Impellizzeri, C. Castagna, G. Abt, K. Chamari, A. Sassi and S.M. Marcora (2007b) Factors Influencing Physiological Responses to Small-sided Soccer Games, *Journal of Sports Sciences*, 25(6): 659–66

Rees, J.D., R.L. Wolman and A. Wilson (2009) Eccentric Exercises; Why Do They Work, What are the Problems and How Can We Improve Them?, *British Journal of Sports Medicine*, 43: 242–6

Regan, D.P. (2000) Implications of Hip Rotators in Lumbar Spine Injuries, *Strength and Conditioning Journal*, 22(6): 7–13

Reilly, T. (1997) Energetics of High-Intensity Exercise (Soccer) with Particular Reference to Fatigue, *Journal of Sports Sciences*, 15: 257–63

Reilly, T. (1994) Physiological Aspects of Soccer, *Biology of Sport*, 11(1): 3–20

Reilly, T., T. Morris and G. Whyte (2009) The Specificity of Training Prescription and Physiological Assessment: A Review, *Journal of Sports Sciences*, 27(6): 575–89

Rhea, M., B. Alvar, L. Burkett and S. Ball (2003) A Meta-analysis to Determine the Dose-Response Relationship for Strength, *Medicine and Science in Sports and Exercise*, 35: 456–64

Rhea, M.R., S.D. Ball, W.T. Phillips and L.N. Burkett (2002) A Comparison of Linear and Daily Undulating Periodized Programs with Equated Volume and Intensity for Strength, *Journal of Strength and Conditioning Research*, 16(2): 250–5

Rienzi, E., B. Drust, J.E.L. Carter and A. Martin (2000) Investigation of Anthropometric and Work-Rate Profiles of Elite South American International Soccer Players, *Journal of Sports Medicine and Physical Fitness*, 40(2): 162–9

Rienzi, E., T. Reilly and C. Malkin (1999) Investigation of Anthropometric and Work-rate Profiles of Rugby Sevens Players, *Journal of Sports Medicine and Physical Fitness*, 39: 160–4

Rogers, R.G. (2006) Research-Based Rehabilitation for the Lower Back, *Strength and Conditioning Journal*, 28(1): 30–5

Romero-Franco, N., F. Martinez-Lopez, R. Lomas-Vega, F. Hita-Contreras and A. Martinez-Amat (2012) Effects of Proprioceptive Training Program on Core Stability and Center of Gravity Control in Sprinters, *Journal of Strength and Conditioning Research*, 26(8): 2071–7

Ross, A. and M. Leveritt (2001) Long-Term Metabolic and Skeletal Muscle Adaptations to Short-Sprint Training: Implications for Sprint Training and Tapering, *Sports Medicine*, 31(15): 1063–82

Ross, A., M. Leveritt and S. Riek (2001) Neural Influences on Sprint Running: Training Adaptations and Acute Responses, *Sports Medicine*, 31(6): 409–25

Sabick, M.B., Y-Y. Kim, M.R. Torry, M.A. Keirns and R.J. Hawkins (2005) Biomechanics of the Shoulder in Youth Baseball Pitchers: Implications for the Development of Proximal Humeral Epiphysiolysis and Humeral Retrotorsion, *American Journal of Sports Medicine*, 33(11): 1716–22

Saeterbakken, A.H., R. van den Tillar and S. Seiler (2011) Effect of Core Stability Training on Throwing Velocity in Female Handball Players, *Journal of Strength and Conditioning Research*, 25(3): 712–18

Saez de Villarreal, E., B. Requena and J.B. Cronin (2012) The Effects of Plyometric Training on Sprint Performance: A Meta-Analysis, *Journal of Strength and Conditioning Research*, 26(2): 575–84

Santana, J.C., F.J. Vera-Garcia and S.M. McGill (2007) A Kinetic and Electromyographic Comparison of the Standing Cable Press and Bench Press, *Journal of Strength and Conditioning Research*, 21(4): 1271–9

Saunders, N. and L. Otago (2009) Elite Netball Injury Surveillance: Implications for Injury Prevention, *Journal of Science and Medicine in Sport*, 12(Suppl): S63

Schale, A.G., P.D. Blanch, D.A. Rath, T.V. Wrigley, R. Starr and K.L. Bennell (2001) A Comparison of Overground and Treadmill Running for Measuring the Three-Dimensional Kinematics of the Lumbo-Pelvic-Hip Complex, *Clinical Biomechanics*, 16: 667–80

Schick, D.M. and W.H. Meeuwisse (2003) Injury Rates and Profiles in Female Ice Hockey Players, *American Journal of Sports Medicine*, 31(1): 47–52

Schmitz, R.J., S.J. Shultz and A.-D. Nguyen (2009) Dynamic Valgus Alignment and Functional Strength in Males and Females during Maturation, *Journal of Athletic Training*, 44(1): 26–32

Selye, H. (1956) *The Stress of Life*, New York: McGraw-Hill

Serpell, B.G., W.B. Young and M. Ford (2011) Are the Perceptual and Decision-Making Aspects of Agility Trainable? A Preliminary Investigation, *Journal of Strength and Conditioning Research*, 25(5): 1240–8

Shankar, P.R., S.K. Fields, C.L. Collins, R.W. Dick and R.D. Comstock (2007) Epidemiology of High School and Collegiate Football Injuries in the United States, 2005–2006, *American Journal of Sports Medicine*, 35(8): 1295–303

Sheppard, J.M. (2003) Strength and Conditioning Exercise Selection in Speed Development, *Strength and Conditioning Journal*, 25(4): 26–30

Sheppard, J.M. and W.B. Young (2006) Agility Literature Review: Classifications, Training and Testing, *Journal of Sports Sciences*, 24(9): 919–32

Shields, R.K., S. Madhavan, E. Gregg, J. Leitch, B. Petersen, S. Salata and S. Wallerich (2005) Neuromuscular Control of the Knee during a Resisted Single-Limb Squat Exercise, *American Journal of Sports Medicine*, 33(10): 1520–6

Shiner, J., T. Bishop and A.J. Cosgarea (2006) Integrating Low-Intensity Plyometrics into Strength and Conditioning Programs, *Strength and Conditioning Journal*, 27(6): 10–20

Shinkle, J., T.W. Nesser, T.J. Demchak and D.M. McManus (2012) Effect of Core Strength on the Measure of Power in the Extremities, *Journal of Strength and Conditioning Research*, 26(2): 373–80

Sierer, S.P., C.L. Battaglini, J.P. Mihalik, E.W. Shields and N.T. Tomasini (2008) The National Football League Combine: Performance Differences between Drafted and Nondrafted Players Entering the 2004 and 2005 Drafts, *Journal of Strength and Conditioning Research*, 22(1): 6–12

Siff, M.C. (2002) Functional Training Revisited, *Strength and Conditioning Journal*, 24(5): 42–6

Silvers, H.C. and B.R. Mandelbaum (2007) Prevention of Anterior Cruciate Ligament Injuries in the Female Athlete, *British Journal of Sports Medicine*, 41(Suppl. 1): i52–i59

Simenz, C.J., C.A. Dugan and W.P. Ebben (2005) Strength and Conditioning Practices of National Basketball Association Strength and Conditioning Coaches, *Journal of Strength and Conditioning Research*, 19(3): 495–504

Simenz, C.J., L.R. Garceau, B.N. Lutsch, T.J. Suchomel and W.P. Ebben (2012) Electromyographical Analysis of Lower Extremity Muscle Activation during Variations of the Loaded Step Up Exercise, *Journal of Strength and Conditioning Research*

Sirotic, A.C. and A.J. Coutts (2007) Physiological and Performance Test Correlates of Prolonged High-Intensity, Intermittent Running Performance in Moderately Trained Women Team Sport Athletes, *Journal of Strength and Conditioning Research*, 21(1): 138–44

Smith, D.J. (2003) A Framework for Understanding the Training Process Leading to Elite Performance, *Sports Medicine*, 33(15): 1103–26

Sole, G., S. Milosavljevic, H. Nicholson and S.J. Sullivan (2012) Altered Muscle Activation Following Hamstring Injuries, *British Journal of Sports Medicine*, 46(2): 118–23

Soligard, T., A. Nilstad, K. Steffen, G. Myklebust, I. Holme, J. Dvorak, R. Bahr and T.E. Andersen (2010) Compliance with a Comprehensive Warm-Up Programme to Prevent Injuries in Youth Football, *British Journal of Sports Medicine*, 44: 787–93

Souza, A.L., S.D. Shimada and A. Koontz (2002) Ground Reaction Forces during the Power Clean, *Journal of Strength and Conditioning Research*, 16(3): 423–7

Spencer, M., M. Fitzsimons, B. Dawson, D. Bishop and C. Goodman (2006) Reliability of a Repeated-Sprint Ability Test for Field-Hockey, *Journal of Science and Medicine in Sport*, 9: 181–4

Spencer, M., D. Bishop, B. Dawson and C. Goodman (2005) Physiological and Metabolic Responses of Repeated Sprint Activities – Specific to Field-based Team Sports, *Sports Medicine*, 35(12): 1025–44

Spencer, M., D. Bishop and S. Lawrence (2004) Longitudinal Assessment of the Effects of Field Hockey Training on Repeated Sprint Ability, *Journal of Science and Medicine in Sport*, 7(3): 323–34

Sperlich, B., C. Zinner, I. Heilemann, P.L. Kjendlie, H.-C. Holmberg and J. Mester (2010) High-Intensity Interval Training Improves VO_2max, Maximal Lactate Accumulation, Time Trial and Competition Performance in 9–11-Year-Old Swimmers, *European Journal of Applied Physiology*, 110: 1029–36

Sporis, G., I. Jukic, L. Milanovic and V. Vucetic (2010) Reliability and Factorial Validity of Agility Tests for Soccer Players, *Journal of Strength and Conditioning Research*, 24(3): 679–86

Stanton, R., P.R. Reaburn and B. Humphries (2004) The Effect of Short-Term Swiss Ball Training on Core Stability and Running Economy, *Journal of Strength and Conditioning Research*, 18(3): 522–8

Stasinopoulos, D. (2004) Comparison of Three Preventive Methods in Order to Reduce the Incidence of Ankle Inversion Sprains among Female Volleyball Players, *British Journal of Sports Medicine*, 38: 182–5

Stephenson, J. and A.M. Swank (2004) Core Training: Designing a Program for Anyone, *Strength and Conditioning Journal*, 26(6): 34–7

Stevenson, M.R., P. Hamer, C.F. Finch, B. Elliott and M.-J. Kresnow (2000) Sport, Age, and Sex-Specific Incidence of Sports Injuries in Western Australia, *British Journal of Sports Medicine*, 34: 188–94

Steyck, S.D., S.P. Flanagan and W.C. Whiting (2008) The Missing Link: Integrated Core Training, *NSCA Performance Training Journal*, 7(6): 13–16

Stone, M.H. (1993) Literature Review: Explosive Exercises and Training, *NSCA Journal*, 15(3): 7–15

Stone, M.H., H.S. O'Bryant, L. McCoy, R. Coglianese, M. Lehmkuhl and B. Schilling (2003a) Power and Maximum Strength Relationships during Performance of Dynamic and Static Weighted Jumps, *Journal of Strength and Conditioning Research*, 17(1): 140–7

Stone, M.H., K. Sandborn, H. O'Bryant, M. Hartman, M.E. Stone, C. Proulx, B. Ward and J. Hruby (2003b) Maximum Strength-Power-Performance Relationships in Collegiate Throwers, *Journal of Strength and Conditioning Research*, 17(4): 739–45

Stone, M.H., D. Collins, S. Plisk, G. Haff and M.E. Stone (2000a) Training Principles: Evaluation of Modes and Methods of Resistance Training, *Strength and Conditioning Journal*, 22(3): 65–76

Stone, M.H., J.A. Potteiger, K.C. Pierce, C.M. Proulx, H.S. O'Bryant, R.L. Johnson and M.E. Stone (2000b) Comparison of the Effects of Three Different Weight-Training Programs on the One Repetition Maximum Squat, *Journal of Strength and Conditioning Research*, 14(3): 332–7

Stone, M.H., H.S. O'Bryant, R.L. Johnson, K.C. Pierce, D.G. Haff, A.J. Koch and M. Stone (1999a) Periodisation: Effects of Manipulating Volume and Intensity: Part One, *Strength and Conditioning Journal*, 21(2): 56–62

Stone, M.H., H.S. O'Bryant, B.K. Schilling, R.L. Johnson, K.C. Pierce, G.G. Haff, A.J. Koch and M. Stone (1999b) Periodization: Effects of Manipulating Volume and Intensity. Part 2, *Strength and Conditioning Journal*, 21(3): 54–60

Stratton, G., M. Jones, K.R. Fox, K. Tolfrey, J. Harris, N. Maffulli, M. Lee and S.P. Frostick (2004) BASES Position Statement on Guidelines for Resistance Training in Young People, *Journal of Sports Science*, 22: 383–90

Straub, W.F. (1968) Effect of Overload Procedures upon Velocity and Accuracy of the Overarm Throw. *Research Quarterly*, 39(2): 370–9

Swenson, D.M., E.E. Yard, S.K. Fields and R.D. Comstock (2009) Patterns of Recurrent Injuries Among US High School Athletes, 2005–2008, *American Journal of Sports Medicine*, 37(8): 1586–93

Tabata, I., K. Irisawa, M. Kouzaki, K. Nishimura, F. Ogita and M. Miyachi (1997) Metabolic Profile of High Intensity Intermittent Exercises, *Medicine and Science in Sports and Exercise*, 29(3): 390–5

Tabata, I., K. Nishimura, M. Kouzaki, Y. Hirai, F. Ogita, M. Miyachi and K. Yamamoto (1996) Effects of Moderate-Intensity Endurance Training and High-Intensity Intermittent Training on Anaerobic Capacity and VO_2max, *Medicine and Science in Sports and Exercise*, 28(10), 1327–30

Takarada, Y. (2003) Evaluation of Muscle Damage after a Rugby Match with Special Reference to Tackle Plays, *British Journal of Sports Medicine*, 37: 416–19

Takeda, Y., S. Kashiwaguchi, K. Endo, T. Matsuura and T. Sasa (2002) The Most Effective Exercise for Strengthening the Supraspinatus Muscle, *American Journal of Sports Medicine*, 30(3): 374–81

Talanian, J.L., G.P. Holloway, L.A. Snook, G.J.F. Heigenhauser, A. Bonen and L.L. Spriet (2010) Exercise Training Increases Sarcolemnal and Mitochondrial Fatty Acid Transport Proteins in Human Skeletal Muscle, *American Journal of Physiology Endocrinology and Metabolism*, 299(2): E180–8

Talanian, J.L., S.D.R. Galloway, G.J.F. Heigenhauser, A. Bonen and L.L Spriet (2007) Two Weeks of High-Intensity Aerobic Interval Training Increases the Capacity for Fat Oxidation during Exercise in Women, *Journal of Applied Physiology*, 102: 1439–47

Tarnanen, S.P., K.M. Siekkinen, A.J. Hakkinen, E.O. Malkia, H.J. Kautiainen and J.J. Ylinen (2012) Core Muscle Activation during Dynamic Upper Limb Exercises in Women, *Journal of Strength and Conditioning Research*

Taube, W., C. Leukel, M. Schubert, M. Gruber, T. Rantalainen and A. Gollhofer (2008) Differential Modulation of Spinal and Corticospinal Excitability during Drop Jumps, *Journal of Neurophysiology*, 99: 1243–52

Taube, W., M. Gruber, S. Beck, M. Faist, A. Gollhofer and M. Schubert (2007) Cortical and Spinal Adaptations Induced by Balance Training: Correlation between Stance Stability and Corticospinal Activation, *Acta Physiologica*, 189: 347–58

Taylor, J. (2004) A Tactical Metabolic Training Model for Collegiate Basketball, *Strength and Conditioning Journal*, 26(5): 22–9,

Thacker, S.B., D.F. Stroup, C.M. Branche, J. Gilchrist, R.A. Goodman and E. Porter Kelling (2003) Prevention of Knee Injuries in Sports: A Systematic Review of the Literature, *Journal of Sports Medicine and Physical Fitness*, 43: 165–79

Thorpe, J.L and K.T. Ebersole (2008) Unilateral Balance Performance in Female Collegiate Soccer Athletes, *Journal of Strength and Conditioning Research*, 22(5): 1429–33

Tricoli, V., L. Lamas, R. Carnevale and C. Urginowitsch (2005) Short-term Effects on Lower-Body Functional Power Development: Weightlifting vs. Vertical Jump Training Programs, *Journal of Strength and Conditioning Research*, 19(2): 433–437

Trojian, T.H. and D.B. McKeag (2006) Single-leg Balance Test to Identify Risk of Ankle Sprains, *British Journal of Sports Medicine*, 40(7): 610–13

Tse, M.A., A.M. McManus and R.S.W. Masters (2005) Development and Validation of a Core Endurance Intervention Program: Implications for Performance in College-age Rowers, *Journal of Strength and Conditioning Research*, 19(3): 547–52

Twist, P.W. and D. Benicky (1996) Conditioning Lateral Movement for Multi-Sport Athletes: Practical Strength and Quickness Drills, *Strength and Conditioning*, 18(5): 10–19

Tyler, T.F., M.P. McHugh, M.R. Mirabella, M.J. Mullaney and S.J. Nicholas (2006) Risk Factors for Noncontact Ankle Sprains in High School Football Players: The Role of Previous Ankle Sprains and Body Mass Index, *American Journal of Sports Medicine*, 34(3): 471–5

Tyler, T.F., S.J. Nicholas, R.J. Campbell, S. Donnellan and M.P. McHugh (2002) The Effectiveness of a Preseason Exercise Program to Prevent Adductor Muscle Strains in Professional Ice Hockey Players, *American Journal of Sports Medicine*, 30(5): 680–3

Tyler, T.F., S.J. Nicholas, R.J. Campbell and M.P. McHugh (2001) The Association of Hip Strength and Flexibility with the Incidence of Adductor Muscle Strains in Professional Ice Hockey Players, *American Journal of Sports Medicine*, 29(2): 124–8

Valovich McLeod, T.C., L.C. Decoster, K.J. Loud, L.J. Micheli, J.T. Parker, M.A. Sandrey and C. White (2011) National Athletic Trainers' Association Position Statement: Prevention of Pediatric Overuse Injuries, *Journal of Athletic Training*, 46(2): 206–20

van den Tillar, R. and M.C. Marques (2011) A Comparison of Three Training Programs with the Same Workload on Overhead Throwing Velocity with Different Weighted Balls, *Journal of Strength and Conditioning Research*, 25(8): 2316–21

van den Tillar, R. (2004) Effect of Different Training Programs on the Velocity of Overarm Throwing: A Brief Review, *Journal of Strength and Conditioning Research*, 18(2): 388–96

Van Huss, W.D., L. Albrecht, R. Nelson and R. Hagerman (1962) Effect of Overload Warm-Up on the Velocity and Accuracy of Throwing, *Research Quarterly*, 33(3): 472–5

van Ingen Schenau, J.J. de Koning and G. de Groot (1994) Optimisation of Sprinting Performance in Running, Cycling and Speed Skating, *Sports Medicine*, 17(4): 259–75

Vera-Garcia, F.J., S.G. Grenier and S.M. McGill (200) Abdominal Muscle Response during Curl-Ups on Both Stable and Labile Surfaces, *Physical Therapy*, 80: 564–9

Verhagen, E.A.L.M., A.J. van der Beek, L.M. Bouter, R.M. Bahr and W. van Mechelen (2004) A One Season Prospective Cohort Study of Volleyball Injuries, *British Journal of Sports Medicine*, 38: 477–81

Verkhoshansky, Y.V. (1996) Quickness and Velocity in Sports Movements, *New Studies in Athletics*, 11(2–3): 29–37

Verrall, G.M., J.P. Slavotinek and P.G. Barnes (2005) The Effect of Sports Specific Training on Reducing the Incidence of Hamstring Injuries in Professional Australian Rules Football Players, *British Journal of Sports Medicine*, 39: 363–8

Visnes, H. and R. Barr (2007) The Evolution of Eccentric Training as Treatment for Patellar Tendinopathy (Jumper's Knee): A Critical Review of Exercise Programmes, *British Journal of Sports Medicine*, 41: 217–23

Vossen, J.F., J.F. Kraemer, D.G. Burke and D.P. Vossen (2000) Comparison of Dynamic Push-Up Training and Plyometric Push-Up Training on Upper-Body Power and Strength, *Journal of Strength and Conditioning Research*, 14(3): 248–53

Vuorimaa, T. and J. Karvonen (1988) Recovery Time in Interval Training for Increasing Aerobic Capacity, *Annals of Sports Medicine*, 3(4): 215–19

Wagner, P. (2003) A Comprehensive Approach to Shoulder Complex Maintenance, *Strength and Conditioning Journal*, 25(3): 65–70

Wallace, B.J., T.W. Kernozek, J.M. White, D.E. Kline, G.A. Wright, H.T. Peng and C.-F. Huang (2010) Quantification of Vertical Ground Reaction Forces of Popular Bilateral Plyometric Exercises, *Journal of Strength and Conditioning Research*, 24(1): 207–12

Wang, H.K. and T. Cochrane (2001) Mobility Impairment, Muscle Imbalance, Muscle Weakness, Scapular Asymmetry and Shoulder Injury in Elite Volleyball Athletes, *Journal of Sports Medicine and Physical Fitness*, 41: 403–10

Waryasz, G.R. (2010) Exercise Strategies to Prevent the Development of the Anterior Pelvic Tilt: Implications for Possible Prevention of Sports Hernias and Osteitis Pubis, *Strength and Conditioning Journal*, 32(4): 56–65

Wathen, D., T.R. Baechle and R.W. Earle (2000) Training Variation: Periodization. In: *Essentials of Strength Training and Conditioning* (2nd Edition), Baechle and Earle (Eds). Champaign, IL: Human Kinetics

Weyand, P.G., R.F. Sandell, D.N.L. Prime and M.W. Bundle (2010) The Biological Limits to Running Speed are Imposed from the Ground Up, *Journal of Applied Physiology*, 108(4): 950–61

Wikstrom, E.A., M.D. Tillman, T.L. Chmielewksi, J.H. Cauraugh and P.A. Borsa (2007) Dynamic Postural Stability Deficits in Subjects with Self-Reported Ankle Instability, *Medicine and Science in Sports and Exercise*, 39(3): 397–402

Wikstrom, E.A., M.D. Tillman, T.L. Chmielewski and P.A. Borsa (2006) Measurement and Evaluation of Dynamic Joint Stability of the Knee and Ankle after Injury, *Sports Medicine*, 36(5): 393–410

Wilder, N., R. Gilders, F. Hagerman and R.G. Deivert (2002) The Effects of a 10-Week, Periodised, Off-Season Resistance Training Program and Creatine Supplementation among Collegiate Football Players, *Journal of Strength and Conditioning Research*, 16(3): 343–52

Wilk, K.E., K. Meister and J.R. Andrews (2002) Current Concepts in the Rehabilitation of the Overhead Throwing Athlete, *American Journal of Sports Medicine*, 30(1): 136–51

Wilkins, H.A., S.R. Petersen and H.A. Quinney (1991) Time–Motion Analysis of and Heart Rate Responses to Amateur Ice Hockey Officiating, *Canadian Journal of Sports Sciences*, 16(4): 302–7

Wilkinson, D.M., J.L. Fallowfield and S. D. Myers (1999) A Modified Incremental Shuttle Run Test Protocol for the Determination of Peak Shuttle Running Speed and the Prediction of Maximal Oxygen Uptake, *Journal of Sports Sciences*, 17: 413–19

Willardson, J.M. (2007) Core Stability Training for Healthy Athletes: A Different Paradigm for Fitness Professionals, *Strength and Conditioning Journal*, 29(6): 42–9

Williams, G.N., M.H. Jones, A. Amendola (2007) Syndesmotic Ankle Sprains in Athletes, *American Journal of Sports Medicine*, 35(7): 1197–207

Willoughby, D.S. (1993) The Effects of Mesocycle-Length Weight Training Programs Involving Periodization and Partially Equated Volumes on Upper and Lower Body Strength, *Journal of Strength and Conditioning Research*, 7(1): 2–8

Wilmore, J.H. and D.L. Costill (1999) Metabolic Adaptations to Training, In: *Physiology of Sport and Exercise* (2nd Edition), J.H. Wilmore and D.L. Costill (Eds) Champaign, IL: Human Kinetics

Wilson, B.D., K.L. Quarrie, P.D. Milburn and D.J. Chalmers (1999) The Nature and Circumstances of Tackle Injuries in Rugby Union, *Journal of Science and Medicine in Sport*, 2(2): 153–62

Wilson, G.J. and A.J. Murphy (1996), Strength Diagnosis: The Use of Test Data to Determine Specific Strength Training, *Journal of Sports Sciences*, 14: 167–73

Wilson, G.J., A.J. Murphy and A. Giorgi (1996) Weight and Plyometric Training: Effects on Eccentric and Concentric Force Production, *Canadian Journal of Applied Physiology*, 21(4): 301–15

Wilson, G.J., A.D. Lyttle, K.J. Ostrowski and A.J. Murphy (1995) Assessing Dynamic Performance: A Comparison of Rate of Force Development Tests, *Journal of Strength and Conditioning Research*, 9(3): 176–81

Wilson, G.J., R.U. Newton, A.J. Murphy and B.J. Humphries (1993) The Optimal Training Load for the Development of Dynamic Athletic Performance, *Medicine and Science in Sports and Exercise*, 25(11): 1279–86

Winchester, J.B., J.M. McBride, M.A. Maher, R.P. Mikat, B.K. Allen, D.E. Kline and M.R. McGuigan (2008) Eight Weeks of Ballistic Exercise Improves Power Independently of Changes in Strength and Muscle Fiber Type Expression, *Journal of Strength and Conditioning Research*, 22(6): 1728–34

Witvrouw, E., L. Danneels, P. Asselman, T. D'Have and D. Cambier (2003) Muscle Flexibility as a Risk Factor for Developing Muscle Injuries in Male Professional Soccer Players, *American Journal of Sports Medicine*, 31(1): 41–6

Witvrouw, E., J. Bellemans, R. Lysens, L. Danneels and D. Cambier (2001) Intrinsic Risk Factors for the Development of Patellar Tendinitis in an Athletic Population: A Two-Year Prospective Study, *American Journal of Sports Medicine*, 29(2): 190–5

Woods, C., R.D. Hawkins, S. Maltby, M. Hulse, A. Thomas and A. Hodson (2004) The Football Association Medical Research Programme: An Audit of Injuries in Professional Football – Analysis of Hamstring Injuries, *British Journal of Sports Medicine*, 38: 36–41

Woolford, S. and M. Angove (1991) A Comparison of Training Techniques and Game Intensities for National Level Netball Players, *Sport Coach*, 14(4): 18–21

Workman, J.C., D. Docherty, K.C. Parfrey and D.G. Behm (2008) Influence of Pelvis Position on the Activation of Abdominal and Hip Flexor Muscles, *Journal of Strength and Conditioning Research*, 22(5): 1563–9

Yaggie, J.A. and B.M. Campbell (2006) Effects of Balance Training on Selected Skills, *Journal of Strength and Conditioning Research*, 20(2): 422–8

Yessis, M. (1994) Training for Power Sports – Part 1, *Strength and Conditioning*, 16: 42–5

Young, W.B. (2006) Transfer of Strength and Power Training to Sports Performance, *International Journal of Sports Physiology and Performance*, 1: 74–83

Young, W.B. and D. Farrow (2006) A Review of Agility: Practical Considerations for Strength and Conditioning, *Strength and Conditioning Journal*, 28(5): 24–9

Young, W.B., R.U. Newton, T.L. Doyle (2005) Physiological and Anthropometric Characteristics of Starters and Non-starters in Elite Australian Rules Football: A Case Study, *Journal of Science and Medicine in Sport*, 8(3): 333–45

Young, W.B., D. Benton, G. Duthie and J. Pryor (2001a) Resistance Training for Short Sprints and Maximum-Speed Sprints, *Strength and Conditioning Journal*, 23(2): 7–13

Young, W.B., C. Macdonald and M.A. Flowers (2001b) Validity of Double- and Single-leg Vertical Jumps as Tests of Leg Extensor Muscle Function, *Journal of Strength and Conditioning Research*, 15(1): 6–11

Young, W.B., M.H. McDowell and B.J. Scarlett (2001c) Specificity of Sprint and Agility Training Methods, *Journal of Strength and Conditioning Research*, 15(3): 315–19

Young, W.B., A. Jenner and K. Griffiths (1998) Acute Enhancement of Power Performance from Heavy Load Squats, *Journal of Strength and Conditioning Research*, 12(2); 82–4

Young, W.B, B. McLean and J. Ardagna (1995) Relationship between Strength Qualities and Sprinting Performance, *Journal of Sports Medicine and Physical Fitness*, 35(1): 13–19

Yu, B., R.M. Queen, A.N. Abbey, Y. Liu, C.T. Moorman, and W.E. Garrett (2008) Hamstring Muscle Kinematics and Activation during Overground Sprinting, *Journal of Biomechanics*, 41: 3121–6

Zatsiorsky, V.W. and W.J. Kraemer (2006) Timing in Strength Training. In: *Science and Practice of Strength Training* (2nd Edition) Champaign, IL: Human Kinetics

Zazulak, B.T., T.E. Hewett, N.P. Reeves, B. Goldberg and J. Cholewicki (2007) Deficits in Neuromuscular Control of the Trunk Predict Knee Injury Risk: A Prospective Biomechanical–Epidemiological Study, *American Journal of Sports Medicine*, 35(7): 1123–30

Zupan, M.F., A.W. Arata, L.H. Dawson, A.L. Wile, T.L. Payn and M.E. Hannon (2009) Wingate Anaerobic Test Peak Power and Anaerobic Capacity Classifications for Men and Women Intercollegiate Athletes, *Journal of Strength and Conditioning Research*, 23(9): 2598–604

Zuur, A.T., J. Lundbye-Jensen, C. Leukel, W. Taube, M.J. Grey, A. Gollhofer, J.B. Nielsen and M. Gruber (2010) Contribution of Afferent Feedback and Descending Drive to Human Hopping, *Journal of Physiology*, 588(5): 799–807

Zwerver, J., S.W. Bredeweg and A.L. Hof (2007) Biomechanical Analysis of the Single-leg Decline Squat, *British Journal of Sports Medicine*, 41: 264–8

INDEX

9 780415 637930